Conversations

in Nursing Professional Development

Belinda E. Puetz, PhD, RN

Julia W. Aucoin, DNS, RN,BC

Editors

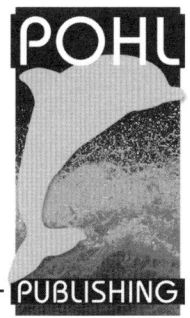

POHL

PUBLISHING

Publisher: Pohl Publishing, Inc.
312 East Nine Mile Road, Suite 11–409
Pensacola, FL 32514

Publisher: Belinda E. Puetz

Managing Editors: Patricia M. Adkison
Keleita L. (Shay) Stephens

Text & Cover Design Susan A. Hoege
Innovative Business Communications
2910 Valley Manor Drive
Kingwood, TX 77339

Copyright © 2002 by Pohl Publishing, Inc.

ISBN 0-9717449-0-6

Printed in the United States of America.

Preface

It has been our pleasure to prepare for you this book on nursing professional development (formerly known as continuing education and staff development). Our intent was to provide you with the most current and useful information available to you in a thoughtful and inquisitive way. The goal has been reached and we had fun getting there. Assembled herein are the thoughts of a wide variety of leaders from all over the US. Many have been colleagues for years and some are new faces, full of innovation and ideas.

We hope you enjoy and use this book frequently in your practice.

— Belinda E. Puetz and Julia W. Aucoin

About the Editors
Belinda E. Puetz, PhD, RN

Belinda has worked in staff development and continuing education since the 1970s. She is the Founder and current Administrator of the National Nursing Staff Development Organization (NNSDO), and the Founder and current Editor of the *Journal for Nurses in Staff Development*, a publication of Lippincott Williams & Wilkins and the official journal of NNSDO. Belinda is the author of three books in the specialty of continuing education and staff development. The prestigious Belinda E. Puetz Award for Excellence in Staff Development was established in 1994 by NNSDO to recognize Belinda's contributions to the organization and to the specialty. Founding Pohl Publishing in 2001 is her latest venture in the field of nursing.

Julia W. Aucoin, DNS, RN,BC

Julie has worked in nursing professional development since it was known as inservice education more than 20 years ago. After sitting for the certification exam in Continuing Education and Staff Development the first year it was administered, Julie began teaching the certification review course with a team of faculty from the National Nursing Staff Development Organization (NNSDO). She now serves on the Content Expert Panel for the American Nurses Credentialing Center Nursing Professional Development certification exam. Julie is a frequent presenter to staff development groups and author of *101 Tips to Better Conferences*, published by NNSDO. She has worked in departments ranging from single person to multi-site in several parts of the country and brings a wealth of experience to the specialty.

Publisher's Note

Pohl Publishing, Inc., is named after my mother, Elizabeth Pohl Puetz. She was the first woman entrepreneur in the family—buying and operating a German delicatessen when she was in her 60s—and she was a great inspiration to me throughout my life. My mother died May 26, 2001, but I hope that my publishing efforts will honor her memory and her legacy to me.

It is fitting that the premiere publication of Pohl Publishing, Inc., be a book on staff development, for publishing and staff development have been two of the major hats I have worn in my professional life. *Conversations in Nursing Professional Development* is set up in question and answer format to simulate asking a staff development/continuing education expert a question and getting an immediate, easy-to-implement answer.

It is my hope that it will be as easy for staff development professionals to use it as it was to produce. I am very excited about the format and plan to use this book as a model for subsequent books published by Pohl Publishing, Inc. on various topics of interest to professional registered nurses.

— Belinda E. Puetz
June, 2002

Table of Contents

Section 1: *Getting Started*

Section 2: *Organizational Structures*

Section 3: *Staff Development Roles and Responsibilities*

Section 4: *Planning, Implementing, and Evaluating Educational Activities*

Section 5: *Accreditation/Approval of Staff Development and Continuing Education Activities*

Section 6: *Approaches to Learning*

Section 7: *New Approaches to Staff Development*

Section 8: *Issues in Staff Development and Continuing Education*

Section 9: *Staff Development as a Career*

Section 1:
Getting Started

Welcome to the specialty of Nursing Professional Development (NPD), formerly continuing education and staff development. We practice as expert interpreters of education principles.

Major differences between nursing professional development specialists and nurse educators are their employment setting and their functions. Traditionally, the nurse educator has been viewed as faculty for undergraduate and graduate nursing students, while the NPD specialist is viewed as the educator for the practice setting. However, both are advanced practice roles based on a common set of competencies, which are grounded in nursing education principles. This section focuses on the variety of skills and responsibilities that are setting dependent.

Chapter 1: *Preparing for the Staff Development Role*

1. *Just what do staff development educators do?*

1. Staff development educators primarily design programs to assess and develop competence of nurses and other clinical care providers in hospitals, long term care facilities, and other healthcare settings. Depending on the complexity, maturity, and state of the healthcare system, some staff development programs provide a full spectrum of comprehensive services and products to an integrated healthcare system with reports of selected staff development outcomes provided for the organization's governance boards. Other programs may be limited to those required by regulatory agencies that license or accredit healthcare organizations. Yet others may be a mix of orientation, new product and procedure skills training, continuing professional education, and leadership development. Staff development educators may lead or work in many roles providing staff development services within healthcare organizations. Staff development roles are defined by the organization's leadership, frequently the chief nurse executive and/or executive team, and should be guided by staff development specialists and experts, contemporary literature, and successful programs with established track records for improving clinical competence.

2. *How can I try out some aspects of the role?*

2. Nurses who would like to try out facets of the staff development role have quite a few options. First and foremost, just letting the unit manager and the staff development specialist know of your interest will start you in the right direction. They will likely have a prioritized list of upcoming staff development activities; choose something from that list. You can also:

- Volunteer to organize and provide a unit-based learning activity on a topic that interests you

- Get involved in unit-based competence assessment activities by volunteering to be an assessor

- Design and try out a competence assessment tool for a skill specific to a unit's requirements working with the unit manager and staff development specialist

- Serve on a planning committee for a continuing education program

- Become an instructor for BLS, ACLS, PALS or other related courses necessary for continued competence development in your clinical specialty

- Seek preceptor training and improve your teaching, coaching, and counseling skills

- Volunteer to organize a unit-based staff development work group to design and implement an annual program of educational activities

- Volunteer to provide unit-based or organization-wide orientation program improvement activities

- Learn about educational and staff development program planning and design

- Learn about requirements for quality continuing professional education and approval criteria

- Apply technical or clinical competence to designing computer-based staff development

3. *How long will it take to learn all aspects of the different staff development roles?*

3. The staff development role in healthcare organizations today is dynamic and continually evolving. Role related learning is ongoing, but generally, most nurses new to staff development report that it takes about a year to feel comfortable in a role that provides comprehensive staff development services. Nurses promoted to staff development roles usually have a bachelor's degree in nursing or a related field. If you don't have a bachelor's yet, plan to get one and look for a program that provides some elective courses in educational program planning and design. Some programs offer an opportunity to do an elective internship in a staff development department.

Some staff development specialists, like me, have graduate degrees in adult and continuing education; these programs always have opportunities to apply learning to the real work world of staff development. Seek those out, too. I was able to apply course-required assignments to my staff development role, frequently meeting course requirements and improving the hospital-based program simultaneously. It was a win-win situation. I also was a volunteer preceptor for many graduate students in nursing and other programs. The organization benefited from the projects completed by these students and the students benefited from the real world experience of a busy staff development department.

Some organizations have highly specialized staff

development roles like a computer or Web-based training specialist. These specialists might be called instructional technologists or information architects. These individuals may or may not be nurses, and may work with a clinical specialist to co-author clinical training or a staff development specialist for quality educational design.

4. What are some good resources? Is there a professional group for this role?

4. Of course, the professional society for nurses in staff development, the National Nursing Staff Development Organization is an excellent resource; go to its Web site at **www.nnsdo.org** and visit the resource center. Members of NNSDO are willing to talk with nurses interested in this practice and even to mentor novice staff development specialists. Check with NNSDO to see if a local chapter exists in your geographical area— these are locally affiliated groups. If you're employed, nurses in your own staff development department are good resources. Some staff development specialists in local hospitals and healthcare facilities are willing to provide an informational interview to help you learn more about the role. Several textbooks are available, including mine, published by Lippincott as a second edition in 1998 titled *Clinical and Nursing Staff Development: Current Competence, Future Focus*. In addition, the *Journal for Nurses in Staff Development*, published since 1985, is an exquisite resource for learning about the status and progress of this specialty practice. And finally, a literature search on adult learning, human resource development, organization development, quality improvement, and competence assessment and development are additional resources that will provide theories and principles that underpin nursing staff development.

5. Are there other professional groups for this role?

5. The American Nurses Association once had a Council for Nursing Professional Development (NPD). Now, the original and dedicated members of this former group organize an annual conference. Also, the American Society for Training and Development is an active organization that publishes a useful monthly journal and has chapters in many metropolitan areas. Finally, the Health Care Educators Association, formerly the American Society for Health Education and Training, is helpful to educators in hospital or healthcare system education roles.

6. *What are some professional meetings that staff development nurses usually attend?*

6. The most important one is the annual convention that NNSDO conducts each year in July; check the Web site for specifics. The NPD annual meeting is also a good convocation for many staff development and continuing education nurses. Staff development nurses providing services to nurses in specialty services, for example, perinatal, perioperative, oncology and such, will find the meetings of the related professional organizations helpful for keeping clinically up to date.

7. *Can I get certified in nursing staff development?*

7. Yes, the American Nurses Credentialing Center (ANCC) offers a certification exam in Nursing Professional Development. This comprehensive exam provides recognition to those who have demonstrated knowledge about this specialty practice. NNSDO provides certification preparation review courses before each convention; these courses can also serve to provide a comprehensive and intensive orientation for a new staff development nurse.

8. *Are there formal academic programs to help me prepare for a role in staff development?*

8. The program of study I found most helpful was one that focused on adult and continuing education. It was also designed for individuals who were working in the field. Many universities will allow graduate students to design programs to prepare them for specific roles in education and health care. Some even offer certificate programs that include a series of specialized courses and a project to complete. Check with a local university or college counselor to see what options might be available.

9. *How is the staff development role different from being an instructor or professor at a college or university?*

9. The responsibilities in staff development are different and the role is quite a bit more dynamic in most cases. A staff development specialist may be responsible for conducting a two-day workshop on critical care nursing one week, an nursing internship course the next, and perhaps a CPR course for learners from various backgrounds the next—sometimes the staff development specialist may provide this variety of services in one week! A faculty member usually has a clinical assignment with a group of students over a period of time in one or two settings and may have responsibility for selected lectures related to the assigned area of nursing. Depending on their experience and status, professors often have responsibility for several courses, overseeing several clinical rotations and may provide clinical instruction for a group or two as well. I think the main difference lies in the nature of the learner.

Student nurses in academic programs are participating in a planned course of study toward a specific degree and must meet certain requirements. Nurses employed in various clinical settings must demonstrate competence and continue to learn vast amounts of new information, knowledge, and skills to provide quality care to patients. The staff development specialist is challenged indeed to assess needs and provide, or organize others to provide, the most relevant information and skill training using efficient and effective strategies.

10. *What can I do in my clinical role to see if I'd like to be a staff development specialist?*

10. Volunteer to do a unit-based learning activity based on an identified problem that is high risk, high volume, or problem prone. Volunteer to help with an upcoming course or workshop on a topic of interest to you; prepare and deliver it and ask for feedback on your presentation. Better yet, simply ask the unit manager or the staff development specialist in the facility what you can do to help—there's always plenty to be done and volunteers are often tapped for new roles as they are created.

11. *Can I create a new role?*

11. Yes, many experienced staff development nurses can tell stories about how a new program or continuous quality improvement project was initiated that called for an individual to be dedicated to changing behaviors requisite to the organizational change desired. Volunteering for a task force charged to change an organizational issue or start a new initiative or program often will provide additional information to help create new roles. Staff development specialists reinvent their roles on a regular basis based on the needs of the organization and its vision. There is no better way to help improve organizational services than by being part of the solutions task forces convened for that purpose. New roles emerge from these activities—the key is to connect the new role to the planned change and then make it happen!

12. *Educators and staff development nurses seem to get cut sometimes. Do I need to worry about job security?*

12. Yes, unfortunately in the past few years of efficiencies and downsizing, educators and staff development nurses were cut, often inappropriately. In today's rapidly changing environment, given increased technology and continuous infusion of new knowledge and evidence to guide clinical practice, we need more educators. It is up to us to demonstrate the contribution that the competent nurse makes to the bottom line of quality patient care. Staff development services are critical to an organization's commitment to quality patient care. We can use established formulas and published information to make that case. Staff development nurses are also a resilient group, with a high tolerance for ambiguity. Creative use of scarce resources often underscores the nature of this rewarding work.

13. What are some of the aspects of the role that some staff development nurses don't like?

13. Some staff development nurses say they don't like the repetitive nature of some aspects of staff development: monthly or biweekly orientation classes, for example, or required classes to meet regulatory body requirements. The unpredictability of the programs you might be offering in several months, depending on changing patient needs, troubles some working in this field. While the work is rewarding, as mentioned earlier, creativity and a high tolerance for ambiguity are characteristics that will serve the staff development specialist well in these unpredictable times. Most do like the control over their schedule this work often provides.

14. What do staff development nurses not do?

14. Wash windows. Seriously, a staff development specialist can solve just about any educational problem and coach others to resolve problems that are not their responsibility. It is the clinical manager who is accountable for the competence of staff assigned to the unit. Often in collaboration with the staff development specialist, the unit manager may develop specific performance improvement plans for individuals. The staff development specialist contributes to the evaluation of the individual, but the clinical manager conducts the overall performance evaluation.

15. How do the one-person staff development departments do it all?

15. With help from the many nurses interested in helping others stay current and competent and the managers dedicated to the same mission! A one-person department may seem overwhelming, but it is often those departments, usually in small facilities, that are most creative about involving many in the staff development program. Those staff development specialists become masterful at identifying talent, creating opportunities to develop that talent, and coordinating the myriad tasks for successful staff development programs.

16. Can I do research as a staff development specialist?

16. Yes, NNSDO can even provide a list of research priorities of highest interest to the field. I usually advise nurses to investigate a problem of high interest to the employing organization. Graduate students can be placed with staff development specialists in local facilities and assist with research projects that will provide quality data with which to make good decisions. A good place to start is with a comprehensive needs assessment of the organization on which to base a sound and contemporary staff development program. Resources mentioned above can help design and plan the needs assessment and evaluation projects necessary to quality staff development programs.

RESOURCES

Case, B. (1997). *Career planning for nurses*. Albany, NY: Delmar.

National Nursing Staff Development Organization. (2001). *Getting started in nursing staff development*. Pensacola, FL: Author.

Kelly Thomas, K. J. (1998). *Clinical and nursing staff development: Current competence, future focus* (2nd ed.). Philadelphia: Lippincott.

Chapter 2: *Getting a Staff Development Position*

1. *What can I do to acquire some experience in staff development if I do not have any?*

1. There are a variety of things you can do to gain relevant staff development experience:

   - Volunteer or get appointed to a conference or workshop planning committee.

   - Join a hospital committee. Hospitals or multi-site facilities frequently have education planning groups or steering committees where staff nurses or managers serve in advisory capacities. These committees expose you to discussions and opportunities to get more involved in education-related activities.

   - Join a local chapter of a national specialty nursing organization. These chapters provide education for their members. Offer to teach or arrange continuing education offerings related to your specialty.

   - Avail yourself of preceptor development training and mentorship of new employees.

   - Offer to supervise student nurses in clinical settings or to serve as a role transition preceptor for senior level students.

2. *I want to move to a different city or state. How can I find out about any available staff development positions?*

2. - Check to see if there is a local affiliate of the National Nursing Staff Development Organization (NNSDO) or similar organization. Call the contact person and arrange to talk at length about local employment opportunities; ask for advice and any other contacts to call.

   - Contact several national recruiters or "head hunters." Send them your résumé and let them know of your interests and areas of expertise. Indicate flexibility and willingness to be considered for positions other than staff development educator. Many positions have education/staff development responsibilities without the title.

   - Check the American Hospital Association (AHA) Hospital guide and/or do an online search to locate potential employers. Arrange a visit to the area and set up appointments to talk with the recruiters.

   - Read classified sections under healthcare, nursing, education, and professional listings of the area's Sunday newspaper(s). Larger public libraries and the Internet may provide access to these newspapers.

Some newspaper or grocery stores sell a variety of major market newspapers.

- Go to the facility and read the Human Resources postings or check them on the Internet Web sites (if available). You can ask a friend who works in the facility to routinely review the openings for you, but it is best to add your own efforts as well. Tell friends and colleagues you are looking and interested—many positions are not open very long.

- Send your résumé to hospital or agency recruiters or an HR department; some are kept for only a few months and others could be discarded if there is no open position at the time the résumé arrives. Do not depend on your résumé to make it to the hiring person. It is wise to send a résumé directly to the hiring person with a cover letter indicating your interest.

- Many recruiters will advise you to make appointments to discuss career opportunities and seek advice from experts in the field. You are not directly interviewing for a job in this discussion, but if the conversation goes well, other leads and referrals may result.

3. *How should I prepare for an interview?*

3.
- Find out as much as you can about the potential employer. If the potential employer has a Web site, visit it in advance. Request a copy of the annual report which lists the organization's priorities. Look at the stories and the financial figures. Search for the organization on the World Wide Web to see if there were newspaper articles about the employer published. The tenor of the articles will also alert you to community issues or perceptions.

- Bring copies of any relevant materials that can strengthen your candidacy. This might be a flyer about one of your speaking engagements, positive performance evaluations, a publication reprint, and letters of reference.

4. *Whom should I list as a reference for an interview?*

4. Some people who might be listed are:

- Your current manager or boss (if he/she knows you are looking and you have some indication he/she will say positive things about your performance)

- Another respected staff development educator or director who is familiar with your work

- An individual you have precepted and/or that preceptee's faculty advisor

- A former boss who positively evaluated your work

- Someone from Human Resources who is familiar with your work. Many staff development positions are now interwoven with Human Resources, and evidence of a good working relationship would be most helpful.

5. *How should I respond if I am asked about covering a specialty that I do not know much or anything about?*

5.
- Be honest but willing in your response. For example, "I have not previously had the opportunity to work in XYZ area, but I would welcome the opportunity to acquire skills in that area. An example of how I did this in my current position or the past would be…"

- If you do not believe that you want to take the position being discussed, thank the interviewer and tell him/her you want to think it over. You may not have other options and learning new skills may not be so bad. If after some thoughtful consideration, however, you are still not interested, say so by thanking the recruiter or manager, and telling him/her that you prefer to seek, explore, or accept a different opportunity or position.

6. *How can I tell what the scope of the work will be in a position I am offered or am considering?*

6.
- Ask to see the job description, in advance if possible. If the position is not what you want or are willing to do, you could save everyone time by not even interviewing for it.

- Ask to speak with the person who formerly held or currently holds the position, unless it is a new job or has a revised scope of responsibilities. Listen and learn from that person's successes and failures.

- Ask the person to whom you will report what are the most important priorities he/she will expect you to accomplish in the first three months. Also ask how success will be evaluated or measured.

7. *What personality traits should I emphasize in the interview?*

7. Any of the following are ideal to mention as long as they actually do apply to you:

- Flexibility and credibility

- Dependability

- Ability to work with minimal direction, to see the big picture in an organization, and to tolerate ambiguity

- A sense of humor

- Ability to make the best of less-than-ideal situations (i.e., making lemonade out of lemons)

- Ability to nurture others and take pleasure in seeing others develop and grow through your mentorship or interactions

- Honesty and trustworthiness

- Attention to detail and ability to follow detailed projects through to completion

- Commitment to the organization's mission and values

8. Whom should I ask to meet prior to accepting a position?

8.
- Your potential boss or bosses and any peers would be most important to meet.

- If you will be providing education for a group of units, the managers from those units or at least a representative would be helpful to meet.

- If you have not met the recruiter, make a point to do that.

- Many times there will be committees interviewing candidates. If there are no staff nurses on the committee, make a point to meet some. The cafeteria and coffee shop are good places to start conversations. Ask to have a tour of the area or unit and talk to all staff you encounter.

- Speak to support staff as well. Their experience with education and orientation or the lack thereof may be very different from what you are told.

9. What are the most useful ways to learn about the culture of an organization?

9.
- Ask how decisions are made and implemented.

- Look at who is or is not involved and included in the interview process.

- Bring up conversations with staff. In the cafeteria, join someone and say you are thinking of applying or accepting a position in nursing or whatever is the case, and ask what his/her experience working there has been.

- Ask how system changes occur or have been accomplished.

- Ask how many, or if, hours are budgeted for education or staff development nonproductive time.

- Ask a manager how the staff was prepared for the

Healthcare Insurance Portability and Accountability Act (HIPAA) implementation or most recent Joint Commission on Accreditation of Healthcare Organizations (JCAHO) visit.

10. What questions should I ask?

10.
- To whom does the person in the position report?
- If there will there be multiple bosses, who has the most influence or power?
- How long was the previous person in the position?
- Why was this new position created?

11. What red flags should I watch out for?

11.
- No budget
- No access to support staff or an adequate computer system
- Minimal or no budgeted staff time for staff development or continuing education, yet there is an expectation it will occur

12. What questions should I be prepared to answer?

12.
- How do you handle interpersonal conflict or multiple demands?
- How do you prioritize assignments or tasks?
- How do you deal with ambiguity?
- Be prepared to give examples!

RESOURCES

www.hipaacode.com

www.jcaho.org

www.nnsdo.org

Journal for Nurses in Staff Development (published by Lippincott Williams & Wilkins, Philadelphia, PA)

Case, B. (1997). *Career planning for nurses.* Albany, NY: Delmar.

Chapter 3: *Staff Development in Hospital Settings*

1. What kinds of activities must be done in a hospital?

1. Many of the activities that are done in the hospital setting (e.g., critical care courses, preceptor preparation, management training) are dependent on the expectations of the facility. However, responsibilities that are fairly generic to all settings are:

- Orientation (in some cases both general hospital and nursing or just general orientation with nursing/ departmental orientation provided in some other forum)

- Needs assessment

- Coordination of BLS/ACLS/PALS courses

- Provision of product inservice offerings based on changes in technology

- Management/leadership training

- Provision of education/training in Joint Commission on Accreditation of Healthcare Organizations (JCAHO) and/or Occupational Safety and Health Administration (OSHA) standards for patient safety

2. What is my role?

2. As the staff development educator, you are responsible for training and education based on needs that come as requests from the institution or management, or as the result of mandatory standards from JCAHO, OSHA, and/or other regulating bodies. You will help to define the need, communicate with the manager, provide the education or training, and keep records. In some cases, you may be working only with nursing-related departments, and in some cases you will be working with the entire institution.

3. What credentials are necessary for my role?

3. Educational requirements vary from institution to institution. A Master's degree in nursing education or management is generally preferred, but in many institutions, a Master's degree is not required. You must have an unencumbered license from your state Board of Nursing and current competency in Basic Life Support. Certification in what was formerly known as Continuing Education and Staff Development (now called Nursing Professional Development) by the American Nurses Credentialing Center (ANCC) is not required but indicates that you have demonstrated expertise and are recognized in your field at the national level.

4. *What is the role of the educator in JCAHO preparation?*

4. First of all, as an educator, you must be familiar with the JCAHO requirements. You will be responsible for providing the appropriate information during education and/or training and for preparing the staff to respond to questions, if asked, by the Joint Commission surveyors.

You probably will be responsible for developing a method (e.g., posters, self-learning manuals, a class) for addressing the annual mandatory issues with the staff and for working with content experts to develop these.

5. *What is my role in ensuring competency?*

5. You will be working with managers in nursing and perhaps other departments to develop tools (e.g., forms, checklists, demonstrations) for evaluating competency. The educator frequently provides the education/training for new skills or procedures and may then be responsible for working with managers to evaluate competency (e.g., checking skills in a skills fair).

6. *How should I keep track of my activities/ productivity?*

6. How you keep track of your activities/productivity will depend on the expectations of the institution and your supervisor in addition to your personal needs. A calendar with room for notes is almost indispensable. I find it helpful to jot down information during the day as it happens, or make notes at the end of the day, so I can keep all the information straight! Some hospitals require the educator to keep a monthly log or calendar of activities, including classes taught, requests for consultation, networking, projects you are working on, and the like. As an educator, you may be a salaried rather than hourly employee, and you may find yourself putting in hours different from the usual "7–3." You will have projects that you are working on over a period of time, and keeping records of progress made will be important.

7. *Should we be doing some kind of accounting of the Profit and Loss of programs?*

7. There are many hidden costs in providing staff development in hospitals, and many staff development departments do not generate revenue. However, it is beneficial to be able to "validate your existence" to upper management (who are ultimately responsible for "the bottom line" of the organization) that in-house staff development/education is cost effective. You may need to convince upper management that providing in-house programs is a benefit to the employees, assists in retention, and is cost effective. Hospitals cannot afford not to educate staff.

8. How can I determine the return on the investment of my time and energy?

8. So often this return is difficult to determine in terms of tangibles. The primary way to evaluate a return on the investment is by outcome measurement, but that is difficult to do in a method other than following employees around to observe their performance. The primary return on your investment would be determined by a behavioral change based on education/training. However, the satisfaction of seeing the 'light go on' when an employee finally grasps the concept you are trying to get across can be a very big return, and yet it is impossible to quantify.

9. What should I keep in my personal files?

9. I believe that you should keep your résumé up to date, including awards, organizations, and committee memberships. You should also keep documentation of your personal competency, as well as records of personal compliance with JCAHO/OSHA requirements. In addition, you probably want to keep records of communications that have taken place about projects you are working on or about consulting you are doing. You might want to document department goals as well as performance improvement activities. You will be developing a network of contact persons—in-house and in the community—and you want to be able to contact them easily. I keep phone numbers of anyone who I talk with or who calls me—I never know when having that number will come in handy!

10. What are some good references to have in my personal library?

10. Professional journals certainly help you keep up with current issues and trends as well as provide resources for some programs. Textbooks on a particular field of interest are helpful to have (I like to highlight when I read!) and may be provided by the hospital or available in the library.

11. How can I get support from staff for things they don't buy into?

11. First and always, be positive in your presentation. Seek to understand the rationale behind the request for the education/training and use that information in teaching the audience. Explain the advantages to them as well as to the institution; with that knowledge frequently comes cooperation. Be careful not to display any negative feelings.

12. How can I make adults be accountable and "act like adults"?

12. Well, first of all, we cannot make adults do anything. However, our role in helping staff to be accountable is to understand (and sometimes set) the standards for the institution or department. Next, stick to those standards and not fluctuate according to "circumstances." For instance, if you set a time to begin class, consistently start at the advertised time. If you sometimes start on time, but not always, participants will not feel accountable for being present on time.

13. What if I am the only educator in my department?

13. Education departments can vary from one-person departments to departments of many people. Maybe you are fortunate to at least have a secretary! To be the only educator in a department means that you will be able to do only the very basic education functions and probably none of the development programs. This makes it tough. First, however, you will need to understand the goals of administration for you and the department, considering the mission of the hospital. When you know these goals for the department, then you can better prioritize what you have to do. Be prepared to be asked to do any and every thing—your assignments may change from day to day.

As educator in a one-person department, you will find it helpful to develop educational liaisons, or an education committee, to help define who needs to be included in each program. For example, if the hospital is having complaints about IV starts, by meeting with a committee you may discover that radiology also needs to be included in an IV program, not just nursing personnel.

14. How do you manage to keep all the staff newcomers as well as existing staff up-to-date?

14. Our jobs would be simplified if retention were not a problem! But the truth of the matter is that employees come and go. Information can be included in orientation for the new employees. You can never over-communicate with staff because of the complexity of healthcare organizations and the fact that we are 24/7 organizations. Existing staff can be communicated with via memo, self-learning modules, mailbox inservice programs, e-mail, phone, newsletters, quarterly town hall meetings, and the like.

15. Everything seems to be an education problem; what is a management or systems problem?

15. The question to answer is, "Is this deficiency (problem) performance-based or compliance-based?" If it is performance-based, training might be needed. If it is compliance-based, it is a management issue.

Eighty percent of the time problems are systems related; 10% of the time problems are personnel related; and 10% of the time problems are because of lack of education. Managers usually find it easier to refer to a problem as an education issue because of the energy and time it takes to work through the other 90%. In our role as consultant, as we collaboratively look at the desired outcome, we can assist the manager to see that education is only part of the solution.

16. What records do we need to keep?

16. If programs provide contact hours for continuing education, you need to keep documentation that supports the planning, implementation, and evaluation of this activity. JCAHO and OSHA will require completion/compliance information, (e.g., what percent of staff, by department, have completed annual safety review or hospital orientation).

You will want to have a file system so that you can retrieve information about programs presented including rosters, attendance slips, and some indication of the reason for conducting the program, whether it was for a change of product, a new system, or other reason. If you have access to computerized records for the information, this is ideal because you can then identify access by program, by department, or by individual. It is best that you document the outcomes achieved as well.

17. What about competency? Do employees need to have a competency sheet for each competency or a reference to a master sheet?

17. As competency is just a snapshot of meeting a standard, reference to a master sheet is sufficient; to have a separate sheet would create files that could become unwieldy. Preservation of the master sheets (or standards), however, is a must.

18. How can I effect any behavioral change?

18. We can educate on the right way, but whether learners comply and change their behavior is the result of motivation—external or internal.

19. If I create tools for departments to use, how can I get them to use them?

19. One of the best ways to get their buy-in is to involve representatives from the departments in the process of design and development. Otherwise, you can offer them the tool, with explanations and the rationale for use, and if they choose to not use it, it becomes a management issue.

20. How can I make the same old content stimulating?

20. I find this sometimes a real problem because of the required repetition of programs. However, by reading journals (which often have ideas and suggestions), networking with others, and letting that creativity flow it is possible to stay stimulated. If the instructor is bored by the program, it will come across as "boring" to participants.

In my department, when we think that we are becoming stagnant, we often ask another educator to sit in our presentation, to critique it, and offer suggestions for revitalization. We use a lot of games as the basis for teaching/learning. Television game shows are wonderful to adapt to various types of content.

I attended a national program a few years ago, and the speaker stated, humorously, that she worked by the CASE Management process—*C*opy *A*nd *S*teal *E*verything. And she made no apologies for it—saying we are all in this together and doing the same things, so why not share? We don't have time to keep reinventing the wheel.

21. How can I get management support for a project/idea?

21. Communication to management should include the advantages of the new idea and possibly a cost/benefit analysis both for the manager as well as for the organization. I would discuss with the manager what his/her perception is of what the finished product should look like. What outcome does he/she want? Be sure to communicate frequently with the manager as work on the project progresses. Then, I would use this feedback to develop the product.

22. How can I/we work within our hospital's limited financial resources to produce both quality and quantity?

22. One of the best suggestions I can give you is to make an effort to get to know the vendors that the hospital uses for products and services. They frequently can offer financial support for programs (check with the hospital administration or purchasing department to see if you have to go through any "channels" before seeking financial donations). I have discovered that there are a lot of "freebies" out there; you just have to ask. Also, keep your eyes and ears open for resources for free books, literature, handouts, and the like.

23. What needs to be included in orientation?

23. The content of orientation is driven by regulatory agencies such as JCAHO and OSHA, including safety information and confidentiality. Other content in orientation (e.g., customer service) will be driven by its degree of importance to the hospital. Some content needs to be provided to all employees regardless of the department in which they will be working, and some content is department specific and can be addressed within the department. Decisions will also be made based on time constraints and what is "need to know" versus "nice to know" content.

24. How do you get ideas for programs? How do you begin the process of developing a program?

24. Sometimes programs and/or ideas are assigned based on organizational needs. In planning a program, it is sometimes necessary to determine the gap between what administration sees as the need and what the end-users see as the need. I always want to contact the content expert on the topic in order to develop the objectives for the program: what is the purpose of the program or what situation prompted the request?

Developing a new program can be fun also. Keep your eyes and ears open. You will hear conversations, especially from new nurses, on information that they need. Literature searches can provide "hot topics" in health care. Convene a panel of "experts," who can talk about what they see for the future in health care; that will also give you many ideas.

RESOURCES

Annual convention of the National Nursing Staff Development Organization—**www.nnsdo.org**

TrendLines—the NNSDO newsletter

Journal for Nurses in Staff Development—**www.jnsdjournal.com**

Training & Development Magazine, the journal of the American Society of Training and Development—**www.astd.org**

Chapter 4: *Staff Development in Other Settings*

1. What settings other than hospitals use staff development?

1. Settings are as numerous and varied as there are ways of offering healthcare services. Some that quickly come to mind are:

- Long term care
- Home health
- Hospice
- Clinics and outpatient services
- Community colleges and universities
- Day care centers for Alzheimer and dementia patients
- Rehabilitation centers
- Professional associations
- Businesses and industrial settings that have employee health programs
- Pharmaceutical and medical products companies

Don't forget the publishing arena as a vehicle for staff development for a broad audience. Publishing opportunities include:

- Texts
- Journals
- Monographs
- Internet sites devoted to health care
- Newsletters

2. What kinds of activities do these settings need?

2. All staff development settings have at least one thing in common: programs should be based on identified learning needs. Safety and accreditation agency mandates exist in all areas and need to be adapted for particular settings. The basic starting points for determining activities are:

- Know the audience
- Know the setting
- Know what learning needs exist. Do written surveys, talk to management, and most importantly, talk to staff to "get a handle" on what needs exist. Review risk management data and feedback from performance evaluations.

3. *How can I function as staff and staff development educator?*

3. There is no simple answer to this question! The best advice I can offer is to establish, as clearly as possible (and preferably in writing), how many hours per week are to be budgeted as staff and how many are to be budgeted as staff development. Make sure that planning time, curriculum development, and evaluation activities are included in the budgeted staff development hours. Persons unfamiliar with the education process may not realize that these activities are as critical as the actual program implementation. Also, determine (again in writing) what is expected of you when there is a problem with staffing. If someone calls in sick are you going to automatically be expected to become staff even though you need to be staff development on that day? The more clearly you identify expectations the better.

4. *How can I get administration to value staff development more?*

4. You can't "make" administration value something that is not critical to the strategic plan. First, review your organization's mission, vision, values, and strategic plan. Where and how are staff development and staff education mentioned? (If it's not mentioned you can bet it's not valued and probably won't be.) Next, identify the top priorities of the organization and what education will be necessary for staff, patients, and community. When you write a staff development business plan, make sure you demonstrate how the department will contribute to the strategic plan, particularly in terms of dollars and cents.

5. *How do I coordinate staff development activities among a variety of settings and geographic sites within the same health system?*

5. First, determine who among the staff has expertise and contacts in particular settings. You may wish to assign staff to certain sites and have them assume responsibility for those sites. It will give them a sense of ownership and the employees at those sites an ability to bond with a specific contact person or persons. Establish regular meetings with staff so that no one feels left out. I highly recommend that the healthcare system in question develop a means of video conferencing among sites and an effective Intranet system. This will help keep staff in touch with you and with each other and also be a vehicle for offering a program simultaneously among sites.

6. *What qualifications do I need to coordinate staff development in other settings?*

6. Your most important asset will be an education background with expertise in staff development, inservice, and continuing education. I recommend a graduate degree in education for the staff development manager in addition to management experience. You are assuming a position that does not mandate clinical expertise in all settings as much as an ability to apply the education process to achieve outcomes throughout the health system.

7. How do I write a staff development plan for other settings?

7. The basic principles for writing a good staff development plan are the same regardless of setting. Know and understand the components of the organizational strategic plan. Get a copy and know exactly what education is expected to accomplish in terms of staff performance and the bottom budgetary line. I recommend the following components as an outline for a good staff development plan.

- Executive summary

- Departmental description

- Departmental structure

- Products and services

- Market and competition analysis

- Action plan

- Financial plan

8. What types of staff development programs are required/mandated in settings other than hospitals?

8. These are specific to the population served at each setting. Familiarize yourself with the following:

- Federal, state, and local mandates

- Accrediting agency mandates

- Safety training

- Disaster training (Make sure you know the particular potential environmental and political/social conditions that could result in emergency conditions in the areas served.)

- Mandates resulting from particular specialties (such as accredited trauma center requirements)

9. What staff development programming is especially important for continuing education/professional development of staff?

9. Again, this depends on the specialty area and the populations being served. In addition to the requirements discussed in Question 8, you'll need to know the strengths and weaknesses of the staff working at the various locations. You can retrieve this information from a variety of sources, but you'll need the cooperation of management and staff and a means of ensuring confidentiality when discussing data from risk management reports and from performance evaluations. You need not actually see performance evaluations, but you

should set up a time to discuss with managers what recommendations they have given staff about areas for improvement. This does not require that you know which employees need help in specific areas. After making appropriate programming available, it is up to the manager and the employee to make sure he/she receives the needed education. Here are some potential sources of information:

- Risk management data

- Quality improvement reports

- Performance evaluations

- Professional associations, journals, the Internet, and other sources of printed and verbal information about advances in specialty areas.

10. How can I differentiate between an educational need and a process or system problem?

10. We have all been in the position of having to prepare an educational program that we believe is inappropriate. First, find out who believes that the problem is educational and why. Review any and all available data including risk management reports. Is there a trend in the types of problems? Do the individuals have the necessary knowledge? Can you identify a flaw in process? An educational need is indicated if there is a true lack of knowledge or a change in process or treatment modalities. If data point to a flaw in the system I would recommend that it be referred for review to the quality improvement committee.

11. How can I determine the staffing needs for a Staff Development Department in other settings?

11. Find out what expectations the organization has for the Staff Development Department. What resources will you need to fulfill your part of the strategic plan? What resources can be shared from the overall organization or corporate setting? Talk to other educators in similar settings to establish a benchmark for staffing. Make sure you plan for both current and future needs.

12. How do I evaluate the impact of staff development?

12. Evaluation must include assessment of impact on productivity and the bottom line. I recommend the 5-level process.

- **Reaction** or the so-called happiness index. Were the learners satisfied with the instructor, methodology, environment, and handouts? This is usually accomplished with a written survey. (Do not forget the potential for completing evaluation forms and sending them via e-mail for distance learning students.)

- **Learning** demonstrated via an increase in knowledge or skill. This may be accomplished by a pre and posttest or return skill demonstration.

- **Behavior** can be demonstrated by an actual change or improvement in the work setting.

- **Results** are demonstrated by actual hard data. Sources include risk management reports, quality improvement findings, or a decrease in cost or increase in profit.

- **Return on Investment** involves clear financial data showing that the costs involved in designing and implementing the education program do not exceed the benefits. Ideally, there should be a link between the program(s) offered and monetary savings to the organization or an increase in the profit generated by the Staff Development Department.

13. *What might I expect as the chain of command (reporting mechanism) in other settings?*

13. This varies according to the tradition of the setting and the needs of the organization. If part of a large health system you may report to a Vice-President or Director of Education responsible for the entire system. You may have a dual reporting mechanism to such a director and to a member of the executive staff in your particular setting(s). Human resource directors or nursing administrators may also act as immediate supervisors.

14. *How do I go about finding the right "time slot" to offer programs?*

14. This question has plagued staff development specialists in all settings since staff development became a specialty. The following questions may help you decide.

- What are the hours of operation of the setting?

- Are there certain days of the week or times of day that most staff are available?

- Do you have the capability of using distance learning techniques such as computer-based learning, videos, or self-learning packets?

- What programs are mandated by accrediting agencies and/or organizational needs?

- In long term care, when are residents in activities? In home health, when do staff leave to begin daily visits?

15. *What teaching strategies and delivery methods are appropriate for other settings?*

15. Appropriateness depends on the setting, its services, and its staff. Consider a variety of methodologies including:

- Classroom learning

- Video-conferencing

- Audiotapes

- Videotapes

- Computer-based learning

- Self-learning modules

- E-mail

- Inter and Intranet

16. *What are some good resources for staff development in other settings?*

16. I would recommend the 2nd edition of the *Core Curriculum for Staff Development* published by National Nursing Staff Development Organization (NNSDO) as the primary resource. Also, see the resources listed at the end of this chapter.

17. *How can I establish a network of resource persons to help me in this role?*

17. There are a variety of ways to network. My favorites are the following:

- Local chapters and national professional associations such as NNSDO and associations devoted to specific specialty areas

- The local Chamber of Commerce

- Alumni associations

- Authors of journal articles, textbook chapters, books, or Internet sites that you particularly admire

- Other staff development specialists in similar settings

- Local newspapers for announcements about programs or events sponsored by similar groups or organizations. These are great places to meet colleagues!

18. *How can I best interview for a staff development position in other settings?*

18. Familiarize yourself with the setting and its services. Know the education mandates established by the setting, its parent organization, if applicable, and local, state, federal, and specialty accrediting agency mandates. If possible, study the strategic plan and mission, vision, and values statements. Come prepared to discuss how you can make education a major contributor to the achievement of the strategic plan.

RESOURCES

Avillion, A. E. (Ed.). (2001). *Core curriculum for staff development* (2nd ed.). Pensacola, FL: National Nursing Staff
   Development Organization.

Kirkpatrick, D. L. (1994). *Evaluating training programs*. San Francisco: Berrett-Koehler.

Tiffany, P., & Peterson, S. (1997). *Business plans for dummies*. Foster City, CA: IDG Books Worldwide, Inc.

Section 2:
Organizational Structures

As health care has advanced, so too has the scope of nursing professional development (NPD) responsibility. While some NPD specialists are still responsible just for nursing ("just" is used lightly, as nursing is ever changing its scope and responsibilities), others have responsibility for the education of more than 10,000 employees. This can seem daunting just as it is to work in a single person department. Responsibilities and scope vary by the type of department, number of employees, and organizational mission. In this section, explore the complexities of a nursing, hospital, and health system scope.

Chapter 5: *Nursing Staff Development*

1. How do you determine priorities of learning needs, especially clinical versus non-clinical?

1. You must consider many factors when prioritizing, including:

- Organizational goals and objectives
- Regulatory agency requirements
- Quality patient care outcomes
- Criticality of the need

You also must be able to balance the educational needs, time, and resources with the needs of the staff, the unit, and the organization.

Often the organizational goals and objectives directly relate to quality patient care outcomes. That pushes the learning need near the top of the priorities.

2. How do you determine which clinical competencies to assess?

2. You need to focus on competencies that are:

- New skills
- New products
- Rarely performed skills
- Skills with high risks

3. How do you determine which non-clinical competencies to assess?

3. Corporate initiatives provide the main areas of concentration. Each unit must then identify how that area of concentration affects it. For example, customer satisfaction for an educator may be measured by program evaluations and direct observation. Customer service for a staff nurse may include patient interviews.

4. Is there only one person in each area who can check off competency assessments?

4. No, thank goodness. However, someone has to be responsible for being an expert in the skill/process. If implementing a new product, the vendor may be the content expert. Ask the vendor to teach and verify the competency assessment in a "Train-the-Trainer" format. I encourage you to have *at least* one "back up" evaluator. The "back up" should be someone knowledgeable and comfortable with the skill. It is difficult to pull an assessor from another area to check off a person's competency because one had the day off.

5. What are some of the strategies you use when frequent orientations are requested?

5. With staffing at a critical stage, orientations have become a touchy issue. To be cost effective, the educators would like to present materials to as large a class as possible. To meet the needs of the organization, more frequent orientations are requested. Sometimes you bite the bullet and offer more frequent orientations. Along with a two-day general orientation for all staff, nurses also attend a two-day nursing orientation that is offered one to two times per month. Computer classes are offered several times throughout the month.

For casual nursing staff (working one to two shifts per pay period), we currently offer an abridged eight-hour evening orientation (offered over two four-hour evenings.) Along with the evening classes, the nurses must also complete self-study packets with post-tests. (The nurses are paid their salaries for the estimated time needed to complete the packets, since the information is required for their positions. The estimated time for the packet completion was established by the person who developed the self-study.) All the competencies are not covered in the abridged Evening Orientation; therefore, the preceptors on the nursing units take the responsibility of ensuring that all competencies are completed by the orientee. The nurses also attend required computer courses.

6. What should be included in orientation for agency nurses and travelers?

6. Agency nurses and travelers attend one day of general orientation. This day includes an overview of history, mission, corporate compliance policies, and basic safety for the institution. If possible, the nurses also attend the two-day nursing orientation. If it is not possible to attend the two-day program, the preceptors review the content with the nurse one-to-one on the nursing units. As with any new staff nurse, the agency nurses and travelers also attend computer classes and review specific equipment/policies for the area with preceptors.

7. How do you manage nursing faculty orientation/competencies?

7. Similar to the agency nurses, nursing faculty attend one day of general orientation. The faculty members work with preceptors at least one day to be oriented to the specific nursing unit. Annually the faculty are updated on corporate-wide safety issues using self-study and post-tests.

8. What is your responsibility in meeting the educational needs of nursing students (especially those being precepted by staff)?

8. • I coordinate student placement in the organization. This allows the schools to have one contact person for multiple clinical sites. I try to match the schools' clinical requests with available sites without having too many students in an area at one time. Of course, the clinical manager has the final decision about how many students are allowed on the unit.

- For precepted experiences, the manager offers the opportunity to staff who have been trained as preceptors. Once a preceptor volunteers, I notify the appropriate faculty member.

- The faculty members meet with the preceptor to explain expectations and goals for the semester.

- The precepted student then contacts the identified preceptor. The preceptor and student plan the specific period of time the student will be on the unit for clinical experiences.

- The preceptor and student meet to develop learning experiences congruent with the student's goals and objectives.

- The preceptor also provides specific and effective ongoing feedback to the student and faculty throughout the experience.

9. Should you be involved in educating Unlicensed Assistive Personnel (UAP)?

9. Yes, the education of unlicensed assistive personnel (UAP) is very important to overall patient care. Some methods that we use specifically for UAP are self-study "newsletters," topics on video, and an Annual Teaching Day with topics geared toward UAP. The UAP are also invited to general inservice and continuing education programs offered to other staff.

10. What teaching methodologies do you use to reach all levels of staff?

10. Use as many teaching methods as possible. We use —

- Computer-based instruction (with sound and Spanish available)

- Fair settings

- Short didactic topics in department meetings

- Skills competencies with return demonstration

- Newsletters

- Learning packets with post-tests

- Dialogue groups to discuss nursing issues

- Workshops with lecture, discussion, small group work, experiential learning

I also know of institutions using closed-circuit television for continuing education for the staff. The programs run throughout the day (and night).

11. How do you schedule education so all staff can attend?

11. Offering programs at a variety of times is optimal, but be aware of workload and staffing patterns. 3:00 a.m. may be a quiet time on the unit, but there may be only one RN on duty. He/she would not be able to leave the unit for a 50-minute class. Ask the manager and staff the best time for them. (This assessment might also get their buy-in.) Think about alternative ways to cover the unit—such as having a staff member come in early. The shorter the program, the better—but make sure you have enough time to cover the necessary information.

12. What are some methods to advertise educational opportunities?

12. We use a variety of strategies including:

- Flyers posted at many places and sent by interoffice mail

- E-mail

- Word of mouth

- Talk about upcoming programs in classes with similar target audiences

- Leadership meetings

- Weekly corporate-wide newsletter

- Unit-based bulletin boards

- Education Calendar (the calendar covers educational opportunities over a 3-month period)

- Education Catalog (the catalog gives a brief description of the courses and the frequency of the offerings)

13. How do you motivate others to help you meet the educational needs of your area?

13. As positive reinforcement, I often send thank you notes or e-mail. I also send e-mail to the person's managers/supervisors to let them know of the staff member's contribution and copy to the staff member. I like to include comments from the evaluations, too.

Some staff are uncomfortable because no one ever taught them how to teach. With new educators, it is important to take the time to explain the educational process and walk them through their first few experiences. Help them trouble shoot and anticipate possible difficulties. Always give feedback. The better prepared the new educators, the better experience it will be for everyone concerned.

14. *How do you keep track of all the records/competencies/educational history?*

14. In a perfect world, we would have one computerized system, which would include all educational history, competencies, and credentials. The staff would be self-motivated to enter any programs attended outside of the organization. I don't know about you, but I don't live in a perfect world!

We have at least two basic systems in place. One system involves a database of the programs offered within the organization. Anyone offering a class in the organization can turn in a roster of the participants for entry into the database. The database is a part of the Human Resources Information System.

Along with this organization-wide computer program, many areas have area-specific databases. The area-specific databases usually include unit-specific programs and educational programs attended outside of the organization. These databases are usually maintained on a spreadsheet in the computer or on paper.

15. *What educational opportunities should be centralized in nursing services versus decentralized to the unit?*

15. Centralized education should include topics that cross several lines of authority.

For example, new nurse orientation is centralized because it includes topics and skills used by most RNs in the organization. American Heart Association classes are also centralized for staff because many areas require the courses.

Decentralized education should be used for area-specific information. For example, a procedure that will be performed only in one area of the hospital should be decentralized.

16. *What continuing education topics should you offer versus outside agencies (e.g., colleges/universities)*

16. This decision should be based on several factors:

- Availability of content expert(s)—Is there someone in the organization who can offer the program, or do you need a nationally known speaker?

- Potential costs—Can you afford the content expert? Would it be better to co-sponsor the program?

- Number of people who will attend—If only a handful of staff have the need or interest, it may be better to send the staff off-campus.

- Classroom space—Can you accommodate the number of people interested in the topic?

17. How do you get content experts for programs?

17.
- First, look within the organization—not just the nursing staff. The ancillary staff and physicians may have a wealth of knowledge that they would be honored to share with interested staff.

- If you cannot find a qualified content expert in the setting, ask the staff if they know anyone who would be a good speaker. Then investigate content experts in area colleges, universities, or Area Health Education Centers (AHECs).

Helpful Hint: As you search for content experts, also make sure they like to teach. If they don't like to teach, it will come across in their presentations.

18. How do you get buy-in from management for education?

18. In order for managers to have buy-in to education, they must understand the importance of the education and applicability of the content. They want to know what's in it for them, for the staff, and the patients.

Managers have more buy-in when they have some

- Ownership of the process

- Input into planning

- Respect for the merit of the process outcome

- Accountability for the process outcome

It is important to have the managers involved early in planning stages of the educational process—even if this simply means notifying them of upcoming programs and asking for their feedback. Sometimes it means asking for their opinions of topics, presentation method, or speaker.

19. What are some tricks/methods for maximizing small budgets to achieve desired big budget outcomes?

19. When it comes to providing a professional program on a shoestring, the little things mean a lot—and the little things don't have to cost a lot.

- Ask, "Do we need a binder or will a folder work just as well?" Participants just want to keep their materials in a relatively neat manner.

- Consider a theme. One of our programs uses a travel theme within the state. We decorate with posters and travel brochures. We give away the current state maps and travel guides. All of these items are free from the travel bureau.

- Offer prizes. We use leftover advertisement novelties

from the organization. I am always surprised how many people are excited over "winning" a stress ball, including me!

- Put some candy on the table. The participants appreciate this added jolt of sugar.

20. How do you get additional funding for programs?

20. There are a few methods to obtain funding for programs.

- Vendors may support classes. Pharmaceutical companies especially help foot the bill if physicians plan to attend the program. The support may come in the form of meals, folders, novelties, or honoraria for speakers. (They may even help you find content experts!)

- Consider co-sponsoring a program with the local Area Health Education Center, another hospital in the area, or a local college or university.

- Grants are available from a variety of sources—within the county, state, and nation—sometimes within your own institution.

21. As staff development professionals, we should be instrumental in recognizing staff. How do you celebrate nursing achievements?

21.
- In the corporate-wide newsletter, positive patient comments are noted on a weekly basis. Newly awarded certifications, publications, and awards are also noted in the newsletter.

- Some areas have "employees of the month." They are celebrated with a cake, engraved plaque, and a visit by the vice president.

- Many staff enjoy one-to-one acknowledgment of achievements. This can include quietly praising a person or sending a card.

- We have several statewide nursing recognition programs, such as opportunities through the North Carolina Center for Nursing (**www.ga.unc.edu/NCCN/**) and the Great 100 (**www.great100.org**). We encourage staff to nominate others for these recognition programs.

22. How do you differentiate between an education problem and a management problem?

22. An educational need can be met through some form of instruction. If the staff member *cannot* demonstrate or explain a procedure or concept, it is an educational need. If the staff person *can* perform the skill and explain the concepts, then there is *not* an educational need. Something other than a lack of knowledge is keeping this person from performing at the expected level (e.g., lack

41

23. What should you consider when orienting a new graduate?

23. As with any new employee, you will want to do a needs assessment.

(of supplies, ambiguous expectations, or inadequate support.)

- Where did he/she have clinical experiences?

- Has he/she worked in health care before?

- What strengths does he/she bring to the work place?

- What areas does he/she need to develop?

Along with skills and procedures, don't forget to role model and encourage time management, prioritization, and critical thinking skills.

24. What should be included in an internship program?

24. Internship programs vary in length—6 weeks to one year. The coordinator of the program must plan for didactic and clinical components. The preceptor should validate skills, reinforce the knowledge learned in class, and serve as a positive role model for the new nurse. The preceptor should encourage socialization within the unit and the hospital by introducing the new employee to the staff, physicians, and others within the organization. Many internship programs provide time for the new nurses to discuss their progress, similar to a support group. This allows time for the new nurses to share positive and negative experiences and learn from each other.

Resources

Abruzzese, R. S. (1996). *Nursing staff development: Strategies for success* (2nd ed.). St. Louis: Mosby.

Fey, M. K., & Miltner, R. S. (2000). A competency-based orientation program for new graduate nurses. *Journal of Nursing Administration, 30*(3), 126–132.

Flynn, J. P. (Ed.). (1997). *The role of the preceptor: A guide for nurse educators and clinicians*. New York: Springer.

Kelly Thomas, K. J. (1998). *Clinical and nursing staff development: Current competence, future focus* (2nd ed.). Philadelphia: Lippincott.

Chapter 6: *Hospital-Wide Staff Development*

1. *My department has assumed hospital-wide responsibility for education and I'm not sure where to start. The various hospital departments aren't sure how to use my services either. What can I do?*

1. Clearly define the services you can provide. It is equally essential to hear the various departments' perception of their current education needs; however, describing the types of services you can provide may serve as a great starting point.

Don't be shy about offering expert consultation services. Staff development educators are proficient in developing orientation, inservice and continuing education programs to meet diverse learner needs, and in the evaluation of competency. Do any of your new customers need assistance in these areas?

Re-examine programs you currently offer. Would any of them, such as preceptor training, be applicable to disciplines outside of nursing? If so, share a list and description of the classes. Start with the mandatories such as Management Training Classes, CPR, and other classes designed to meet regulatory agency or organizational requirements.

2. *The current Staff Development Department consists of nurses. Is it realistic to expect that we can effectively respond to the needs of other disciplines?*

2. It is realistic to expect that the department will effectively respond to the needs of other disciplines. However, it is not realistic to expect, nor is it necessary for the educators to be content experts as related to all disciplines. Remember, although you may not be the clinical expert, you are an education expert. Characteristics of the successful educator do not change although the scope is broadened. Put your leadership, management, and communication skills, in addition to your political savvy, to work for you. Your ability to assess learning needs and develop, implement, and evaluate programs will be a valuable resource. All disciplines can benefit from your knowledge of adult learning principles, knowledge of current trends in health care, flexibility, and acceptance and respect for individual differences and diversity.

3. *How can I keep abreast of the needs of all of the disciplines for which I have assumed responsibility?*

3. If you have not already done so, get to know your new customers. The key to success will be in building relationships with the various departments. One way to do this is by establishing a multidisciplinary hospital-wide education committee. This committee will prove helpful in facilitating communication among the groups, clearly identifying education needs, streamlining efforts in meeting these needs, and decreasing the duplication of efforts. Keep the communication going!

4. Each discipline is requesting their "own classes." How can I decrease my chances of becoming overwhelmed or feeling spread too thin?

4. Work smarter, not harder. Use posters/flyers, closed-circuit television, self-instructional materials, computer-based instruction, newsletters, and portable educational carts as applicable. If possible, use the "Train-the-Trainer" model and product reps for product training. The Train-the Trainer model will also be valuable in the introduction of new "work area specific" skills. Examine the feasibility of each teaching strategy in relation to available resources, the information you are trying to teach, and the level of learners.

If classes are needed, be sure to develop them to include only the essential "need to know" information. Identify concepts generic to all disciplines and teach in large groups, if appropriate. Solicit members from the inter-disciplinary education committee to facilitate sessions in their work areas to cover discipline specific content. The focus should be shifted from being that of a teacher to being an education consultant or facilitator.

5. What are my responsibilities in the orientation of new employees from the various disciplines within the hospital?

5. Coordinating/facilitating the hospital-wide orientation is a major focus. Be sure that the program includes broad concepts, which are essential to all new hires. These topic areas are usually limited to those required by regulatory agencies and organizational requirements, including payroll and benefits discussions. Department and work area specific types of detail would not be appropriate. If not already in place, serve as a consultant to the various departments as they develop their own department specific orientation programs.

6. Now that I am trying to manage hospital-wide education needs, I need more staff, but I do not have the money in my budget for additional staff. What can I do?

6. Depending upon the education need, there are several ways to maximize available resources. First, re-evaluate what you are currently doing. Are you employing creative teaching strategies as much as possible in order to decrease actual classroom time?

If more manpower is really needed, the resources are probably there but they have to be sought out. Try bartering. If hospital staff assist with CPR training, how can you/or the institution reward them? Is there a clinical ladder in place? If so, are staff rewarded for teaching? If the answer is no, could this be incorporated? Is assisting with educational programming recognized in the Performance Review Process?

If you work in a department that offers major conferences, can staff be rewarded for teaching by allowing them to attend a conference for free?

7. *In addition to changes in required "people resources," where else might I feel the impact of my increased responsibility for hospital-wide programming?*

7. Your budget! The volume of learners will increase and you will need to consider this even when budgeting for programs you have routinely offered. Will the audio-visual equipment already in the department be sufficient for the increased customer base? Both operational and capital budgets may be affected. Space needs will also need to be reassessed because of an increase in the numbers of customers served.

8. *I am receiving feedback from nurse managers stating that there is less visibility of the clinical educators since we assumed hospital-wide responsibility. What should I do?*

8. Communication is essential. Be sure managers are kept abreast of the educators' involvement in projects that are beneficial to patient care. This is especially important when initially changing from a Nursing Staff Development to a Hospital Staff Development Department. Be sure the "new" role of the educator has been clearly defined and communicated to the leadership group.

   If educators have specific units for which they are responsible, it is beneficial for them to establish formal meetings with the nurse manager and to attend staff meetings whenever possible. To enhance visibility with staff, try making unit visits really count. Can you have lunch with the staff? Is there a particular time when the unit is less busy and you could have time to actually talk to the staff to assess their needs? Is there an education committee on the unit? If yes, become an active part. If not, with the manager's support, spearhead the development of the committee.

9. *In a hospital-wide education department, are there any benefits specific to nursing?*

9. Yes, because a large percentage of hospital education department educators are nurses, programs will incorporate a nursing perspective and thus, improve patient care. Using multidisciplinary resources benefits the nursing department by providing more programming for nurses than a nursing staff development department could provide alone. Multidisciplinary programs will also stimulate a collaborative practice environment.

10. *What types of programs should be centralized? Decentralized?*

10. To decide whether a centralized or decentralized approach would be best for a program, it is helpful to consider how many learners you have to reach and what resources in terms of personnel, equipment, and supplies will have to be used.

   Programs such as orientation and other regulatory agency and organizational requirements, hospital-wide continuing education programs, and management development are a few examples of programs that lend themselves to a centralized approach. Because these programs are attended by large numbers of diverse learners, clerical and support services are usually more extensive. Clerical staff can be assigned to support designated functions, thereby enhancing their proficiency in the assigned areas. Depending upon the class, offering it centrally avoids the need to transport heavy equipment and supplies from location to location. Also, the opportunity exists for collegial support among educators.

A decentralized approach may prove most effective when responding to learning needs that are highly specialized such as those related to one discipline, or one unit within a discipline. The number of learners will be smaller thereby decreasing the need for extensive clerical support. This approach affords greater flexibility and allows the educator to more easily schedule times to meet the needs of the staff.

If the program is truly decentralized and offered in the work environment, the educator is challenged to keep the focus on education and off of the activities going on simultaneously in the work environment.

11. *There are multiple house-wide education programs being scheduled and staff development is expected to take the lead on all of them. How can this be managed?*

11. Prioritize! Be sure to consult with administration as a part of the prioritization process. Be honest and realistic, however; do not promise what you cannot deliver. If trade offs will have to occur in order to move forward with the education programs, clearly define for administration what the trade offs will be. Benefits and risks will have to be weighed. Be flexible; be creative.

12. *It's not time to embark upon a formal evaluation of my department's effectiveness in providing hospital-wide education, but I would like to perform a "spot check" just to make sure I'm on target. What can I do?*

12. Ask! Don't be afraid to ask your customers for constructive feedback. Since it is not time for a formal evaluation, employ informal strategies such as face-to-face dialogue in multidisciplinary team meetings or develop a brief survey consisting of two to three simple questions to which customers can respond.

13. *Nurses are coming to programs; however, attendance of learners from other disciplines has been minimal. Why might this be the case?*

13. If you haven't already, review evaluations from past programs. Have you received feedback from other disciplines stating that the programs "do not relate to me" or "too focused on nursing?" Take an open, honest look at the class. Is it relevant to other disciplines? Be sure you have included case examples relevant to staff from various disciplines. Using all nursing examples in a class with multidisciplinary learners can be a turn-off. On the front end, be sure to use multidisciplinary teams when developing courses/programs.

Touch base with the departments to gain insight to other possible pitfalls that may be affecting attendance such as competing priorities, conflicts in scheduling, relevance of the topic, and/or marketing effectiveness. Be prepared and willing to make program changes based upon feedback.

Resources

Abruzzese, R. S. (1996). *Nursing staff development. Strategies for success* (2nd ed.). St. Louis: Mosby.

Bland, C., & Michael, S. (1997). Redesigning the role of the centralized educator. *Journal of Nursing Staff Development, 13*(5), 279–281.

Cracolici, F., Gianella, A., Sullivan, D. T., & Frazier, J. (1996). Nursing staff development goes hospital-wide. *Journal of Nursing Administration, 26*(11), 6–9.

Hardt, M., Yanko, J., & Brandstock, J. (1996). Broadening the educator's role: The use of support staff in implementing staff empowerment. *Journal of Nursing Staff Development, 12*(6), 300–305.

Kelly Thomas, K. J. (1998*). Nursing staff development: Current competence, future focus*. Philadelphia: Lippincott.

Mateo, M., & Fahje, C. (1998). The nurse educator role in the clinical setting. *Journal for Nurses in Staff Development, 14*(4), 169–175.

Chapter 7: *Health System Staff Development*

1. What is the definition of a "Health System"?

1. A health system is comprised of multiple clinical entities that operate at varying degrees of independence. Usually, a health system has a corporate structure that governs the overall activity of the entities. The advantages of a health system are that it can:

- Respond quickly and effectively to community healthcare needs
- Ensure consistent quality standards throughout the system
- Increase access to care
- Enhance quality of care available to all members of the community
- Integrate and coordinate services across facilities and organizations where appropriate
- Achieve operational and cost efficiencies
- Cover continuum of care
- Focus on wellness and prevention
- Establish effective communication channels
- Heighten awareness of mutual dependency
- Create new partnerships

2. When education departments "merge" or "integrate," how is this best accomplished?

2. Integration of departments is best accomplished when a process is put in place that is well planned, sequential, facilitated by neutral parties, and ensures accountability. Ernst and Young, LLP, facilitated the process at Duke University Health System. An overview of the Transition Process is as follows:

- Transition Task Force Selection Process (12 months prior to "go live")
  - Operating Philosophy
  - Assessment of Integration Opportunities
  - Strategic Operating Model
- Transition Task Force: Establish Integration Teams (11 months prior to "go live")
  - Identification of Integration Teams
  - Team Charters
- Integration Teams: Develop Initial Business Case (9 months prior to "go live")
  - Current State Assessment

- Future State Vision & Gap Analysis
- High-Level Implementation Action Plan

• Transition Task Force: Prioritize Integration Opportunities (7 months prior to "go live")
  - Integration Criteria
  - Ranking of Initiatives
  - Management Subcommittee Approval

• Office of Operations Integration: Establish the Infrastructure (6 months prior to "go live")
  - Internal Infrastructure
  - Implementation Work Plan
  - Performance Measurement System

• Resources and Act Teams: Implementation Planning (3 months prior to "go live")
  - Day One Policy Review
  - Detailed Implementation Plan
  - Business Case with Performance Targets

• **Day One:** Plan and Design Teams: Plan & Prioritize for Future Integration
  - Future State Development
  - Initial Business Cases and Implementation Plans

Following a planned, sequential process allows those involved to focus on the opportunities that are inherent in working collaboratively. The facilitation by a neutral source, when possible, assists the team with moving forward and letting go of political, historical, or personal agendas.

3. *How do I deal with common education needs of several healthcare entities?*

3. Needs assessment is a decision-making tool used by educators to determine the educational needs of staff. In health care, needs assessments can be derived from a number of sources including self-perceived needs, organizational needs, emerging trends and issues, and needs arising from performance improvement activities. According to Queeney (2000), method selection should be tailored to:

1. the nature of the need(s) being assessed

2. a realistic inventory of available resources, including budget, expertise, time, and facilities

3. the population being assessed.

Common educational needs of several entities are easily identified via simple, low cost methods such as questionnaire, focus groups, and manager input. It is helpful to the educator to focus questions on the complexity level of the intervention that is desired. This makes the program planning process much easier. Typical programs that address common educational needs include such topics as basic physical assessment, patient education, and regulatory issues.

4. How do I deal with different education needs of several healthcare entities?

4. Managing multiple education needs across healthcare entities can be particularly challenging. The clinical educational needs of the tertiary care hospital, for instance, may be quite different from those of the community hospital or long-term care facilities. It is advisable that the educator uses the expertise of the staff in each setting to determine the complexity and content of different educational programs. Offering a core set of programs that serve the entire system provides the departmental infrastructure. Programs are then developed which build on either clinical skills (according to Benner's Novice to Expert Model) or specialized site needs. Educational interventions based on regulatory or accreditation needs are integrated throughout most offerings and emphasized by faculty.

Additionally, a critical issue in managing educational needs across a healthcare system involves the collaboration and partnering with other entities, agencies, or departments. Thriving in this new healthcare environment requires that educators think more creatively than ever about collaborating with others to deliver education. For example, state agencies are often willing to partner and share costs to develop programs which benefit the staff in their facilities. Developing community advisory boards and keeping those relationships open and flexible can yield programming that is both very effective and cost efficient.

5. What should we consider to avoid duplication of services?

5. Duplication of services is a drain on both human and fiscal resources. It is essential that educators constantly communicate among entities and collaborate on offerings when possible. If performance gaps exist in all entities, the educators are able to plan jointly to manage the needs.

Also, simple measures can be taken to save educator time and departmental dollars. These measures include joint brochure development and/or marketing, printing course materials collectively to decrease costs, and rotating geographic locations to increase access to all learners. Having a centralized registration and tracking system in place decreases the need for administrative staff at each entity.

6. What are the advantages of a centralized education services department serving a health system?

6. The advantages of a centralized educational services department include:

- Increased efficiency (develop centrally; deliver locally)
- Economic advantages (economies of scale)
- Quality control and accountability
- Standardization across departments

7. How are staff educators assigned?

7. Staff educators are assigned according to their core functional service area:

- Staff Education
- Patient/Family Education
- Community Education
- Information Systems Education

The largest number of FTEs supports the staff education function, which includes Orientation, Life Support, Clinical Education, and Professional Educational Offerings.

All educators can teach in the Life Support component of the departmental activities.

8. How often should staff from all facilities meet?

8. Staff educators should meet on a monthly basis as a group. Core service staff should meet on a weekly basis.

Meeting	Frequency
Full Staff Meeting ....Monthly	
Core Service Area Meeting .... Weekly	
Clinical Teaching Block Meeting .... As needed	

9. How does the department director deal with multiple accountability at each site?

9. Dealing with multiple geographic sites and the accountability of educational delivery can be extremely difficult to manage. The organizational structure of the department becomes a key factor in keeping communication open, managing day-to-day operations, and evaluating the effectiveness of educational interventions. Having strong management presence at each site is essential. The entire leadership team should meet no less than bi-weekly and discuss an agenda including, but not limited to:

- Position Management
- Budget
- Operations
- Issues/Concerns

Additionally, all educators file quarterly reports into a database. These reports indicate the work accomplished at each site. At the end of the Fiscal Year, the reports are compiled into an Annual Report of the Educational Services Department and distributed widely across the system.

10. How is equity at each site accomplished?

10. "Equity" in educational delivery is difficult to quantify. Within the Duke Health System, the distribution of both human and fiscal resources is determined by the number of staff based at each site, the complexity of the training that needs to occur, and the educational space within each location. The department should be able to "flex up" and provide episodic support during times of specific needs, such as rolling out new standards or equipment within an entity.

11. What kinds of team building activities are helpful to the education services staff?

11. Staff educators are typically a motivated, creative, and intelligent group of professionals. The most basic need of educators is having access to the equipment and materials that they need to do their jobs. This includes a pleasant office and teaching environment, electronic communication capabilities, and instructional supplies and materials.

They also need professional development and teambuilding activities exclusively for them. Staff can be nurtured and developed in a number of ways. Annual staff retreats give the educators the opportunity to focus on past accomplishments and look toward the future in planning programs and events for the next year. Attending specific continuing education conferences brings renewal to the staff and motivates them by bringing fresh new ideas to their repertoire of skills. Occasionally staff groups will engage in mobile team building initiatives such as physical challenge courses.

12. How do I manage three or more geographic sites?

12. As mentioned before, a strong organizational infrastructure, visible management presence, and communication among staff are helpful in managing multiple geographic sites. If the entities are standardized regarding policies such as time and attendance, it relieves a portion of the burden associated with personnel management. Clear and constant communication from the leadership team to all of the staff creates a positive working relationship among all department members.

13. How does the department director collaborate successfully with other departments within the health system?

13. Health systems represent complex organizations. Often, they are associated with academic health centers and universities. This complexity can make the environment difficult to navigate for the educational services director. It is essential that the director be part of the leadership team of the organization and that the individual determines the stakeholders within the organization who can help meet the educational services mission of the department. Examples of such stakeholders would be the chief nursing executive, operating officers, accreditation and regulatory affairs officers, deans of health professions schools, and department directors.

It is sometimes helpful to generate memoranda of understanding, service level agreements, or other contractual models in writing to ensure that each partner is clear on the specific responsibilities during a collaborative project. It is always appropriate to involve other departments in program planning if they are interested in being active participants in the program planning and development or in sharing in the outcomes.

14. What kind of pricing structures should we consider?

14. Pricing structures in continuing professional education vary greatly. Deciding on the cost of educational programs and interventions is largely determined within a health system by an examination of how the department is funded. If a department is subsidized by the system and perhaps leverages an educational allotment per entity, then pricing for orientation and core programs would not become an issue.

For conferences where expenses such as site hotel,

speaker honoraria, and catering are needed, the educator may use a formula based on the projected costs (direct and indirect) and expected number of participants to determine the registration fee.

15. How do I use a "Balanced Scorecard" approach in staff development?

15. According to Kaplan and Norton (1993), the "balanced scorecard provides a framework for managing the implementation of strategy while also allowing the strategy itself to evolve in response to changes in the organization's competitive, market and technological environments" (p. 134).

The application for a balanced scorecard approach in staff development involves development and communication of the departmental vision and mission and the delineation of measures and targets within the following four quadrants:

- Internal Growth/Learning Perspective

- Customer Perspective

- Internal Business Perspective

- Financial Perspective

16. What process should we use to prioritize the work of the department?

16. The work of the department is broken down into the work of the core service functional areas of (1) Staff Education, (2) Patient/Family Education, (3) Community Education, and (4) Information Technology Training. Staff Education needs in the area of Life Support are performed by all staff members. Departmental staff members sit on committees within the health system to represent the Education Department. Orientation, Life Support, and Core Curricula are routinely managed each month. Clinical and professional skill-building courses are offered quarterly and advertised via an Intranet site. Emerging needs related to regulatory, societal, research, equipment, or accreditation needs are managed as they develop. Committees develop training and rollout plans based on staff educator input.

17. What kind of performance improvement activities should the department engage in?

17. Initiation of performance improvement teams can greatly affect the work of the Educational Services Department. Teams can work together to analyze workflow and to plan for process improvements that are often efficient as well as cost effective.

The minimum that should be done is listed in the table below:

What is evaluated?	When is evaluation done?
Departmental Policies & Procedures	Annually
Budget	Monthly
Personnel	Ongoing with Annual Review
Equipment	Annually
Participant Evaluation Feedback	Each Program
Educational Programming for Year	Annually

18. What health system educational programs are easily managed via Computer Based Training (CBT), the Intranet, and the Web?

18. The programs most easily delivered via CBT, the Intranet, and the World Wide Web are often the activities that are needed for mandatory compliance among staff. Access to a workstation with content delivered electronically offers the bedside staff member the opportunity to use a break period to engage in a continuing education activity. Some research has shown that staff use the materials at intervals during a shift and prefer this method to leaving the unit in some instances.

Additionally, courses that can offer remediation for staff needing additional resources in specific clinical areas are very well accepted using this medium.

CBT, the Intranet, and the Web offer staff educators an additional delivery method for training and development. A "blended" approach using synchronous and asynchronous learning might be the most effective method of all.

19. What type of learning management system is appropriate when multiple sites are involved in record keeping?

19. Various learning management systems are currently on the market. While each may have desirable features, it is often difficult for the Educational Services Director to find one that has all of the features and fits into the budgeted needs of the organization. The following are features that are desirable:

- Course Registration

- License Renewals

- Mandatory Course Lists

- Staff Profiles

- Print Name Badges

- Attendance Statistics

- Sign-In Sheets

- Mailing Labels

- Instructor Database

- Budget Reports

20. How important are various types of accreditation?

20. Accreditation is very important within a health system education department. Provision of contact hour certificates is essential to most healthcare professionals, whether it be for relicensure, credentialing, and/or certification. The type of credit that is sought is most easily determined by the target audience that the department serves. For instance, if the majority of the participants are nurses, the credit approval would be sought through the American Nurses Credentialing Center (ANCC). The Continuing Education Unit (CEU) is also widely accepted as credible and adhering to principles of practice in continuing professional education. Hospitals and other healthcare agencies can also make use of their own internal recognition of course participants.

It is helpful for a Department Director to be able to articulate the differences in units of measurement (e.g., contact hours, CME, CEU) used by professional accrediting bodies.

RESOURCES

Abruzzese, R. S. (1996). *Nursing staff development: Strategies for success* (2nd ed.). St. Louis: Mosby.

American Nurses Association. (2000*). Scope and standards of practice for nursing professional development*. Washington, DC: American Nurses Publishing.

American Nurses Credentialing Center. (2001–2002). *Manual for accreditation as an approver of continuing education in nursing*. Washington, DC: Author.

Benner, P. (1984). *From novice to expert: Excellence and power in clinical practice*. Menlo Park, CA: Addison-Wesley.

Kaplan, R. S., & Norton, D. P. (1993). Putting the balanced scorecard to work. *Harvard Business Review, 72,* 134–137.

Kelly Thomas, K. J. (1998). *Clinical and nursing staff development: Current competence, future focus* (2nd ed.). Philadelphia: Lippincott.

Nowicki, C. R. (1996). 21 predictions for the future of hospital staff development. *The Journal of Continuing Education in Nursing, 27,* 259–266.

Queeney, D. S. (1995). *Assessing needs in continuing education.* San Francisco: Jossey-Bass.

Section 3:
Staff Development Roles and Responsibilities

While the *Scope and Standards of Practice for Nursing Professional Development* (NPD) (American Nurses Associates [ANA], 2000) introduced six roles for the NPD specialist—educator, consultant, researcher, change agent, facilitator, and leader, we have included three additional functional roles in our discussion: manager, clinical educator, and patient educator. The nurse working in NPD may have a single function, to teach classes, or may wear many hats and serve as an internal consultant, patient educator, or program manager. The terms roles and functions are interchangeable in this section, as the job description tends to be expansive rather than restrictive. In the collegiate setting, the NPD specialist is often assigned the responsibility for leadership and facilitation of many university initiatives. Multitasking, fluidity, and creativity are themes of these roles.

8. **Educator**
   Michele L. Deck, MEd, BSN, RN, LCCE

9. **Manager**
   Theresa A. Herb, MEd, RN,C

10. **Consultant**
    Marilynn J. Jackson, PhD, MA, RN

11. **Researcher**
    Patricia Welch Dittman, MSN, RN, CDE

12. **Clinical**
    Margaret H. Sturdivant, MSN, RN

13. **Patient Education**
    Karen D. Stallings, MEd, RN

14. **Change Agent, Facilitator, Leader**
    Mitzi T. Grey, MEd, RN,C

Chapter 8: *Educator*

1. *How do I motivate participants?*

1. Some proponents contend there is only one person you can motivate successfully: you. Start by examining your attitude toward the class before you get there. Do you believe the message and its importance? Do you model what you teach? Have you adequately prepared for class to make it the best it can be for the participants? If you can answer yes to all of these questions, then look to the other side of motivation. You can create the environment for learners to motivate themselves. What are the components of a motivating environment? It must be positive and interesting and recognize the value of the learners in the process. Involving the learners is a key element. Another is gaining the learners' commitment by asking what they want to gain in the class as well as showing appreciation when they try. There are many elements, and these are a few of the key ideas.

2. *How do I deal with difficult learners?*

2. This situation has haunted educators over the years. I have a few secrets that work with these learners without anyone knowing that is your goal. The first is to mix the group so that "dynamic duos" and "terrible trios" can't sit together. Mix groups in a way that looks random but ensure they can't sit together or be on the same team. You might mix groups using different colors of construction paper, mixed candies, or playing cards.

I also like to give each group sitting together a team identity, making all of them responsible for the behavior of their members. This way peers manage each other and the whole class doesn't know who your problem child is. I avoid eye contact with the difficult learners when lecturing. Some educators try to give more attention to the difficult learners trying to convince them to change their attitude. I would rather focus my energy on everyone but the negative and difficult learners. This makes it possible for me to pretend all is well because I am making eye contact with the positive people.

3. *How do I maintain energy to deliver the message?*

3. The first key to maintaining energy is to find it. If you get nervous or a little anxious before you stand in front of others, harness that energy and put it into the delivery of the presentation. Begin with a smile and a positive statement, such as "Good morning! I'm so glad to see your smiling faces this morning!" and mean it. I also suggest you take excellent care of yourself when teaching. Get enough sleep, eat well, rest when you can, and completely relax when it is over. Be very kind to yourself, because, to maintain energy, you must provide yourself with the right fuel. That fuel is good food, critical information, and a positive attitude.

4. What ideas do you have to keep things interesting?

4. It is so important that what we are teaching interests us that we want to seek opportunities to love what we do. If you have taught the same content over and over again, maybe it's time to change it, or look for a new activity or prop to add. The minute you are bored or tired of teaching a class, change it. If not, all of the learners will know from your nonverbal communication how you feel. If you don't love the topic or the teaching, the audience won't love it either or appreciate the message. Create ways to keep it interesting for you.

5. How does the educator role relate to other roles?

5. The educator role has to be a partnership with all the different people throughout the organization. Make yourself available as a resource on more than just CPR. As you expand the relationships you have with key members in the organization, the better you can understand the learning needs and how they match the strategic language and commitment of the organization. Creating and maintaining these relationships with all levels of people is critical to success.

6. How can I get people to attend inservice programs?

6. You might want to invite them in a fun, clever way that gets their attention. Instead of just sending out a registration form, you might make it an announcement, such as . . . Mary Jones has been selected as a contestant on "Who wants to be a million . . . air infection control maven?" Make people curious and they will be more likely to come. When they arrive, make the learning fun and rewarding, and you will have plenty of participants.

7. How can I get them back from breaks on time?

7. I find a four-tiered approach works well. First, divide the class into small groups and make one member responsible for bringing everyone in the group back on time. Second, use a clock that all can see and select an odd time to return, such as 3:12 p.m. I like to use a clock called a teach timer. It can display the time on an overhead projector so everyone can see from the back of the room. The third approach is to offer an incentive to come back on time (all groups here at 3:12 are eligible to answer a trivia question worth 2 points). The fourth approach is to follow your own rules and start on time even if everyone isn't back. That shows respect for the ones who are on time.

8. How do I teach a large amount of content in a short amount of time?

8. I think the best way to do that is to set the stage from the beginning and use some colored tape flags. Distribute red tape flags and tell your learners to mark the page numbers you announce with red flags because this is "need to know" content and will be taught in class time. Distribute yellow tape flags and ask them to mark other pages you announce as "need to find information." When they leave they can "let their fingers do the walking through the yellow pages" because this is reference information they might need to find when they get back to the job. Distribute blue tape flags and ask them to mark the rest of the sections not currently flagged. This information is called "the nice to know information." They can read this in their spare time; you will not address it in class. It is critical that you can differentiate these before class because it is not all "need to know."

9. How do I make boring, mandated topics interesting?

9. I like to use interactive activities that teach the content without lecture. I might use some of the current popular game formats. Put learners in teams and ask them to compete to learn or review the information that is mandated. Make the process of learning the topics or reviewing the topics fun and light hearted.

10. What are some ideas I can use to spice up computer training?

10. Purchase three colors of paper or plastic cups, so that each participant can receive one red, one green, and one yellow cup. Ask the participants to stack the cups so that the green is on the top of the stack. They are to keep the stack on top of their monitor or in an area where you can see it. As long as they understand what you are teaching and are successfully progressing, they are to leave the green cup visible at the top of the stack. This means "I understand and am with you mentally." If they get stuck or need attention immediately, they are to put the red cup on the top of the stack. This means, "I need help right this minute." If they have a question that can wait until the end of your current explanation, they are to place the yellow cup on the top of the stack. This means, "When you have a minute, I have a question." This will allow the instructor to monitor everyone's progress in a timely fashion and ensure all are on board with the learning.

11. How do I keep them awake and alert?

11. I suggest that you vary the method you use to teach every eight to twenty minutes. This can serve to refocus the group and reenergize them. I would use some activities that require physical movement to teach or reinforce the message of the class.

12. *How can I get them to implement what they have learned in my classes?*

12. Get the unit manager's support before you plan the class and agree then how it will be evaluated and validated. Make the plan to follow-up a part of the class before it begins and announce it (these are the expectations). After class, meet with managers and check in to see if they are following up on learners. You can also design a contest where learners tell you a story of how they have used what they learned in class. Conduct a prize raffle for all entrants and give away something desirable. Make the contest follow up explanation during the class as well. Give positive feedback and recognition to all who participate.

13. *How long does it take to develop a new class?*

13. I always find this question interesting because the real answer is it depends. It depends on the length of the class, the detail, and whether or not you know the topic. I can give these general guidelines: Conservatively, it is a four to one ratio (1 hour class, 4 hours to develop), or liberally, for high tech course design it can take up to 100 hours to develop and implement 5 minutes of content (decision based software design to finished product use and upkeep).

14. *Whom should I involve in the planning of classes?*

14. I like to involve three sets of people. I include some of the potential audience members, some of their bosses, and some of the people below them on the organizational chart. Sometimes asking people one level above and one level below learners gives you a more complete picture of the learning needs that exist than if you just asked the learners themselves. This also creates participation and commitment from those you involve as advisors and helpers.

15. *How do you teach a class where you know they know more about the topic than you do?*

15. I would enlist the group's help in teaching the subject. If I had known this ahead of time, I might ask each person to take one bit of content and be willing to teach it to all in a five-minute format. That shows you honor their experience, and you see them as credible and important. If someone asks a question you can't answer, admit it, and ask the group for help. I think people respect you more when you are honest versus trying to appear to know everything when you don't.

16. *I've been asked to teach about infection control again to the same group;*

16. Become a partner of the unit manager to tackle this problem. I would meet with him/her and discuss exactly what the situation is with infection rates on the unit. I would also determine whether the people have a

I have done it four times this year. They have the knowledge, but aren't using it. What do I do?

knowledge deficit in this area or a compliance issue. If the people can tell or demonstrate proper infection control measures in a class situation or elsewhere, it is a compliance issue. It is our job to support the manager in taking the necessary actions to ensure people are using proper technique or dealing with the consequences of continuing to use poor practice. Sometimes an educator can be called in to reiterate policy or procedure, but we don't have the power to enforce those. I would do what I could to support the actions of the unit manager. Without action, there will be no change.

17. *How do I teach a class that has a variety of people in it such as nurse aides, nurses, managers, and board members?*

17. I think it is important to conduct an opening activity they can all participate in, in small teams, that makes them realize their commonalities and minimizes their differences. This gets people to connect and feel comfortable, no matter what their job title might be. One example of an opening activity is to give them two minutes to find something they have in common. It can have nothing to do with work or their jobs and is a bit unusual. I ask them to turn their commonality into a group name and then refer to the group by that name throughout class. When they meet in the halls later, they can smile and feel they know someone not in their department, and a good relationship has begun with them.

18. *How do I teach groups that have different levels of experience on the topic?*

18. If the group is a mixed one (some have never heard the information, others know it better than you), capitalize on the people who are experienced. You might ask the class to line up by amount of experience with the topic, from "I've never heard this before," through to "I've learned this topic every year for the last 20 years." Let them find where they go in the single file line by mingling and talking for two minutes. When the line is complete, select one person from each end of the line (most experienced and least experienced). Have those two people pick two more people from the line in the middle and form a group that sits together. Continue in this fashion until all are selected. Once you have groups defined, invite them to work together throughout class to help everyone learn the information. At intervals, give them 90 seconds to check in and teach back to each other in the groups. This way the experienced people feel valued and the less experienced people feel mentored and helped by all. The midlevel people sometimes act as the balance between the two ends of the continuum.

19. Is fun in class appropriate when teaching serious topics?

19. I think having fun while learning a serious topic is critical to getting people to remember it! If anxiety is high about a learning topic or situation, retention is low. The brain downshifts when under stress, which makes higher thought impossible. Learner anxiety is a barrier we must eliminate to set the stage for effective learning. One way to do that is to create joy and fun in the learning process. That doesn't mean you must be a comedian or make light of a serious topic. It means getting the learners involved in a learning activity that teaches or reinforces information; that activity generates fun in and among the participants.

20. How do I handle a person who wants to argue with me in front of the class?

20. I always try not to argue in front of a class. When someone challenges me in front of the group, I become a diligent listener until I hear him/her mention something that will benefit everyone. Then I phrase what was said in a positive light, and then say thanks for the contribution. To best illustrate this, let me describe just such a situation.

A few years ago, I was presenting at a national conference and had about 400 attendees in my session. My topic was opening activities to use in CPR class. I was about half way through the material when someone in the back stood up in the middle of my sentence and said, "It is ridiculous for you to say we should use opening activities in CPR class. We don't have enough time as it is to teach everything we are supposed to in the time they give us!" I asked her what her name was with a smile on my face and she said, "Judy." I said, "What a great point you have brought up, Judy! How many others of you feel you are pressed for time when teaching a large amount of content in a short amount of time?" Several people raised their hands. I continued, "Would it be helpful if I shared three ways you can find the 2 to 5 minutes it takes to do one of these activities?" There was audience approval, and before I shared those I said, "Let's all give Judy a hand for raising such an important issue!" Everyone clapped and she sat down. I thought to myself that she had really helped to make my session a better one than it was before she stood up. I try not to get caught up in the negative emotion and look for the seed of good. This is hard to do but possible with practice.

21. How do I handle learners who continually interrupt me when I'm trying to teach something?

21. I like to use an idea that is called, "Put your two cents in." When I discover I have an over talker, I distribute two poker chips to each learner at the first break or activity when the focus is not on the lecture. I then announce that I would like to invite everyone to "Put your two cents in" in the class. Each chip will buy them 30 seconds of uninterrupted storytelling time during class time. When both chips are spent, the speaking time is up. I encourage everyone to spend his or her chips wisely throughout class time. The chips are not meant for questioning, just examples or war stories. I handle all the questions with an "ask it basket." I distribute blank index cards to everyone and place a basket or gift bag on the side of the classroom group, in easy reach for both of us. I ask them to write down any questions they have and then drop them in the basket immediately. At intervals, I go to the bag and remove a question or two and answer them. The learners like this idea because it makes all the questions anonymous, so there is no fear in asking any question. I like it because it allows me to pace questions throughout the class.

22. *How can I stay prepared for the educator role?*

22. Read journals and books; take courses and attend conferences; network with other educators. Learn, practice, and experiment.

RESOURCES

Deck, M. (1995). *Instant teaching tools for healthcare educators.* St. Louis: Mosby.

Deck, M. (1998). *More instant teaching tools for healthcare educators.* St. Louis: Mosby.

Chapter 9: *Manager*

1. What does it mean to be a manager?

1. To me, it means to direct or administer. Someone can manage something without having an official management title. Being a manager requires the skills of planning, organizing, controlling, directing, implementing, and evaluating to reach an end goal. A manager is responsible for the outcome. If you manage an educational activity, you deliver learning; if you manage an educational department, you deliver many learning opportunities in an organized fashion that assist the institution to meet its mission, regulatory requirements, and strategic initiatives.

2. What type of person best fits the role of instructor or educator in a staff development department?

2. The best instructor or educator is a person who is an expert clinical practitioner with strong facilitator skills. This person is knowledgeable in the area of clinical practice and educational design. This person also is flexible, organized, questions, embraces change, tolerates ambiguity, challenges self to learn, and is dedicated to the profession. I feel strongly that a staff development instructor or educator is a facilitator of learning for staff at all levels, from the orientation of new staff to the development of expert staff.

3. How does the manager role relate to the other roles in education?

3. Managing an educational program is an administrative role for the process of producing an educational activity. You become the one in charge who relates to the faculty, the participants, and the approval agency and who is essentially responsible for the education.

If you are managing a department of education, you relate to the education staff as a leader, coach, role model, supervisor, as a teacher, and facilitator of learning. You also are the one who sets direction and expectations, who holds people accountable, and, at times, who acts as a colleague when teaching with others.

4. Who are the customers of the education department?

4. The obvious ones are the learners and the manager who schedules the learners to attend educational programs. Just as important though, if not more so, are the patients, the person in the top administrative position for patient services, the physicians, and the staff and administrators of any other departments that relate to patients. Educational activities should always relate back to patient outcomes and the mission of the organization.

5. What styles of management would be applicable to an educational manager?

5. When managing, it is best to use all of the styles—authoritative, democratic, laissez-faire, and participative—and adapt them to the specific situation.

- **Authoritative:** Use this style when the situation calls for direction and control. In designing the program that must meet certain regulatory requirements, you become directive and authoritative because you know what criteria the educational activity must meet.

- **Democratic:** Use this style when working with a group of people who are working toward the same goal. A planning committee designing an educational activity is a good example of using this style.

- **Laissez-faire:** Use this style when the group members can make the decision themselves. During an educational program when the same person is speaking all morning, have the participants decide when to take a break. In this style, all the decision making and control lies with the group.

- **Participative:** Use this style when you want input from the group, but when you will be making the final decision. Others participate in the process; you consider the suggestions; and then you make the decision. The best example of this is when staff, unit managers, and others interview candidates for education positions in a centralized education department. I ask them to assist in the selection process by interviewing the candidates and giving me feedback about each candidate; however, the final decision is mine to make.

Working with educated health professionals, I believe the participative style is the most effective for the majority of educational situations.

6. What policies and procedures should be in an education department?

6. These would include:

- job descriptions for the various roles;

- philosophy of education and organizational structure as well as policies and procedures for programmatic expectations;

- confidentiality of education records;

- contact hour approval;

- expectations for orientees, for preceptors, for leadership staff; and

- competency plan, which would include documentation (basic, annual, and ongoing).

Other policies and procedures may be for a lending library; requirements for completing an educational activity; American Heart Association (AHA) requirements of training center management and AHA Conflict of Interest; expectations of BLS, ACLS, PALS Instructors; fees and disclaimers; manikin cleaning; Quality Assurance of AHA programs; and Internal Dispute Resolution. Policies and procedures would also describe the expectations of staff to attend continuing education programs (include amount paid, time off, and any requirements when they return); course completion requirements; reimbursement for lectures; faculty affiliation; and student clinical practicum. Other policies and procedures are related to continuing education activities and would include CE criteria, CE records, commercial support, co-sponsorship, verification of attendance, and evaluation.

7. Can you think of circumstances in which the manager of education becomes involved with discipline?

7. The manager of the activity would become involved if anybody acts out during the educational activity, if participants do not meet the knowledge or skill requirements of the educational activity, and if participants do not attend all of the educational activity.

The manager of the department would become involved in discipline of staff who are not performing according to department standards as defined in the policies and procedures. The manager may also become involved in staff's ability to complete course requirements to work in certain clinical areas.

8. What reports does the manager generate?

8. The manager is responsible for all sorts of educational and management reports, depending on the requirements of the institution. Examples include number of educational programs; number of program hours; number of programs offered as a result of quality improvement efforts; number of participants and number of RN participants; number of new hires; and reports for contact hour approval, which would include a qualitative evaluative summary, not just a quantitative evaluative summary. Other types of reports would include reports for the American Heart Association Training Center designation, cost analysis of specific programs, budget summaries, number of staff in department, and educational programs related to community service. A manager would also generate ad hoc reports for committees and special assignments from top leadership. A report that I have recently completed is the tracking of new graduate nurses. In the past, it was a report just for numbers for orientation purposes. Now, it is a report that incorporates length of employment for retention purposes.

9. *What reports do the instructors and educators generate?*

9. They contribute the detail to all of the reports that the manager generates as listed in the answer to the previous questions. They also report the number of participants at programs, number of orientees, number of preceptors, number of students, and number of pass/fails. They generate individual and unit competency reports with staff and specific programmatic reports. They also contribute reports about the qualitative evaluation of the educational activity both from the learner's perspective and from the instructor's perspective, that is: Did learning take place? Did the speakers say what they said they were going to say? Did the learners leave with more knowledge? Did the learners like the program? Did the instructor believe the program met the original intent?

10. *How does education relate to practice and to quality improvement?*

10. Education, practice, and quality improvement are all interrelated—I see them in a continuous circle. They complement each other, they require each other, and essentially one doesn't exist without the other.

11. *How does an education department link education to outcomes?*

11. I can think of two ways to link education to outcomes. First, by designing an educational program based on the learner need in relation to what is expected in the educational activity. The need can be identified by the institution (adding a new program, a new patient population, or a new practitioner) and using a planning team of the learners to determine the educational objectives. You can't ignore what the learners already know and what they don't know. Identifying the knowledge deficit helps determine the objectives of the learning activity. This way the learners determine the education needed to produce the new program, care for the new patient population, or complete the orders by the new practitioner.

The second way education relates to outcome is by conducting a qualitative review of the educational activity. This would determine if the learners gained knowledge and are able to apply that knowledge in their practice. Data from customer survey reports, staff performance, and quality improvement projects also provide a link to outcomes and should be used by the education staff when planning educational activities.

12. *How do you determine the learning needs of the staff?*

12. In multiple ways: by asking them, by asking their supervisors, by asking their peers, through quality improvement reports, and through patient satisfaction reports. I use formal and informal ways—practice issues, new practices, research, and input from other disciplines. You can also determine learning needs through formalized testing, observation in clinical practice, and documentation audits. As the instructor or educator, you are the facilitator of learning and that very much includes the learners being in charge of their own learning.

13. *How would I learn or teach curriculum development?*

13. You would identify the target audience, identify the learning needs, and identify the objectives, content, timeframe, faculty, teaching method, and evaluation. After determining the learner, the next step is to ask yourself and the learner planning team, "what do the learners need to know or perform when they leave the educational activity?" and that forms the basis for objectives. And from there, everything else flows. So, start with learners, then proceed to objectives, then have a feedback loop so evaluation takes place and you can determine if the learners have met the objectives. That's the best advice I give new staff—start with the objectives.

14. *Where do I begin in planning an orientation for a new instructor or educator to the education department?*

14. Well, it depends upon the person's own level of knowledge in educational design. I begin by setting priorities for the educational needs in the assigned area(s), and then structure an orientation for the instructor to assist him/her to meet those educational needs in the area. For example, if the clinical unit has many orientees scheduled to begin, then the priority would be to teach the instructor or educator about orientation. If the new educator's unit has certain new patient populations coming in, then the priority would be to teach the instructor or educator how to do inservice classes. If the priority is competency, then I would orient to competency forms, documentation, and various ways to meet the competencies.

In general, all new education staff should know about:

- the philosophy of the department

- the expectations of the role

- how to complete the required reports

- office, administrative, and conference details

- routine meetings

- department supplies
- educational materials available

They should come to the position with presentation skills; however, it is important to assess and coach them, if needed. Other aspects of the orientation would include the way to:

- determine a needs assessment,
- evaluate performance,
- evaluate an educational activity,
- schedule programs,
- use audiovisuals specific to the institution,
- apply for contact hours,
- administer an educational activity, and
- set priorities.

An additional part of orientation to the education role would include discussion about:

- nursing practice standards;
- committee assignments;
- the library;
- the inservice program recording numbering system;
- budget;
- responsibilities for the educational programs of BLS, ACLS, PALS, and mandatory topics; and
- goals for the next three months, then six months, then a year.

Don't forget to welcome new members to the education department—the details of office space, coffee, and lunch dates. Welcome them the same way you expect them to welcome new staff.

15. How do you manage multiple orientees at the same time?

15. Very carefully! I do this by planning a specific schedule for each individual orientee, moving orientees to their off shift, by working with a committed leadership team on the clinical unit, and by coaching preceptors. But even before that planning, the institutional commitment to a preceptor program is critical for orientation success, so develop a formal preceptor program. Alspach's (2000) *A Preceptor Training Program for Professional Healthcare Staff* is a great reference.

In managing multiple orientees, it is also important to take the time to get to know each one individually—

personally and professionally. A way to get to know orientees is through their nursing practice stories, through their learning needs assessments, or tests in basic knowledge. Another way is by having self-directed study packages for the specific clinical areas so each orientee can proceed at his/her own pace and the instructor or educator could work clinically with the other orientees. Additional ways include scheduling clinical time with each orientee and making that a priority, and by using effective evaluation tools that look at the orientee's progress at weeks one, two, four, six, and eight and so on. Finally, remember to document on all of the orientation forms so you know where everyone is in the progression through orientation.

16. *How do you manage the frustrations when a low number of staff attend the educational activity after you've designed the program from an identified need and did all the work in planning?*

16. Recognize that this is a frustrating situation and that sometimes the best-laid plans can go awry. Learn from this experience and use it to evaluate: Did you use the right steps in curriculum development? In addition, survey the staff and survey the unit leadership to help better understand why the program was not well attended: Are there some underlying reasons why staff did not attend? Take a close look at the teaching methods: Could the learning need be met in a different way?

Additionally, I suggest taking a step away from the program and discussing the issues with an education colleague in a day or two. Then, get right back out there and facilitate learning needs.

17. *How do you know the cost of programs?*

17. By doing a cost analysis. I highly recommend using an excellent chapter (Chapter 8) on budget and cost information written by Donna Richard Sheridan and Patricia Frost-Harzer in *Nursing Staff Development: Strategies for Success* (Abruzzese, 1996).

18. *How do you budget for a staff development department?*

18. You need to have an operational budget that takes care of the day-to-day costs of running an education department. This would include any revenue and any expenses of personnel including salaries and benefits, purchased services, and office and program supplies and materials. Personnel expenses would be the majority cost of anyone's budget, so include all part-time and full-time employees along with salary information and benefits. Some institutions work with capital budgets, which would be used for any major equipment costs, usually more than $500 or as the institution defines.

19. How do you manage multiple programs at the same time?

19. First, by not scheduling them to occur at the same time! However, since different learners have different learning needs, this may occur. Multiple programs can be managed by soliciting assistance from colleagues, from leadership staff on the unit, and by other staff. An educational planning committee can easily manage speakers and a program while the instructor or educator prioritizes where his/her education abilities are needed the most.

The best way to do this is by keeping focused on the goals of each of the programs. Spend most of your time planning what needs to be done and when it needs to be done. Put this plan in writing for yourself, and then communicate the plan to all involved parties and your colleagues in education. Organize topics when possible to combine audiences and delegate tasks to the learners.

20. How does the manager of education relate to the manager of the nursing unit?

20. As a partner, because both are committed to the same goal of quality patient care. The education manager supports the unit manager in making quality patient care happen through established competencies and sound educational activities, which then relate to practice and quality improvement.

21. What organizational structure is the most efficient for an education department?

21. I believe that a structure that is both centralized and decentralized is the most efficient structure for an education department. In the centralized part of the structure, designated instructors support the entire hospital, nursing (or other discipline), and general or basic information for orientation or the inservice program. In the decentralized part of the structure, specific educators and instructors have positions in the education department that support the differing educational needs of specific units. These educators and instructors have assigned clinical units and assigned programmatic responsibilities. Both types of positions should report to a director or manager of education. For example, a centralized instructor would be responsible for facilitating learning about documentation, computers, and basic procedures. The decentralized educator or instructor assigned to a specific unit would add to the learning by applying this information to the specific type of patient population in the clinical area. The decentralized educator or instructor should have a very close working relationship with the manager of the unit. The manager of the unit gives input into the educator or instructor's evaluation that is completed by the director or manager of education. When there is a need for house-wide education on a topic, then both centralized and decentralized instructors participate.

The director or manager of education oversees this centralized and decentralized structure and should report to a person in the top position for patient services and serve on any policy-making boards. In a small organization, one person may manage all of the education. However, this depends upon the organization.

22. Where should the education department be placed in the organizational structure?

22. I believe the manager position should be at the highest level possible where the clinical decisions are made. If the institution's structure reports to the Human Relations department, then there needs to be a link to the clinical areas through the Clinical Practice Committee or the Patient Services Structure. I have a direct reporting relationship with the chief nursing officer and relate to the directors of clinical areas in managing a centralized–decentralized education department, and I work collaboratively with Human Resources on orientation and competencies.

The bottom line is that the education department needs to know what the issues are in the organization in relation to hiring, performance, quality improvement, regulatory requirements, and patient satisfaction. Education can then support the institution's goals and strategic initiatives.

23. I have never managed before; should I apply to be the manager?

23. It depends on the organization, and the requirements of the job. Ask yourself: Does the institution promote career development and is it open to coaching and mentoring new managers? Think seriously about the skills you have and those you currently use that can easily translate to the role of a manager, and then compare what skills you have to offer in the manager role to what is expected. Talk to those who would be peers of this manager and talk to staff who would be responsible to this manager to get their expectations of the manager. Then determine where your strengths are and what areas you need to develop and list these during the interview process. I would also suggest beginning course work on leadership topics and healthcare administration.

24. All other departments have a manager with an MBA. I have an MSN or MEd. How will I hold up against them?

24. I think you would do just fine provided that you continue your education in business administration and healthcare topics. Each person brings certain expertise to the table, and a nursing or education degree is very valuable in light of the current healthcare environment with the need for quality patient care. Someone at the table must be able to talk intelligently about what is needed to deliver safe, effective patient care.

25. The previous manager works in the department, what should I do?

25. Be professional. In time, initiate a conversation with this person to establish a working relationship that will be conducive to both personalities. Always use tact and acknowledge the former manager's past accomplishments publicly. At the same time, set new goals, new direction, and new expectations for yourself and for staff.

26. I hear that being a manager can be a no-win situation, as you are caught between the needs of the employees and the desires of administration. How do you deal (or cope) with it?

26. I just don't agree with this statement. The role of the manager is to create a win-win situation and that is why the role is so challenging and rewarding. If administration has a clear mission and set of values that have been communicated to all staff and the manager is committed to the mission and values of the organization, then the manager should not be in no-win situations. The decisions that are made would be ones that benefit the organization. I see the manager as the administration. If situations are arising in an organization that cause conflict between staff and administration, then it is the manager's responsibility to communicate upward and work together to resolve them as a representative of administration.

RESOURCES

Journal for Nurses in Staff Development, published by Lippincott Williams & Wilkins

Abruzzese, R. S. (1996). *Nursing staff development: Strategies for success* (2nd ed.). St. Louis: Mosby.

Alspach, J. G. (2000). *A preceptor training program for professional healthcare staff.* Aliso Viejo, CA: American Association of Critical-Care Nurses.

Alspach, J. G. (1995). *The educational process in nursing staff development.* St. Louis: Mosby.

Avillion, A. E. (Ed.). (2000). *Core curriculum for nursing staff development.* Pensacola, FL: National Nursing Staff Development Organization.

Kelly Thomas, K. J. (1998). *Clinical and nursing staff development: Current competence, future focus* (2nd ed.). Philadelphia: Lippincott.

Sheridan, D. R., & Frost-Harzer, P. (1996). Documenting effectiveness: Budget and cost considerations. In R. Abruzzese, *Nursing staff development: Strategies for success* (2nd ed., pp. 122–141). St. Louis: Mosby.

Chapter 10: *Consultant*

1. What does it mean to serve as a consultant?

1. The defining step in consulting is that of *being asked*. Your consulting services may be offered or described so that the interested party knows you are capable of doing, and interested in providing, but the service should never be provided unless the client requests it. I consider a consultant one who will assess a situation or problem from a variety of objective perspectives and then present options for action. The role of consultant implies an ability to offer advice in the form of suggestions for steps that will continue and support a current, desired behavior, or are solutions for a given problem. Resources as alternative suggestions are included, as many times the consultant will be the conduit between the right resource and the given situation.

2. What is the difference between an internal and an external consultant?

2. In your role as staff development educator, you will have many opportunities to wear different hats—that's what makes your job both a challenge and a frustration! You will be asked to develop courses, provide standardized training, conduct employee orientation, and so on. What distinguishes the role of internal *consultant* will be the times that you are asked for advice, for an assessment of a given situation, with the presentation of options to alter, improve, or resolve the existing condition within your place of employment. Consulting can be an exciting bonus to your work, giving you the opportunity to be creative, while perhaps not being the one to implement the suggested action. In contrast, you may want to offer your services to an outside agency, working independently or representing your employing organization as an external consultant. Be sure to make the representation clearly understood at the outset, and to discuss any external opportunities with your boss, making certain there is no misunderstanding. Related questions will discuss contracts, fees, and what to ask the client. However, with the exception of fees, all of the following responses will relate to both internal and external consulting roles.

3. How does the consultant role relate to the other roles?

3. Acting as a consultant employs all of the other roles you might play, as many times you will negotiate, coach, educate, facilitate change, or provide feedback in a consulting capacity. The important distinction is noted above, whether the role is to be internal or external. The majority of the time, consulting will be limited to the internal approach, unless you are actively seeking to work outside the employing organization. You may also

have created a model or learning process that is highly successful, and you wish to share it with others. Often, poster sessions at major nursing conferences are excellent opportunities to showcase your work. However, be prepared for the requests to follow to help another organization implement your model or apply your process, making you, therefore, an external consultant.

4. What if my advice isn't followed?

4. This is always a source of frustration for every consultant, and the best advice I can offer is to simply "get over it." Your goal is to provide alternatives, to present a point of view that may not have been considered, or to suggest resources and actions that, *in your opinion*, would best serve the existing situation. However, there is no guarantee that those you are consulting with will be able or willing to act on your advice, or find your approach the best; you need to realize that their limitations are not a reflection on your ability.

5. What situations should I avoid involvement in?

5. As a rule, I avoid situations where there is no win. By that I mean those circumstances where what is requested is not possible, where there is a controversial or adversarial approach from leadership, and where there are not sufficient resources to achieve the desired results. I have turned down projects in which there was no realistic opportunity for the organization to benefit from what was requested (e.g., presenting a customer service program for staff when management refuses to attend or actively support the proposed model). Know your limits! It is unlikely that a one-time program will change the behaviors of the team, particularly if only a small percentage attend. Why would you want to be part of such an endeavor?

6. What should I negotiate as my ongoing role in a project?

6. Limits will be based on the time you have available and the importance of the project. It is important to realize that unless you want to become a continuing player in the project, you need to structure your role in order to develop the client's ability to implement the necessary actions and to function without you. The start-up of any consulting effort will naturally be more time intensive, with the realization that there should be a gradual transition to infrequent follow-up in progressively longer intervals. It is always a good idea to define expectations at the outset, so that you are not in a protracted effort and believe you are functioning as one of the staff and no longer in a consultant role.

7. Is it possible to function as a consultant outside of my employing organization?

7. It is entirely possible, fun, financially and personally rewarding, *if* your employing organization allows such opportunity, and you are not taking away from fulfilling the obligations you have to your employer. External consulting helps you broaden your perspective, and in turn, benefit the employer as you continue to develop your creative abilities and share them internally with the organization.

8. How do I decide what to charge if I am doing external consulting?

8. Another tough question! Consulting is a highly competitive field, and sharing "going rates" is not something freely done. Take your lead by doing some research; call consultants and ask for quotes on what their fees are for certain projects (e.g., daily rates, workshop presentations, keynote addresses, problem assessment). Most consultants will have an hourly or a daily rate, and it will vary considerably based on the type of work/field the consultants are in, their experience, and their degree of recognition. Generally, those consultants who have published books or articles in their field, and who have presented at national conferences are more highly paid than local consultants. However, you have to start somewhere, and many will tell you that the first jobs were often free, just to get the experience and exposure.

9. What initial questions should I ask the client?

9. As in any endeavor, I begin by defining the desired outcomes, or results, that the client (either internal or external) is looking for in terms of the project. I put that at the top of the list, and proceed from there with the following list:

- Exactly what results are you looking for?

- How long do you expect this will take (or when do you want to be done)?

- How do you see my role/what do you expect me to do for you?

- What do you see as the main problems, and what have you already done about them?

- Do you have a budget for the project?

- Who is involved in the decision making/who are the key players?

10. What should go in the contractual agreement?

10. I would include all of the responses to the questions asked above, being very specific and organized as follows:

- Agreed upon results/outcomes or goals

- Timeframe in terms of specific start and end dates

- Billing in terms of fees to be paid (including expenses) and when

- Resources needed from the client (e.g., copying, clerical support, office space).

- Cancellation statement discussing any penalty for canceling, and any options for substitutions or rescheduling if you are unable to fulfill the agreed upon duties.

- The organization contact person, or "point person," who will oversee the organizational perspective in terms of posting announcements, scheduling meeting rooms, copying handouts, and so on.

11. What if the client is unrealistic about what can be done or how long it will take?

11. This may be another time that you step out of the situation, if the client is not responsive to your assessment and expertise regarding what is possible. Most clients are initially unrealistic, thinking the project will take less time, fewer resources, and cost less than what you propose. If the client is unwilling to adjust based on your recommendations, you may offer specific examples of similar projects, and invite inquiry with past clients. Lacking those, this may be the time you say no thanks, and look for a more reasonable client. With progressive experience you will be able to gauge the time and cost of certain endeavors, but if you are just starting out, it is best to get advice from another consultant. Find someone who is willing to mentor you, and ask questions!

12. Where do I find a mentor?

12. If you have ever booked a speaker for a presentation at your organization, or used consulting services, this may be a good place to start. Not all consultants are going to be receptive to giving free time for the development of someone who will become a competitor, so you may only be able to get some quick advice on your initial request. Consider asking the consultant if he/she offers coaching services, and then be willing to pay for a couple of hours of coaching. Get questions ready beforehand, submit them to the consultant prior to the coaching session, and take good notes during the session. Consider taping the coaching session, if that is acceptable to the consultant.

13. *What questions would I ask a mentor/coach?*

13. You might consider the following:

- How do I define my area of expertise? Should I limit my approach or be a generalist?

- What is the best way to get exposure?

- How do I market myself?

For additional insight, ask any of the questions that are in this chapter, and it will be like getting a "second opinion"!

14. *How do I use my knowledge and skills to further my professional goals (possibly with another company/ department), but avoid a conflict of interest with my current employer?*

14. This can be a very delicate situation if not handled up front and honestly. If you are considering using your skills to do work for another department or company, it is prudent to let your immediate manager/ supervisor know. You will want to include personal/ professional development goals in your evaluation, and if additional consulting is a goal, be sure to discuss it with your boss, and determine what the organizational parameters are that would affect your actions. Some organizations are delighted at the additional exposure, and realize that they will also benefit from your enlarged scope of experience. However, if you are doing work for a competitor, this will take careful consideration and discussion with your boss.

15. *How do I balance the consultant role with my other duties/roles?*

15. The majority of staff development educators have an overwhelming plate of responsibilities that include many repetitive functions such as monthly and annual presentations of required programs for regulatory compliance. No doubt, a consulting opportunity will offer variety, and may be tempting to consume more time on what may be the "fun stuff" as opposed to the daily challenges of an internal staff role. If you are clear about the desired outcome of the consultant role, it becomes easier to allot time in a judicious manner. If several of your duties are repetitive, consider delegating to others where possible. Creativity is the cornerstone of growth, and your talents may be more beneficial to the organization if you allow time in your day for consulting projects as well as the required daily duties. Only you and your supervisors will be able to determine the "correct" balance.

16. *How do I deal with a person/group who shows resentment of my role?*

16. Unfortunately, there will be those who do not fully support your efforts. They have their own reasons, be it jealousy, envy, anger, or a violated sense of "fairness" in which they may believe the situation to be unfair in terms of your being in a position to advise them. In these cases, you are dealing with feelings, and it is very important to remember that there is no right or wrong feeling. It will be much better to spend your time trying to understand the feeling, rather than to judge it. As with all conflict and resentment, the cause generally has to do with a sense of loss of respect or control, and if you can acknowledge that and find a way to give respect or control back to the individual, you will create a better working relationship. I always find it helpful to acknowledge what I am sensing, rather than to avoid or pretend otherwise. You may say, "I know you were not expecting me to be called in to assist, and that might be surprising or unsettling to you. I respect your feelings, and would certainly appreciate your input on this project…"

17. *If I do work as a consultant outside of my current position, and assuming there is a positive outcome to celebrate, what can I share in terms of my role in the client's success?*

17. Client confidentiality is an important factor to respect and to clarify. You are doing work as a guest within someone else's organization, and they will want you to respect that the work is confidential, unless specifically stated otherwise in the contract or agreement. If the project you assist with is successful, they may be very happy to have their name linked to any article or publication you may create describing the efforts. However, it is *always* necessary to obtain written permission, whether you are planning on using the client for a reference of your work, or as an example of an intervention process that is successful. Equally important to remember is that you did not do this alone, and that there should be recognition for all of the work done by the organization in achieving the outcomes you are now celebrating.

18. *What criteria should be used to determine the best learning method when considering the client's time and money constraints?*

18. More than likely, the client will have limitations that will pose a challenge in terms of both these resources. Time and money are at a premium, and organizations need effective stewardship of both, looking to you as the consultant/expert to know about the optimum approaches for the most reasonable use of resources. If both are severely limited, and below market rate, you may not be willing to take on such a challenge. Be honest about what is possible, both in terms of time and money, and based on either your first hand experience or careful research of similar projects. Again, consulting is about providing the client with a series of options, and recommendations for what would be the best choice in your opinion. The "best choice" of learning methods does not always mean the most expensive. You may not be the one who has the primary role in this project, serving only as the initiator who "trains the trainers" and allows the internal staff at the organization to take on the majority of the work.

19. Is it reasonable to expect support and assistance from the client in terms of clerical needs and management follow-up?

19. I have found it not only to be reasonable, but to be an absolute necessity. You will need to be very clear at the outset regarding what specific services you are providing, and what expectations you have of the organization. Be sure to include this list in your performance agreement, or contract for services, itemizing clearly what you will need from the client in terms of computer support, timely copying and distribution of materials you may provide for preparation, announcements of your visits, and if staff preparedness is necessary. Resources are wasted if there is no follow-up, if materials have not been copied or provided in sufficient time to allow staff to prepare, and if attendance is minimal due to poor planning. However, you need to recognize that your work is not the only project on the organization's plate, and the organization will have many more compelling issues that may keep it from adhering to the agreed upon expectations. Help everyone complete the project by creating and following a specific, *detailed* timeline and employing frequent reminders, conference calls, and e-mail to clarify the steps of the project.

20. How do I deal with managers who want to use education as a punishment for a difficult or challenging employee, putting me in the middle as the "consultant" who must recommend educational interventions for this employee?

20. The relationship of the educator and the manager can fill several volumes, and in fact much has been written about the issue. I am not sure how the perception of "education as punishment" was created, but would suspect that the manager is hoping that additional education will delay or eliminate the need for disciplinary actions. The best first step would be to meet with the manager and clearly define the problem, listing the desired outcome, and then suggesting options for achieving those goals. It may be through this mutual planning and problem solving session that you are really coaching the manager to a better process and increasing the chances that this employee will either improve or find that the current position is not the best fit. You may want to consider the following problem solving format, and present this tool as an option to the manager, using it to frame your discussion with him/her.

- What are the specific details (i.e., what tells you there is a problem with this employee)? Consider the frame of reference of the manager, the attitudes and assumptions that he/she might be making, and potential reasons why the current situation may exist.

- What is good about the problem? (Listing 3 good things can free up creative thought and help everyone to see the problem from a different perspective, reducing the "ain't it awful" syndrome.)

- What should be happening? (This is where the manager defines the desired goal—the situation as he/she would like it to be.)

- Do I need to do something about this? (This is a time to look at who the behavior directly affects, and how the manager sees accountability in correcting this situation.)

- What can be done to correct this situation? Short and long term goals, a timeline, and specific measurements of success are essential components of this step.

For more details about this process, be sure to see the discussion in *Clinical Delegation Skills* 2nd Ed., (p. 318–320) by Ruth Hansten and Marilynn Washburn, Aspen Publishers, 1998.

21. How do I set limits for an educational consulting project when I am not involved in the planning process, but am expected to go forward even though I don't agree with the methods or the goals?

21. If this is an external opportunity and not related to your employment, you will have more choices. My first recommendation would be to carefully consider what you would gain by participating in this project. Not being part of the planning and not agreeing with the methods and/or the goals would be very good reasons to refuse the job. However, if you feel committed to being a part of this process, start by being very clear about what you are willing to do, how and why, and most importantly, share your ideas for successful outcomes. Provide examples of projects in which you have been part of the planning and what strategies you have used in the past that have worked. Be sure to be positive; do not continue to announce that you disagree with the process chosen, and do NOT use the excuse that you were not part of the original planning process. Remember, if you choose to participate, then you have already accepted the terms of the existing situation.

However, if this is part of the job you are asked to do by your employer, you are faced with making the best of a potentially difficult situation. Whatever the reason you were not part of the initial planning, you are now part of the project, and have the opportunity to offer neutral suggestions focused on making the best outcome possible. As stated above, the worst thing to do would be to remind everyone that you have come to the middle of the event, that you are not supportive of the efforts chosen, but that you have to be here anyway. Maintain your objectivity, and when you offer suggestions for changes or next steps, be specific, and have examples of where such strategies have worked before. Be very clear about how you see your role at this point in the project, outlining how you see yourself as best assisting the current situation. You may just find that this project provides opportunities for creative planning and showcases your abilities as an unbiased consultant!

Resources

Briles, J. (1994). *The Briles report on women in healthcare*. San Francisco: Jossey Bass.

Puetz, B. E., & Shinn, L. J. (1997). *The nurse consultant's handbook*. New York: Springer.

Robinson, D., & Robinson, J. (1995). *Performance consulting*. San Francisco: Berrett-Koehler Publishers.

Schwarz, R. (1994). *The skilled facilitator*. San Francisco: Jossey Bass.

Wilson, C. K. (1992). *Building new nursing organizations*. Gaithersburg, MD: Aspen Publishers.

Training & Development Magazine would be an excellent magazine to subscribe to—all issues have something that takes you "outside the box" of health care and gives you a fresh perspective on consulting.

Chapter 11: *Researcher*

1. Why are nurses reluctant to read, use, or conduct nursing research studies?

1. Many barriers prevent nurses from engaging in and using nursing research in their practice. Some of these barriers include the misconception that only nurses with master's or doctoral degrees can understand and conduct research. The use of scholarly language such as methodology, conceptual frameworks, or theory can be intimidating to those who have not been exposed to this knowledge. Nurses also believe that they do not have the time to read nursing research, implement the findings, and/or monitor the success of the research. Hospitals have historically been reluctant to implement changes suggested or proven by nursing research. I believe that one of the most important educational changes needed in nursing research is to become more user friendly to the bedside nurse and to teach them how to properly implement research findings into their daily practice.

2. What is nursing research and why is it important to practice?

2. Nursing research is a formalized approach into the scholarly inquiry of generating and testing nursing theory (Burns & Grove, 2001). The nursing research study should be grounded in the context of conceptual models of nursing and nursing theory. When nursing research is used in everyday practice, it provides answers to questions like what nursing is and can be. When a profession studies what the profession is, it advances the discipline's specific knowledge. Nurses who are familiar with the research process can help mentor other nurses, including incorporating research findings into practice. This can be done in staff meetings where there is a sharing of ideas or problems that can affect the care of patients.

3. What Web sites are the best for information on nursing research?

3. There are many Web sites that provide excellent information on nursing research. Based on the specific area of nursing research you wish to find, information on the sites will drive you through the information highway. I recommend the National Institute of Nursing Research (NINR). This site offers a frequently asked questions page that describes how to get information and what research is currently being funded by NINR. The Web site address is **http://www.nih.gov/ninr**.

Another site for beginners is the University of Rochester Nursing Research online site. This site provides a four credit hour course titled Nursing 301. This course is an introduction to nursing research and the critical reviews of evidence-based literature. There is a bonus to this site called "Research Fables from the Sisters Grimm," which reveals research principles in humorous adaptations from the Grimm Brothers Fairy tales and other famous stories.

The Web site address is
http://www.urmc.rochester.edu/SON/courses/301

Other important sites include:

Sigma Theta Tau
http://www.nursingsociety.org

Clinical Nursing Research
http://www.sagepub.co.uk/journals

Nursing Research Electronic Journals
http://www.nursing.uc.edu

Western Journal of Nursing Research
http://www.sagepub.co.uk/journals

4. Is there a role for conducting nursing research via the Internet?

4. Conducting nursing research via the Internet involves designing a study that incorporates all the components of research and Internet processes. You would first need to design a Web page describing the study and recruit participants. Once the Web page is established you would have to address the process to retrieve data by e-mail and analyze and return results to participants.

Advantages to conducting nursing research via the Internet can be reaching a larger number of participants using numerous search engines and anonymity.

Data collection must include permission from the participants for sharing their name, address, or e-mail addresses. Questionnaires can be sent out via e-mail or traditional mail, or through a polling site such as **www.hostedsurvey.com**. Advantages sought in the data collection phase are direct communication between participants and the researcher with no gatekeeper; individuals don't have to experience discomfort with face-to-face interactions and most important an international sample can be recruited.

Disadvantages are that Internet research is not appropriate for all types of nursing research. Qualitative research can require the immersion of the researcher in the participant's world (the lived experience). This could not be accomplished via the Internet. It is also not a truly representative sample in that the Internet user tends to be more educated.

5. What computer programs are essential when dealing with nursing research studies?

5. A variety of computer software packages that help you with the clerical preparation of the research proposal. I would suggest either Microsoft Word (Microsoft Corporation, 2000) or WordPerfect (Corel Corporation, 2000) for word processing applications. Both provide numerous functions and assist with deletions, spacing, formatting tables, and graphs. These applications can also assist with developing a table of contents, spell check, and grammar check.

References can be typed in the traditional manner or be compiled in a bibliographic database. Some examples of bibliographic databases are Reference Manager (Institute Information Systems, 1997), Procite, or Endnotes (Niles Software, 1999). These applications also provide the ability to import citations from external sources, obtain online bibliographic searches, and customize reference types.

Incorporating nursing care data into a structured coding system is needed for recording patient care problems; nursing actions and evaluation of these actions are essential to nursing research. Coding is the process of translating verbal data into categories or numeric form. This can also be accomplished by transferring the data from written documents to computerized files for future analysis. The American Nurses Association (ANA) has supported the standardization of nursing care terms for computer-based patient care systems. The ANA accepted seven systems of terminology for describing nursing practice: North American Nursing Diagnosis Association (NANDA) taxonomy of nursing diagnosis, International Classification of Nursing Practice, Omaha Home Health Care, Patient Care Data Set, Nursing Outcomes Classification, Nursing Interventions Classification, and Georgetown Home Health Care Classification.

Data Coding for quantitative studies is often in a numerical format. This can be summarized and displayed via tables and graphs. All-purpose data management programs like Excel (Microsoft, 2000) are compatible with common statistical packages so that the researcher can analyze the coding data. There can be mistakes in data importing so some programs allow for the data to be repeated twice before data are accepted. As for qualitative studies, computerization has assisted with the time consuming task of coding the text data. Ethnograph (Seidel et al., 1994) interfaces with the most popular word processing software. Another qualitative computer software package is NUD.IST (Non-numerical Unstructured Data Indexing Searching and Theorizing) (Gahan & Hannibal, 1998)

Both data analysis components of the qualitative and quantitative studies can be derived from any common statistical package. Some of the most commonly used are Statistical Analysis Services Institute (SAS Institute, 1999), Ethnograph (Seidel et al., 1994) and NUD.IST (Gahan & Hannibal, 1998)

6. *How can Quality Improvement or Total Quality Management be used as a research tool in healthcare organizations and nursing?*

6. There is a movement to urge practitioners to engage in evidence-based practice that could close the gap between research and practice. Integrating clinical quality improvement strategies with research methodology can assist with meeting the challenges that healthcare systems face today. The foundation of evidence-based practice de-emphasizes making decisions based on ritual or custom but rather applying research findings to specific situations. In health care, the aim of Continuous Quality Improvement (CQI) is to use the best available evidence consistently to support practice standards, thus, to assure the best possible patient outcomes. The phases of the CQI process include benchmarking, planning, and implementing change for an improved outcome. The phases or steps are similar to the quasi-experimental research design.

The benefits of using CQI initiatives are the ability to involve a variety of healthcare practitioners to ask clinically relevant research questions and ultimately to improve the standards of practice. CQI is customer driven and should also incorporate patients' feedback as customers of the facility. The design enables large sample sizes and improves confidence in possible changes that are made from the measured outcomes.

When healthcare professionals use the findings of research to help their clinical decision making, the patient outcomes are optimized. This is done through broadening their own knowledge base, enhancing cooperation in solving problems, and strengthening the bond between research and clinical practice with the ultimate goal of improving patient outcomes.

7. Most of the staff are associate degree graduates; how can I get them involved in the research process?

7. Associate degree nurses are exposed to nursing research in their two-year academic preparation. For the most part they have not actively participated in the research process, but should be able to define a problem using the nursing process. I would start with a CQI initiative that means something to them. This way they will feel part of the decision making process and will see results. The best way for nurses to buy into the benefits of research is to see how it positively affects their practice or the care that they give to patients. The next important step is the share the data. This means to share the results that you studied before the change and after the change. This gives the data collectors (nurses) the answers to: Where we are? Where are we are going? Once they are knowledgeable, they will take ownership.

8. How does the researcher role relate to the clinical and nursing staff development role?

8. The research role or, as I consider it, the research priority of the staff development specialist is to answer the question: Do we make a difference in the community we serve? Depending on the healthcare setting there are many avenues. If you are responsible for the education of new employees, you may want to look at transfer of learning. You would pick a measurement tool that addresses the transference of learning in a reliable way. I would suggest that you use a tool that is already tested for reliability and validity. The patient educator might want to assess patients' knowledge on a particular disease or coping with that disease and how does the disease affect their life views. Nursing research studies have demonstrated that self-learning through computer-assisted, home studies, and other learning packages is more efficient. If we remind ourselves that adults learn in different ways, we can see where research has proven that active involvement in the educational process is important to the adult learner. This could include a preceptor/mentor approach to orientation or a patient class that encourages return demonstration and participation of the patient and family. It is through the constant evaluation process that we look through a different lens for an innovative way to provide service, stewardship, and data that steers us in the right path for the future (Kelly Thomas, 1998).

9. Is there a group or committee that can act as a resource to a new nurse researcher?

9. The National Nursing Staff Development Organization (NNSDO) and other clinical specialty associations sponsor research committees to act as guides through the research process. The NNSDO Nursing Research Committee has chosen to heighten awareness of nursing research through publications, grants opportunities, and providing ongoing support for research education during the NNSDO convention. The Nursing Research Committee believes that the most important contribution is to promote the need for research-based practice among clinical and staff development educators for competence development and assessment (Kelly Thomas, 1998).

10. What is the difference between basic research and applied research?

10. Basic research is concerned with generating new knowledge and it is referred to as "pure research." The purpose of basic research is to test a theory or to generate a new theory. Whether the basic research goal is to generate or develop theories, the application of the research results does not occur immediately. Many years can pass before the usefulness of research is determined or acknowledged by society (Nieswiadomy, 1998).

Applied research is directed toward generating knowledge that can be used. It is research that seeks solutions to immediate problems. The majority of nursing research studies has been applied research. The reason appears to be that the results of these studies can easily be applied to the clinical setting (Nieswiadomy, 1998).

Research studies may contain elements of both basic and applied research because it may be that the theory tested will have immediate implications for nursing.

11. Can you explain the difference between qualitative and quantitative research and does one type have an advantage over the other?

11. Qualitative research is concerned with the subjective meaning of the experience to an individual. Quantitative research is concerned with the objectivity, tight controls over the research situation, and the ability to generalize findings (Polit & Hungler, 1997).

In the past, nurse researchers have primarily conducted quantitative research. Because quantitative research involves the traditional scientific approach, many nurse researchers chose this form of research, which is accepted by many other disciplines and easier to fund. Some members of the research community do not consider qualitative research to be scientific because it does not have a numerical, data-driven result.

Although we do not know the number of nurses conducting qualitative research today, we do know that the number of qualitative nursing research studies published have increased. Marilyn Leininger, one of the grand theorists of nursing, has involved herself in the qualitative researcher role. As an anthropologist she valued the research data and information that the qualitative researchers could obtain. Living in the lived experience of the subject is what the qualitative researcher does; this type of research yields different information than the quantitative process. Consider the patient with chronic pain. Quantitative research would be concerned with the level of pain that the person is experiencing. Qualitative research, on the other hand, would be interested in the experience of living with chronic pain. Both of these approaches to research studies help broaden the scientific community's knowledge about the study subject matter.

12. What responsibilities does the nurse researcher have to the research participants?

12. The nurse researcher is ultimately responsible for the ethics of the study. The first thing that needs to be done is the formation of the ethical codes and guidelines. The ethical guidelines used in nursing research as well as research in other disciplines were developed after World War II. The atrocities committed in the German prison camps led to the Nuremberg trials. The 1947 Nuremberg Code resulted which concerned itself with the ethical study of human behavior. The code has several criteria for research:

1. Researchers must inform subjects about the study.

2. Research must be for the good of society.

3. Research must be based on animal experiments, if possible.

4. Researchers must try to avoid injury to research subjects.

5. Researchers must be qualified to conduct research.

6. Subjects or the researcher can stop the study if problems occur (Nieswiadomy, 1998).

There have been many other codes developed since the Nuremberg Code was developed. The United States Department of Health and Human Services (DHHS) published guidelines in 1971, 1981, 1986, and 1991. Any institution that receives federal money for research must abide by the DHHS guidelines or risk losing federal money. The federal government guidelines resulted in the creation of Institutional Review Boards. These review boards must review every research proposal. In 1985, the American Nurses Association Research and Studies Commission published the *Human Rights Guidelines for Nurses in Clinical and Other Research.* These guidelines discuss the rights of the research subject and the nurse involved in research. The research subject must be protected from harm, ensured privacy, and have his/her dignity preserved. Some institutions have nursing research committees that review research proposals but it is imperative that researchers become familiar with the requirements of the institution that will be used for data collection.

13. **Are there specific elements that must be in an Informed Consent?**

13. The major elements that must be discussed in an Informed Consent are as follows:

1. Researcher is identified and credentials presented.

2. Subject selection process

3. Purpose of the study

4. Study procedures

5. Potential risks

6. Potential benefits

7. Compensation, if any

8. Alternative procedures, if any

9. Anonymity or confidentiality assured

10. Rights to refuse to participate or withdraw from study without penalty

11. Offer to answer all questions

12. Means of obtaining study results (Nieswiadomy, 1998)

14. **I have been asked to participate in a nursing research study. What questions should I ask to make sure that it is something I want to get involved in?**

14. I would suggest the following guidelines when critiquing the ethical aspects of a study. If the primary researcher can answer these questions and you feel good about the information you received, then I would feel comfortable with your involvement.

1. Was the study reviewed by an Institutional Review Board?

2. Was informed consent obtained from the subjects?

3. Is there information about provisions for anonymity or confidentiality?

4. Were vulnerable subjects used?

5. Does it appear that subjects might have been coerced into acting as subjects?

6. Does it appear that the benefits of participation in the research study outweigh the risks involved?

7. Were subjects provided the opportunity to ask questions about the study and told how to contact the researcher if questions arose?

8. Were the subjects told how they could get the results of the study (Polit & Hungler, 1997)?

15. *How do I benefit from nursing research when I am in a small community hospital and we do not have a nursing research committee?*

15. There are many roles for nurses in nursing research. The two primary roles are as consumers or producers of nursing research. Both of these roles are at different ends of the continuum. Consumers of nursing research read studies to typically keep up to date on new information or skills that might be relevant to their practice. This is a great role for the educator. Producers of nursing research are nurses who actively participate in the design and implementation of a research study. Recently, we have seen a shift from the nurse in academia to the nurse at the bedside becoming more involved in nursing research. Here are a few suggestions to get some benefit from additional exposure to nursing research:

- Establish a Journal Club that meets on a regular basis and critiques research articles

- Attend research presentations at professional conferences

- Collaborate in the development of an idea for a research project

- Join a nursing specialty group's nursing research committee

- Incorporate the research findings into practice by discussing new found information with the policy and procedure committee

- Offer to participate in the institution's Institutional Review Board

- Offer to assist in the data collection role for Performance Improvement, Continuous Quality Improvement, or any study that looks at improved patient outcomes

16. *We have just been approved by the hospital's Institutional Review Board (IRB) for a research study. What inservice education should I do with the staff?*

16. Once the study has been granted ethical approval from the Institutional Review Board (IRB), the staff who will be involved in the project will require training regarding the following:

- The purpose of the study

- How to properly use the intervention/device

- Maintaining safety and accuracy according to the manufacturer's guidelines

- Data collection procedures

- How to obtain informed consent

- How to manage and report complaints, adverse events, or departures from the study protocol

17. *Are there nursing research studies that discuss staff nurse fallacies about nursing research?*

17. Several nursing research studies have been done on the topic of rewards and obstacles for nurses conducting research in a clinical setting. There are fewer research studies that present the common beliefs among staff nurses that produce barriers to conducting nursing research. Some of the erroneous beliefs are as follows:

1. The best design is experimental or quasi-experimental.
   * Nurse should choose from a variety of research designs. The trend is to use a design that captures the environmental effects even if there is less control.

2. A researcher must control all variables.
   * Variables can be controlled statistically.

3. The best measurement is physiological.
   * The best measurement is holistic (a combination of physiological, social, and psychological).

4. Clinical expertise is a prerequisite.
   * The most important qualification is research expertise.

5. Hire someone to collect and analyze the data.
   * Novice researchers should complete their own data collection and analysis because it is how the researcher learns.

6. The literature search should be limited to the exact study.
   * The literature search should encompass conceptual similarities even if the studies were conducted on a different sample or topic (Morrison, 1998).

18. Is there a simple way to teach staff nurses how to review and evaluate a nursing research study?

18. Professional nurses should be expected to read and evaluate nursing research. Many nurses report feeling intimated by nursing research. These two issues work against each other, causing the nurse to feel frustrated when asked to critique a nursing research article for use in practice. The ASK (Applicability, Science, Knowledge) model offers the basis needed to review potential clinical significance in a nursing research study. This practice model was designed for use by nurses to determine whether research findings were safe for use in their own practice. This model calls for the practitioner to ask questions under the three categories.

Applicability:

1. Is this study relevant to practice?

2. Do the findings suggest that the interventions tested made statistical or clinical improvement in practice?

3. Does the benefit to the patient outweigh the risk of implementation?

4. Is the change cost effective in terms of human and material resources?

5. Is the potential outcome for the patient or organization worth the effort to implement the change? (Evans & Shreve, 2000)

Science:

1. The science of the research study is evaluated using standard criteria regardless of the practice area.

2. "**SPRMA**" or "**SPRTMA**" are acronyms created to assist reviewers in remembering the key components of research.

   S – Statement of the Problem

   P – Purpose

   R – Research Question

   M – Methodology

   A – Analysis

   SPRTMA is the same except it includes the **T** – Theoretical Framework (Evans & Shreve, 2000).

3. There are many excellent nursing research textbooks

that discuss the science of research. The two that I use all the time are:

Burns and Grove (2001) – *The Practice of Nursing Research*

Polit and Hungler (1998) – *Nursing Research: Principles and Methods*

Knowledge:

1. Do the results fit the existing knowledge base? Or

2. Do the research findings have meaning to the reader's knowledge base?
   It is that old saying, *"Why didn't I think of that?"*

3. Why wouldn't or shouldn't I use this idea?

19. How can nursing research be made more visible in an institution?

19. That is not an easy question to answer. I think that you first have to know the culture of the institution. Are people accepting of this new research position or department? Can the institution provide both material and human resources to assist in the growth of this new initiative? The three most important goals for a research and development department are to:

1. Influence the existing structures and processes

2. Strengthen the research capacity

3. Implement research findings (Thompson, 2000)

20. Can you compare quality improvement to nursing research studies?

20. In hospitals and universities there is a continuing debate as to the difference between quality improvement and nursing research studies. The main distinction is that nursing research represents the discovery of new methods or confirming existing practice. Quality improvement demonstrates how the standard and quality of care or services are provided. One accepted distinction between the two forms of study is that research is finding out what you ought to be doing, whereas quality improvement is whether you are doing what you ought to be doing (Thurston, Watson, & Reimer, 1993). Which type of study to use should be based on the hypothesis or question being proposed.

Resources

Burns, N., & Grove, S. (2001). *The practice of nursing research: Conduct, critique, and utilization.* St. Louis: Mosby.

Evans, J. C., & Shreve, W. S. (2000). The ASK Model: A bare bones approach to the critique of nursing research for use in practice. *Journal of Trauma Nursing, 7*(4), 83–91.

Kelly Thomas, K. J. (1998). *Clinical and nursing staff development: Current competencies, future focus.* Philadelphia: Lippincott.

LoBiondo-Wood, G., & Haber, J. (1998). *Nursing research: Methods, critical appraisal, and utilization.* St. Louis: Mosby.

Morrison, E. R. (1998). Erroneous beliefs about research held by staff nurses. *The Journal of Continuing Education in Nursing, 29*(5), 202–204.

Nieswiadomy, R. M. (1998). *Foundations of nursing research.* Stamford, CT: Appleton & Lange.

Polit, D. F., & Hungler, B. P. (1997). *Essentials of nursing research: Methods, appraisal and utilization.* Philadelphia: Lippincott.

Thompson, D. R. (1999). Making nursing research visible. *NT Research, 4*(5), 325–327.

Thurston, N., Watson, L., & Reimer, M. (1993). Research or quality improvement? *Journal of Nursing Administration, 23*(7–8), 46–49.

www.nih.gov/ninr

Chapter 12: *Clinical*

1. *In today's healthcare environment, change is the only constant. How do I support this ongoing change in the clinical area?*

1. Stay flexible! Be open-minded! Try to see change as a new opportunity. However, recognize that not everybody has this perception. People resist change for a variety of reasons and may be concerned about a potential threat to their role. The educator works with the management and clinical practice team to identify potential technical/clinical concerns with the proposed change. The educator can play a valuable role in identifying strategies to address concerns.

2. *What is the role of the educator in preparing for a change in the patient population?*

2. The educator plays an essential role in the clinical area preparing for a change in patient population. The educator can explore what resources currently exist within the organization. Once these resources have been identified, an educational plan can be developed to include:

- Inservice classes and other unit activities
- "Shadowing" clinical observation experiences
- Policies and procedures
- Reference material

The activities should be as fun and engaging as possible. Use a variety of strategies to meet the different learning styles of the staff. Inservice classes, videotapes, and articles are just a few of the ways to present the information. We often use crossword puzzles and games with prizes or incentives for completion. Experts from other clinical areas are invited to speak. This includes all members of the healthcare team (e.g., physicians, nurses, dietitians, PT/OT). Reinforce all new policies and procedures during the class.

Shadowing experiences involve one nurse observing an experienced nurse providing care. Set clear expectations of what each nurse is to accomplish. Clinical observation experiences are usually most beneficial for the nurse who will share his or her learning with others. The shadowing experience allows the observing nurse to develop resources of people to call along with the opportunity to explore what resources are currently being employed by those experienced nurses.

3. *How do I obtain the knowledge and skills expected of staff (e.g., new products, patient populations, and technology)?*

3. The educator needs to explore ways to learn new skills prior to introducing them to the staff. This can be accomplished by reading current literature, talking with clinical experts, exploring new products with vendors in a simulated environment, and reading product manuals. The educator then uses this knowledge or skill to explore *what if* case situations to predict learning needs and establish the educational plan.

4. How do I learn a new skill?

4. After reading, viewing videotapes, completing CDs, and discussing the skills with the experts, it is now time to practice the skill. Often the best way to learn a skill is to actually perform the skill. Testing may occur in a lab environment or in the clinical setting with a preceptor. New equipment/product testing is critical before introducing it to the nurses in the clinical area. There are numerous computer-assisted learning activities that provide a "safe" environment to learn the skill before attempting it in the clinical setting.

5. Where do I look for resources in learning new skills?

5. Resources are only limited by your creativity and your budget. Human resources include:

- Healthcare practitioners who currently care for the patient population or use the equipment.
- Librarians
- Other educators

Written resources include:

- Manufacturers' manuals
- Books
- Journal articles
- Contact numbers and names of local experts

Other Resources:

- Web sites
- Videotapes
- E-learning activities
- CD-ROMs

6. How do I develop clinical resources for new expectations?

6. Work with the leadership team, the educational committee, and the clinical practice committee within the clinical areas to determine the best resources to match the specific need. Some resources require financial support but many are free. Are experts available within the healthcare setting? If so, locate and post contact information for staff to have available. Develop "Frequently Asked Questions" sheets and place in highly visible areas. What Web sites are valuable for the clinicians? Make useful Web site links available on the unit's Web site or as shortcuts on computer desktops.

7. What is the educator's role in developing an educational plan for the staff within the clinical area?

7. The educator must work closely with the leadership team and any education committees in the clinical areas in developing the educational plan. Critical steps in developing the education plan include:

- assessing the current skill level of the staff,

- defining the new skills and knowledge required and who will be affected by the change in practice,

- implementing multiple learning activities using a variety of teaching strategies,

- outlining available resources, and

- determining measurements of successful completion.

8. How do I reinforce learning in the clinical setting?

8. The clinical educator is able to reinforce learning in a variety of ways:

- Empowering the education committee and informal leaders to role model new behaviors required by policy changes.

- Clarifying information during meetings (e.g., staff or patient care conferences).

- Assessing critical incident reports and performance improvement data.

- Asking staff how they are adapting to new skills. This method requires a good listener who is able to assist the staff to move beyond some of the normal resistance that often takes place with change.

- Conducting clinical rounds.

9. How do clinical rounds involve the educator?

9. Clinical rounds is a time the unit leadership and educator review current patient care issues and treatment options with an individual nurse. Walking with the nurse to the patient's bedside and discussing the plan of care provides an opportunity to assess the nurse's critical thinking ability. Often time will not allow for more than one or two patients to be reviewed. It is advisable to conduct rounds at varying times that are not publicized in advance. The well-known phenomenon of disappearing staff may result from announced rounds.

10. From the educator's perspective, what are some of the advantages of conducting clinical rounds?

10. Clinical rounds provide the educator a view of the real issues in the clinical setting. For instance, you see the impact a change in the restraint procedure can have on the nurse's ability to care for patients. The challenges of communicating with a patient from a different country or culture become real. The continuous beeping of a new piece of equipment provides the opportunity to assist the staff nurse in learning how to troubleshoot the equipment. You see individual learning needs and trends among the staff that assist in determining future learning opportunities.

11. *How do you use clinical education rounds for needs assessment data and knowledge validation?*

11. **Needs Assessment:**

The best indicators of individual and unit educational needs are the questions asked by the staff nurse. Hearing numerous questions on the same or related topics can help the educator plan a learning experience addressing that need.

Knowledge Validation:

Again, questions are a key strategy to confirm that the nurse has the required knowledge. To validate knowledge, ask questions. Skills in asking open-ended questions that do not lead or influence the person in answering the question are essential for a true measurement of knowledge.

12. *What responsibility do I have with clinical activities?*

12. The educator may volunteer to assist with the clinical care to support staff participation in educational activities. Since the educator is often covering more than one clinical area, staffing responsibilities are not routinely possible.

13. *In what cases should I be involved with staffing?*

13. The educator may assist with coverage during inservice classes or skills validation sessions. Staffing becomes the priority if the healthcare agency is experiencing an emergency such as a natural disaster or inclement weather. Sometimes the educator may choose to be involved in staffing to maintain organization and clinical skills required to provide direct patient care.

14. *Describe the educator's role in preceptor and charge nurse development activities.*

14. The educator actively works with the leadership team including the education committee or clinical practice committee in preceptor and charge nurse development activities. The educator assists with developing activities to meet the needs of these roles. Frequently, communication issues need to be addressed. Sometimes implementation of new procedures/policies presents new expectations for the preceptor or charge nurse. Make sure these expectations are outlined in educational activities.

15. *What responsibility do I have in the assessment of the orientee's clinical skills, knowledge, and ability to fulfill job responsibilities?*

15. Since the educator often has more than one orientee at a time, it becomes essential that the educator work with the preceptor in assessing clinical skills. It is critical to use a tool such as Competency Based Orientation (CBO) or orientation pathway that clearly states what is expected of the orientee and allows for a visible means of tracking progress. The educator should assess the orientee's knowledge and clinical skills through observation, questioning, and review of the nurse's ability to perform the expected job responsibilities. Documentation of the orientee's performance must be maintained on an ongoing basis.

16. *How do you design individualized orientation experiences?*

16. Apply adult learning principles to make the most out of the learning experience for the orientee:

- Review the new employee's past work experiences

- Complete a self assessment tool reflective of required skills and behaviors for the clinical area

- Use assessment, challenge exams, or simulations

After the educator reviews the above information, an orientation plan is developed that maximizes the orientee's past work experiences and knowledge base.

17. *What is the clinical educator's role in managing situations where an orientee is challenged?*

17. It is difficult for all individuals involved when an orientee is not meeting expectations. The clinical educator's role becomes one of support, consultation, and facilitation for both preceptor and orientee. The educator collaborates with the preceptor and orientee in writing the developmental plan and providing effective communication. Written documentation is necessary for all orientee conferences. It is essential to keep the management team informed of the concerns and seek their involvement as needed.

18. *What intervention strategies can be used for someone who is challenged to meet clinical expectations?*

18. Frequent communication is critical in this situation. Daily conferences are essential between the preceptor, clinical educator, and the orientee. Weekly conferences that include a representative from the unit management team are necessary to review accomplishments, unmet expectations, future goals, and expected dates for completion.

- Talk with the orientee to determine his/her awareness of the challenges. Ask the orientee, "Help me understand how you decided to do. . ." The response will help determine at what point the orientee misses the critical behavior. Was it a lack of clinical knowledge or policy/procedure differences from a prior work setting? Does the orientee understand the impact of his/her actions?

- Ask if there are problems with the orientee being overwhelmed with orientation goals. If so, develop daily and weekly goals. Have the orientee keep a journal of clinical experiences.

- Investigate with the preceptor a variety of learning opportunities that incorporate different learning styles.

- Explore the possibility of personality conflicts between the preceptor and orientee that may affect the performance of the orientee.

- Finally, determine if the clinical setting is not appropriate for the individual. Is there another place within the organization that the individual would find a more suitable match for his/her skills?

19. What is the educator's role in relation to evaluations/appraisals for orientees and staff?

19. The clinical educator has valuable information on the orientees' performance at the end of orientation. The orientees' accomplishments as well as areas for development are reviewed with the appropriate individuals. The clinical educator should also provide the management team with feedback on the performance of preceptors. There may be additional opportunities for the clinical educator to contribute to staff performance appraisals.

20. How can you assist with performance problems of staff?

20. The educator helps the management team with the identification and statement of the performance problem that relates to an educational need of the staff member. The educator assists in clearly stating the desired expectations, determining objectives to meet the expectations, and defining means to evaluate the successful accomplishment of the expectations. If the performance problem includes educational components, a developmental plan may include additional readings, class participation, or clinical simulations.

21. What is the role of the manager, educator, and staff in development of an educational plan to address a performance problem?

21. The manager, educator, and staff nurse work as a team to address a performance problem. The manager's primary role is to hold the staff nurse accountable for changing the performance problem and permitting time away from the clinical area if educational classes are determined necessary. The manager and the educator review resources and discuss with the staff nurse the best plan to modify the performance problem. The clinical educator's role is to state the objectives of the developmental plan in measurable terms, identify educational resources to meet the learning need, document the results of the educational interventions, and provide feedback to the staff nurse and the manager. The staff nurse must be motivated to implement the activities and change the problem behavior.

22. What is the educator's role in the professional development of clinical staff?

22. The educator plays a critical role in motivating and encouraging the staff member to set high professional goals. The educator must provide resources and support to staff members to assist them in obtaining these goals. Conference brochures, local workshops, and other written materials are sent to educators. The clinical educator has a responsibility to share this information with others. The nurse interested in advancing may need assistance with a special project or the identification of outside resources.

A staff nurse interested in exploring the possibilities of teaching may ask to present a class. Assistance in presentation skills and content delivery should be provided. Another nurse may seek help in writing an abstract for submission to a national conference. Once the abstract is accepted, assistance will likely be needed for the poster or oral presentation.

23. How do I promote the ongoing development of the proficient or expert staff within the clinical area?

23. The ongoing development of the expert and proficient staff nurses is promoted best by valuing their contributions and identifying growth opportunities. These expert nurses then can mentor the new preceptor or charge nurse. They suggest ways to improve clinical practices. Their clinical knowledge should be shared in formal oral or poster presentations.

24. What is my role in supporting the clinical area goal(s)?

24. The educator's role in supporting the clinical area goals is to work collaboratively with the management team and the education committee to develop an educational plan. Once the management team accepts the plan, the learning activities will be implemented. Skills validations will be accomplished as needed with appropriate documentation. Whatever the goal, communication regarding progress toward goal attainment is critical for all staff.

25. *How do you anticipate the impact on the organization if unit practice changes?*

25. New unit practices have an impact beyond the individual clinical area. In one example, adult surgical inpatient intermediate areas required completion of American Heart Association Advanced Cardiac Life Support (ACLS). The sudden increase in number of people requesting the classes made it necessary for additional classes to be offered. This affected the workload of the ACLS instructors, classroom availability, and equipment supply. Any practice change must be thoroughly examined for unintended potentially adverse affects.

26. *What responsibility do educators have for being responsive to customers?*

26. The most effective learning takes place when there is a need for the knowledge. Being able to provide "just in time" training is the challenge for most educators. The customer wants an educational intervention immediately. Providing a rapid response is critical. Just in time training may include Web-based electronic learning opportunities, an article, videotapes, or other educational activities.

27. *What is the educator's role in promoting and coordinating the clinical areas educational activities?*

27. The educator works closely with unit management and the education committee to determine the needs of the unit. An inservice schedule is defined based upon how often, what day of the week, and the time of day the activity is offered. The educator works with the committees on the development of presentation objectives and speaker selection. If appropriate, continuing education credit is obtained.

28. *How do I design educational activities to provide resources for staff 24/7?*

28. The big challenge facing many educators is how to provide resources twenty-four hours a day for seven days a week. Some examples of how to provide resources for all staff include:

- Written materials
- Videotapes or audiotapes of live presentations
- Web-based courses
- Posters

29. *What responsibility do educators have to make learning experiences fun and informative?*

29. Everyone likes to have fun. When you are having fun your brain is more engaged. Use your creativity to put some spirit into educational activities. Try using crossword puzzles, games, and contests to build excitement. Move beyond the traditional lecture presentation to an exciting theme-related event. A colleague chose to present the annual skills update in a Star Wars format complete with costumes and music. Attendance was 100%.

30. What resources are there for my professional development?

30.
- Join professional organizations such as National Nursing Staff Development Organization (NNSDO), **www.nnsdo.org**, or the American Training and Development Society (ASTD), **www.astd.org**.

- Attend local and national conferences on leadership and staff development topics.

- Read professional journals, books, and other current resources on teaching and leadership skills.

- Participate in an academic class or Web-based course on teaching adults.

- Find a mentor within and outside of the organization.

- Network among other professionals.

- Look beyond nursing staff development resources to other nonhealthcare-related training and development resources.

RESOURCES

Avillion, A. E. (Ed.). (2001). *Core curriculum for staff development* (2nd ed.). Pensacola, FL: National Nursing Staff Development Organization.

Abruzzese, R. S. (1996). *Nursing staff development: Strategies for success* (2nd ed.). St. Louis: Mosby.

Rideout, E. (2001). *Transforming nursing education through problem-based learning.* Sudbury, MA: Jones and Bartlett.

Tappen, R. M., Weiss, S. A., & Whitehead, D. K. (2001). *Essentials of nursing leadership and management.* Philadelphia: F. A. Davis.

Zapp, L. (2001). Use of multiple teaching strategies in the staff development setting. *Journal for Nurses in Staff Development, 17*(4), 206–212.

Chapter 13: *Patient Education*

1. *How do patient education responsibilities relate to my other responsibilities?*

1. The Joint Commission on Accreditation of Healthcare Organizations (JCAHO) standards mandate that staff provide patient education as a component of quality patient and family care. Educators and managers assume responsibility for competency assessment, skill development, and educational resources for frontline caregivers who provide patient education. Many educators assume broader roles in directing the delivery of patient education; for example, leading steering committees, conducting needs assessments, reviewing or developing educational materials, and working with providers in other settings to provide continuity of care.

2. *How can we motivate staff to become involved in patient education?*

2. While the core values associated with patient education have not changed, the way that staff go about teaching must change. The two biggest challenges faced in teaching patients today are first, the need to deliver care in the context of new delivery systems which emphasize a team approach, and second, the need to empower rather than overwhelm patients with information. We know that the anatomy and physiology lesson is not what keeps patients safe when they are discharged. Psychomotor skills and problem solving will help patients integrate new behaviors into their daily lives. Nurses and other healthcare professionals benefit from education and coaching to gain useful tips for patient education. Staff realize that patient education is a professional responsibility yet can increase motivation and pride through successful experience, continued learning, and rewards or incentives for performance. Staff development provides opportunities through:

- continuing education, classes, seminars, and self-directed learning

- peer and colleague support, precepting, and mentoring

- patient education-oriented case studies and care "rounds"

- reward and incentive programs such as clinical ladders and awards

3. *How can patient education approaches be streamlined and what leadership can staff development offer to accomplish this?*

3. Rapidly changing models of healthcare delivery are characterized by short stays and care provided across multiple settings. Most patient education programs are outdated, because the current length of hospital stays does not accommodate ambitious learning activities. In fact, teaching programs often become outdated within one year of their creation! Continuing education and

coaching will help staff revise teaching to focus on survival skills and patient outcomes. Staff are frustrated trying to teach too much in a short period of time. Managers and administrators must provide expert nurses the freedom to develop innovative new programs in partnership with other disciplines, practice settings, and the patients and families who receive teaching. Staff development educators can lead, assist, and advocate for needed resources.

4. What are appropriate goals to set for patient education?

4. Every patient and family should receive education specific to their needs, abilities, readiness and length of stay. Patient education is interactive and empowering; it does not overwhelm the patient and focuses on functional health problems rather than simply diagnosis. Discharge instructions are provided in writing and are patient "friendly." Learning activities, resources, and patient progress are shared with other providers to improve continuity of care.

5. How can I be responsible to implement standards?

5. Staff development can help bridge the gap between education and practice. It improves the competencies of health professionals to provide patient education in a rapidly changing healthcare delivery system. Powerful staff development activities include:

- providing leadership, oversight, or coordination of organization-wide approaches to patient education;

- providing formal, ongoing, and immediate training about JCAHO Standards and Scoring Guidelines for patient education;

- teaching managers, supervisors, staff nurses, and other providers how to meet JCAHO Standards and show evidence of patient learning.

6. How can staff be taught to identify "survival skills" needed by patients and families?

6. Patient and family teaching must be focused on survival skills. What three or four critical behaviors are needed, what problems must they be able to recognize, and how should they get help to handle these problems? Knowledge and skill concerning diet, medications, exercise, activity, and smoking cessation are examples of survival skills. Staff nurses and other healthcare professionals must be teachers, but also be coaches. Patient education can be best supported with realistic teaching plans, critical paths, and teaching tools. Every patient who enters the healthcare system should know why he/she

is "here, at this time." This seems obvious, but we discover that many patients do not know how their symptoms relate to a diagnosis. Patients may not know how a group of symptoms relates to the current problem. By learning why they are here, at this time, patients gain skills in health management. We can take learning a step further by teaching if there is anything the patient could have done to prevent the episode. Patients and families want simple explanations about the diagnosis in terms they can remember and repeat to other family members. Teaching for survival skills can be promoted through staff mentoring and case study discussions as well as with teaching tools.

7. What are management responsibilities related to patient education for the organization?

7. The responsibility to educate patients and families has broad implications for all individuals who hold leadership and management positions in healthcare organizations. Responsibility includes:

- Incorporating patient education in the mission and strategic priorities of the organization

- Ensuring an environment that rewards patient education efforts and outcomes

- Providing an organizational infrastructure to oversee, deliver, and support patient education

- Incorporating patient and staff education into policies, procedures, and protocols

- Ensuring that performance improvement efforts address patient education

- Providing critical resources (e.g., staff and teaching materials) for patient education

8. What strategies can staff development educators use to increase administrative support for patient education?

8. Patient education services often lack structure, function, goals, objectives, and tracking of outcomes. As members of the management team, staff development professionals must interpret an overall approach. They advocate for cost-effective and realistic interventions focused on survival skills. They identify barriers faced by staff who deliver patient education and offer strategies to break down the barriers. They raise awareness for new, innovative approaches that address a continuum of care. They also raise awareness of patient needs or populations that are not served by existing programs, especially non-English speaking patients.

9. *How can staff development educators gain input from frontline staff to improve patient education services?*

9. The perspective of frontline staff is critical to the development of realistic, effective, and creative patient education programs. Staff should be asked to identify gaps in programs or resources and to offer their suggestions for improvement.

- Are patient education resources adequate to prepare patients?

- Are critical paths used? Is interdisciplinary collaboration occurring?

- What information and skills do staff need to be better patient teachers?

- Do staff think that providing good patient education is valued and rewarded by their supervisors?

- What problems or challenges most frequently prevent patients and families from receiving needed education?

10. *What are the most important roles that staff development plays in promoting patient education in an organization?*

10. Staff development improves competencies of staff who teach patients through:

- Formal, ongoing training related to patient education standards and responsibilities.

- Socialization to the work setting to increase confidence and competence through coaching, feedback, and mentoring.

- Improving group performance though teamwork, communication, and recognition of excellence.

11. *What are the greatest barriers to patient education encountered by staff nurses and what can staff development do to address them?*

11. The top four barriers identified by staff are:

- Time restrictions. Teaching is seen as time consuming and unrealistic. Help to streamline teaching plans and develop patient friendly teaching materials.

- Lack of teaching skills. Staff lack confidence and specific content for teaching. A combination of formal instruction (live or self-directed) and long-term support from mentors and role models are needed. Staff who are involved in group teaching often need several techniques and those teaching children or elderly need age-specific approaches. Teaching low literacy learners, non-English speakers, and patients with multiple chronic health issues requires special skills.

- Haphazard teaching efforts. If patient education materials are outdated or unavailable, documentation forms are cumbersome, or teaching efforts of the healthcare team are uncoordinated, staff development can take the lead to promote system changes.

- Patient education is not rewarded or recognized. Patient education efforts should be visible, noticed, and put in the spotlight. Staff development's role includes improving documentation, promoting accountability through performance appraisals, and sponsoring special events to recognize patient education successes.

12. How do Benner's stages of skill acquisition relate to patient education skill development?

12. Despite intensive educational efforts to teach, coach, and standardize approaches for patient education, staff development professionals recognize that staff nurses have different developmental needs in the process of becoming expert teachers (Benner, 1982). The clinical judgment and intuition needed to streamline teaching, provide culturally sensitive care, and engage with families requires that nurses move from a theoretical abstract base to a concrete world. Applying Benner's work, the strategies that most effectively promote patient education can be incorporated in staff development efforts. They are outlined in the next four questions.

13. How can staff development assist "advanced beginner" nurses?

13. The "advanced beginner" must master technical skills and learn to organize care. Attuned to rules and procedures, the nurse depends on a preceptor for teaching and coaching in each situation. The nurse is often overwhelmed with the simultaneous demands of the clinical setting. Staff development efforts involve unit-based preceptors who can focus on awareness of agency standards, resources, standardized teaching plans, and documentation. The preceptor can show how-to aspects of teaching and assess the learning needs of the nurse, such as need for knowledge about certain diagnoses or cultural groups.

14. How can staff development address the needs of "competent" nurses?

14. Nurses in the "competent" stage of practice begin to see patterns and recognize relationships among the various aspects of a situation. They have experienced similar situations and have learned from them. The nurse no longer views the patient and family as adding to the demands of care, but begins to interact with them and personalize care. The nurse is deliberate in planning and goal setting and feels responsible for all aspects of patient care. Staff development efforts include classes or workshops in family assessment, group teaching skills, learning contracts, and case studies. The nurse may be interested in and benefit from leading team conferences, making home visits, and serving on committees to design patient education programs. "Competent" nurses are excellent preceptors for beginners, because they can remember how they learned and are good coaches.

15. What are learning resources for the "proficient" nurse?

15. Nurses confidently individualize teaching, detect subtle clues such as stress, pain, family dynamics, and depression, and are attuned to each situation. Although proficient nurses still need support and resources for complex situations, they are skilled preceptors of others. Clinical career ladders, based on critical thinking, help proficient nurses demonstrate their contributions as patient teachers. Proficient nurses see the value of involving patients and families in the design of patient education services to keep programs patient and family centered. They should be encouraged to respect intuition and put aside the teaching checklist when it does not work. Proficient nurses do a wonderful job facilitating focus groups of patients to gain consumer input when developing patient care maps.

16. How can staff development assist "expert" nurses as patient educators?

16. Expert nurses make the qualitative distinctions that are crucial for patients with complex situations. They are well suited to roles of case manager, clinical specialist, and care coordinator. They are not the best choice for precepting beginners because they are developmentally so far ahead. Expert nurses may be involved with new partners in designing patient education programs. We need to give them permission to work "outside the box" and challenge "sacred cows" to design new prototypes. They often become frustrated by a system that does not work but is slow to change. Support and advocacy from colleagues in staff development are key to supporting these nurses and preventing detachment.

17. What approaches can be used for incorporating Internet patient education resources?

17. The Internet provides access to many resources that empower staff and patients. However, many health professionals are concerned that lack of quality control will lead to misinformation. The challenge for patient education is to take advantage of the opportunities for patient education afforded by the Internet, but also reduce the potential damage of erroneous information by:

- Developing an agency's own Internet resources and pointing patients to this reliable information

- Advocating for endorsement of sites by professional organizations

- Serving as an intermediary between patients and Internet information

18. How can staff development facilitate interdisciplinary approaches to patient education?

18. Patient education is built on the foundations of respecting one another, caring, and communicating, not just with the patient and family, but also among all members of the healthcare team. Staff development can facilitate teamwork though:

- leadership of an interdisciplinary patient education committee,

- interdisciplinary work teams that create or revise teaching programs and tools,

- improved documentation across disciplines and shifts,

- sharing expertise of each discipline in continuing education programs,

- and publicizing the patient education efforts of all staff.

19. How can staff development educators help increase the effectiveness of patient education videos?

19. Professional staff should carefully select, introduce, and follow up teaching when videos and CCTV are used. Videos should not be used to "replace" the teacher. A handout to reinforce key information, help the patient focus attention on key points, and apply the information to a role play, case study, or post-test enhances learning. Skills should be taught with live demonstration and practice rather than video.

20. What types of continuing education are needed to promote patient education?

20. All workshops and classes should address patient education strategies. Realistic approaches, documentation, and cultural considerations can also be provided through unit-based teaching and coaching. When it comes to skills, such as teaching patients how to use a metered-dose inhaler for a growing asthma population, research finds that nurses lack the skill to correctly use the devices and, therefore, cannot properly teach patients. Many nurses lack up-to-date knowledge and skills for diabetes management. Staff development educators must target these priorities for high volume or high-risk populations and assure competence of all staff through demonstrated performance.

21. *How can patient care rounds promote patient education?*

21. Rounds that are oriented to patient education can be a motivating force. Nurses and other healthcare professionals should be asked to prepare information about a patient with whom they are familiar. This material may be related to assessment of educational needs, goal setting, the teaching process, and how teaching might be modified based on the patient and family needs. Survival skills can be highlighted. Patient care rounds are also a wonderful opportunity to model culturally sensitive care and age-specific strategies for elderly clients or children, for example.

22. *Recognizing a growing health literacy problem, what can staff development do to assist with the development of written patient teaching tools?*

22. Researchers consistently find that materials are written far above the reading levels of most patients. Patients may not understand directions, lack self-care knowledge, misuse medications, and under use valuable services. If we want patients to understand and benefit from patient education, we must revise or redesign information to the 5th grade reading level. Healthcare professionals are usually unaware of the gap between patient reading ability and the level of patient education materials. Staff development can step in to help staff evaluate and revise medication sheets, consent forms, education brochures, and discharge instructions. Two popular word-processing programs (WordPerfect and Microsoft® Word) have easy tools to assess reading level of written materials. Patients can also provide valuable input in design and pilot testing.

23. *What JCAHO priorities for patient education should be addressed by staff development?*

23. JCAHO surveyors look for evidence that staff have identified priorities for teaching and have planned individualized care for patients. They look for evidence of the patient and family's response to care. Does the patient record indicate how the patient responded to teaching, what the patient understood? This documentation would indicate whether information was understandable and usable to the patient. Many factors prevent patients from understanding the information given to them by healthcare providers. It may be that the reading level of written information was too high, that language, cultural, or religious factors were issues, or that the patient was in pain and unable to absorb teaching. It is very important that these factors be documented. We must show that all patients receive teaching related to survival skills to ensure safe discharge and continuity of care.

24. *How can patient education managers be most efficient in an environment of cost cutting and declining resources?*

24. It is important to remember that patient education is not a list of instructions, or a videotape, or a closed circuit television system through which we simply deliver information to patients and families. Patient education involves a relationship between patients and families that is long-term, and takes advantage of every encounter in the health system to promote healthy behaviors. Patient education must be revamped to factor in patient acuity and short stays and the need for continuity with providers in other settings. Managers' roles are to develop continuity of care services, shared patient education programs, and user-friendly tools to ensure patient safety.

25. *How can staff development address cultural competence in the delivery of patient education?*

25. Healthcare providers must be prepared to work with people from diverse cultural background, and this diversity is increasing. Staff development professionals need to assist with the development of educational materials in other languages and help staff learn as much as possible about the cultures they serve. Although it is not possible to expect an in-depth understanding of all ethnocultural groups in the United States, staff should explore those cultural groups with whom they regularly interact. Much diversity exists within ethnic groups. Family by family, culture and beliefs affect the way we learn and the way we practice health behaviors. What we need are providers who are open to learning from patients.

26. *How can staff development increase the visibility and value of patient education efforts in an organization?*

26. Patient education is often "invisible" in management's eyes because it is frequently undocumented, unmonitored, and underappreciated for the skill, experience, and creativity it demands. Staff development can improve documentation and visibility of teaching efforts, promote accountability of all staff through performance appraisal, and sponsor special events that recognize patient education successes. An annual "Patient Education Week" that includes displays, guest speakers, special awards to individuals and units, recognition of patient education outcomes and commitment by top administrators, and testimonials from patients and families can also provide a needed boost for staff. More than handouts and videos, well-prepared and motivated staff are the most valuable resource for patient education.

RESOURCES

Benner, P. (1982). *From novice to expert.* Menlo Park, CA: Addison- Wesley.

Joint Commission on the Accreditation of Healthcare Organizations. (1996). *Educating hospital patients and their families: Examples of compliance.* Oakbrook, IL: Author.

Kelly Thomas, K. J. (1997). *Clinical and nursing staff development: Current competence, future focus.* Philadelphia: Lippincott.

London, F. (1999). *No time to teach.* Philadelphia: Lippincott Williams & Wilkins.

Rankin, S. H., & Stallings, K. D. (2001). *Patient education, principles and practice.* Philadelphia: Lippincott Williams & Wilkins.

Stallings, K. (1996). *Integrating patient education in your nursing practice* [Video]. Reproduced with permission of Glaxo Wellcome, Inc. (Produced by Horizon Video Productions, 4222 Emperor Blvd., Durham, NC 27703).

A helpful step-by-step approach for finding and evaluating Internet resources for patients can be found in Rankin, S. H. & Duffy Stallings, K. (2000). Patient education resources on the Internet. In *Patient education: Principles & education* (pp. 297–322). Philadelphia: Lippincott Williams & Wilkins.

Chapter 14: *Change Agent, Facilitator, Leader*

1. *How do these roles relate to the more tangible roles of educator, consultant, manager, and researcher?*

1. I see the role of change agent, facilitator, and leader as an integral part of each of the traditional roles of the educator. When I am providing education to a group of staff, I am leading the program, facilitating the learning activities, and providing the opportunity for a change in behavior to improve performance related to the topic. As a consultant, I may lead and/ or facilitate a group of managers in selecting the best method for addressing a performance problem when education is not the best solution. I am acting as a change agent as I encourage the managers to use other options that will give them better results.

2. *How do I position myself to be a change agent?*

2. One of the best strategies that I have used involves "opening the perspective," either the client's or mine. In order to be a good change agent, you must be able to see the problem or opportunity from many different viewpoints. Gathering information about the various perspectives takes time, but is invaluable in gaining support for the change, helping others understand the issues at hand, and in selecting the best solution and method of implementation.

3. *How do you maintain momentum as a change agent?*

3. I use several tools to keep projects or teams on task including roadmaps, action lists, and team/project evaluations. Roadmaps are timelines for specific tasks with assigned responsibilities. A sample of a time line is found below.

Sample Time Line

Activities	Person	J	F	M	A	M	J	J	A	S	O	N	D
Define purpose and goals		X											
Determine membership, meeting time, & ground rules		X											
Study the process—flowcharting			X										
Interview customers			X	X									
Gather data and graph				X	X								
Analyze data						X	X						
Identify problems and root causes—pareto chart								X					
Gather data, graph, and analyze								X	X				

Continued on page 124

Sample Time Line, continued from page 123

Activities	Person	J	F	M	A	M	J	J	A	S	O	N	D
Improve the process—Select a solution and implement a trial period									X	X			
Gather data, graph, and analyze											X	X	
Redesign or implement													X
Establish a system to monitor in the future													X

At each meeting or planning session, an action list is created to track who has agreed to do what by when. The tool is simple and easy to use. I usually ask one person to maintain the list over time. Action list follow-up is a regular agenda item to check for completion of assigned tasks and to hold people accountable. If the next meeting requires completion of a certain task in order for the group to move forward, I ask the action list person to contact and remind the responsible person before the meeting. We also provide a copy of the action list to those who have agreed to an assigned task at the end of the meeting. A sample action list is included below.

Adverse Drug Event Team Follow-Up Action List

What	Who	By When	Completed
Interview staff nurses about why they are reluctant to report med errors. Aggregate results in pareto chart.	John Irving	Jan 12th meeting	
Investigate the addition of a voice mailbox for anonymous reporting.	Sue Burgis	Jan 19th meeting	
Review the med error report form and simplify. Provide draft before meeting.	Marge Jones	Jan 12th meeting	

Regular team or project evaluations allow the members to identify barriers or roadblocks to progress and reorient the group to the purpose statement, goals, and timeline. The evaluation includes not only timeliness of task completion, but group dynamics also. How well is the team functioning in consensus building and decision making? In what areas can the team improve its own process or work?

Each of these tools' primary purpose is to communicate expectations to the members of the team. Communication and follow up are key to maintaining momentum as a change agent.

4. What can I tell staff who are overwhelmed by all the changes?

4. Adequate planning with any change project requires appropriate implementation timing so that staff do not experience this sense of being overwhelmed. It is the responsibility of a change agent to become aware of other changes coming along so that the adverse effect is minimized. One other strategy that I use to prevent the staff from feeling overwhelmed is to tell them a change is coming at least three times before it actually arrives. In other words, give them as much advance warning as possible. When the change is finally implemented, they often comment, "It's about time."

5. How can I become more integrated into the quality improvement of my organization?

5. Being involved in quality improvement in your organization provides many opportunities for exercising your role as a change agent, facilitator, and leader. My first suggestion is to participate in as much training/education as you can. Attend all the offerings within the organization for quality improvement, data analysis, or facilitator training. Schedule yourself to attend at least one continuing education program offered outside the facility. Become familiar with statistical measurement and data display tools. Volunteer to serve on quality improvement project teams. Review the data that are being collected in your own organization. Increase your group facilitation skills and volunteer your services to managers.

6. In what arenas does an educator serve as a facilitator?

6. One of the primary arenas for an educator to serve as a facilitator is in the classroom. We facilitate learning by creating an environment that is welcoming, free of distractions, comfortable, and interactive. Learning is also facilitated by providing information in a way that meets various learning needs and styles. Another arena where we serve as facilitators is with staff development, whether we are working with staff on skills competency

or managers on identifying learning needs. Some educators serve as facilitators for quality improvement teams or with ongoing committees. In this role, we ensure that the team is making progress, facilitate the decision making process, and collaborate with the team leader in managing group dynamics.

7. What are the important elements of facilitating a team or project?

7. Effective facilitators are experienced and educated in work team dynamics and operations; quality improvement principles, practices, and tools; the organization's selected quality improvement (QI) methodology; consensus building and decision making tools; data collection, measurement, analysis, and presentation; and the facilitation skills of questioning, intervening, and giving feedback. Key responsibilities include:

- Educating team members about the QI methodology, improvement tools and techniques, and performance measurement and analysis

- Helping the team create and sustain effective working dynamics

- Coaching the entire team and individual members in the use of improvement tools, data collection and analysis, improvement idea generation and testing, decision making, and development and implementation of improvement strategies

- Helping the team prepare for formal presentations to leadership

- Meeting with the team leader before and after the team meetings to analyze the effectiveness of the team process and to plan for process interventions

- Providing support and encouragement, and assisting with the removal of barriers or roadblocks.

8. What can you do if you do not agree with the "change" that you are asked to facilitate?

8. I have a great example for this one. An administrator asked me to facilitate a team to purchase a new food delivery option that was supposed to be much cheaper and would eliminate several positions from the food and nutrition staff. I was aware of many negative comments about this delivery option and I did not believe that it would work in the facility. My response was that I would facilitate a team to evaluate the options, but I couldn't guarantee that the administrator's preferred option would be selected. After involving representatives from each facility and unit that would be affected, we taste tested,

analyzed costs, prepared a flowchart on the proposed process, and evaluated several other options. We also visited other sites that had implemented the various options. The team presented all the facts and figures to the administrator with a recommendation. The administrator approved the recommendation which was not the original food delivery option he selected.

9. If I am not a manager or I do not have any staff that report to me, how can I be a leader?

9. If we define leader as one who provides direction or guidance, then we are leaders in all that we do as educators. A leader is responsible for determining focus and direction, removing obstacles, developing ownership, and stimulating self-direction. Is this not what we do with every educational opportunity that we provide to customers? Educators often serve as leaders of teams, committees, or projects. We may also perform a leadership function as we coordinate orientation or life support courses or management development programming.

10. How can I improve my skills as a change agent, facilitator, and leader?

10. My answer to this question is practice, practice, practice. The more opportunities we have to use critical thinking and judgment skills in these areas, the more expertise we develop. I also suggest watching others performing this role to identify effective actions and strategies. Speak with those who have more expertise. Create a mentoring relationship with someone whose skills you admire. Ask for feedback to improve your skills. Each year, I send a survey to my clients asking them to rate me on a Likert scale (3 = always, 2 = usually, 1 = rarely) to see how well I am doing. Sample questions include:

Getting the job done (achievement):

1. Do I have initiative by taking needed actions before being asked or required and by doing more than the minimum?

2. Am I committed to accomplishing challenging problems and following through with a job or task?

Working through others (leadership):

3. Do I use power effectively and appropriately by enforcing rules, addressing problems, and setting standards for behavior?

4. Do I encourage participation, promote cooperation and teamwork, reduce conflict, and keep others informed?

5. Am I interested in helping others to improve more than being judgmental or punitive?

Working with others (interpersonal skills):

6. Am I able to understand the concerns, motives, and feelings of others and to recognize strengths and limitations?

7. Do I involve appropriate people in solving problems?

Thinking through issues (problem solving):

8. Do I look at issues from different perspectives and seek options in solving problems?

9. Do I address and assist in problem solving in the organization?

Managing myself (personal performance):

10. Do I recognize my own strengths and limitations and try to improve?

11. Do I use organizational resources to improve practice?

I use the tallied responses to identify goals for the next year.

11. *What are some common strategies for increasing my role in these areas?*

11. Become involved in committees, teams, and improvement efforts. Interview managers and supervisors to identify learning needs and offer your services. Become aware of the improvement efforts throughout the organization especially organization-wide efforts.

12. *How can I evaluate my effectiveness in performing these roles?*

12. Create an annual summary of all involvement and accomplishments for the last year. Analyze each one to identify which role(s) you played. Ask for feedback from managers, peers, or customers verbally or through a survey. Review quality improvement data from measurements and team evaluations of projects you have participated in.

13. *How do I manage the frustration involved in these roles?*

13. My suggestions range from taking time out to using all the resources you have at hand. I have found that my frustration trigger gets much too sensitive when I fail to take care of myself and use the stress reduction strategies that work for me. Sometimes, just acknowledging the frustration and sharing with a trusted colleague is enough.

14. How can I stay out of trouble in these roles?

14. I am not sure that I can answer this one because one of my mottos is: "It is easier to get forgiveness than permission." This tends to get me into trouble. However, a trusted mentor continues to tell me to communicate, communicate, communicate. If I am sharing my ideas, strategies, and plans with others, then I am less likely to get off track. If I am asking for feedback and using this information, I can ensure that I am improving.

15. What are some examples of success with each of these roles?

15. I was asked to provide an inservice class to the medical unit staff nurses because their medication error rate had climbed dramatically in the last quarter. Initially, I verified that the nurses had demonstrated competency in medication administration during orientation. I met with the manager to gather more information. We analyzed the data and discovered that the errors were scattered among all the staff, were primarily in the morning, and involved omissions. Rather than provide an administration inservice class, I evaluated the medication schedule and observed medication passes. The observation revealed that the nurses had difficulty in administering the 8 a.m. medications timely and correctly because of all the distractions and responsibilities during the 7 to 9 a.m. time period. A run chart of the medications scheduled for administration during a 24-hour period revealed that 48% of the medications were to be given at 8 a.m. and half of these were through an NG tube which always takes longer. Working with the manager, a recommendation to move the qd, bid, and tid times to 9 a.m. instead of 8 a.m. was displayed on a run chart and taken to the staff for input. A trial run for a week resulted in positive results—increased staff satisfaction and decreased medication error rate. And best of all, I didn't have to do an unnecessary and ineffective inservice class!

RESOURCES

Craig, R. (1987). *Training and development handbook.* New York: McGraw-Hill.

Hersey, P., & Blanchard, K. (1992). *Management of organizational behavior: Utilizing human resources.* Englewood Cliffs, NJ: Prentice-Hall.

Katz, J., & Green, E. (1992). *Managing quality.* St. Louis: Mosby.

Kelly Thomas, K. J. (1998). *Clinical and nursing staff development: Current competence, future focus* (2nd ed.). Philadelphia: Lippincott.

Knox, A. (1980). *Developing, administering, and evaluating adult education.* San Francisco: Jossey-Bass.

Section 4:

Planning, Implementing, and Evaluating Educational Activities

Just as there is a nursing process and a scientific method, there is an education process to guide the planning, implementation, and evaluation of education activities. While individual texts have been written for each component, viewing this as a process that flows easily from phase to phase is key to developing activities with useful outcomes. This process is fundamental to the work of the nursing professional development (NPD) specialist, is an important component of the orientation of any novice, and is covered extensively in the NPD certification exam.

Chapter 15: *Assessing Learning Needs*

1. What is a learning needs assessment?

1. The learning needs assessment is the first step in planning an educational offering. The needs assessment may be a formal or informal process that identifies what needs to be taught and is the building block for developing objectives and planning the educational activity.

2. What is the purpose of a needs assessment?

2. The purpose of a learning needs assessment is to discover what must be taught. The needs assessment is a decision-making tool to identify what educational activities should be done to meet the participants' educational needs. Two other purposes are to identify the potential target audience and determine whether the program has merit and should be presented.

3. Why do I need to do a needs assessment?

3. A needs assessment is an essential component which guides the program planning process and prevents the planner from providing a program that doesn't meet the participants' needs.

4. What is the value of a needs assessment?

4. The needs assessment is a valuable tool. Other data often gathered on the needs assessment besides potential program topics are: potential target audience, appropriate settings, data on learners, identifying the learners, and date and time choices for programs.

5. What specific audience should be targeted for the needs assessment?

5. The audience selected for the needs assessment should be the potential learners. This will vary according to unit, department, institution, or geographic area. The needs assessment may also be a convenience sampling (everyone in a department), stratified samples (a certain segment of the potential audience), or a random sampling.

6. What resources are needed to do a needs assessment?

6. Resources required depend on the type of needs assessment that is done. Generally, time and costs are the two essential resources. If you need information right away, a formal mail out would not be appropriate as this takes at least month to develop, disseminate, and analyze data.

7. How do I conduct a needs assessment?

7. There are a number of ways to do a needs assessment. A common approach is a printed survey that is mailed to the potential target audience. Other methods, which are not as time consuming, but equally effective, are staff meetings, questionnaires, brainstorming, interviews,

incident reports, performance appraisal/job descriptions, quality improvement, new procedures and products, and accreditation standards.

8. What types of questions should be on a needs assessment?

8. In a survey or formal mail out, questions are usually asked regarding the individual's basic education, amount of education, length of current employment, position, practice area, hours per week employed, potential location for offerings, cost preferences, potential list of program topics, and blank areas for individuals to fill in other educational needs not identified. The potential list of program topics should either be prioritized by the individuals or they should indicate interest in attending (e.g., would attend, might attend, would not attend).

9. What are sources of information for a needs assessment?

9. The best source for information on needs is the potential learner. Other sources would be nursing administrator, the institution (e.g., hospital, nursing home, home health agency, department, clinic, physician's office, school) professional organization, regulatory agency, and clients of learners.

10. Should demographic questions be included on the needs assessment?

10. I think demographic questions are good to include. Say you receive a survey back from 100 nurses and 75 indicate the need for a pharmacology course. You put on a pharmacology course that includes cardiac and diabetic medications and no one comes. If you had a question relating to what area of practice the nurse is from and were able to identify that these were all OB nurses, you would know to put on a program dealing with OB drugs. Or say a critical care nurse identifies a specific learning need related to hemodymanics, but the other 25 critical care nurses do not see this as a need. Putting on the hemodynamics program for one person would not be appropriate.

11. How do I select a tool that would be right for the institution?

11. There are three routes you can go for needs assessment tools. First, use a tool that has been previously used by someone else. Second, review the literature to find other needs assessment tools. If you use either of these methods, ensure that the tool meets your needs and gathers the data you want. The third option is to develop your own tool. When developing your own tool, pretest it to ensure you are getting the right information. Items should be short and simple and worded positively; limit choices to 5; and choices should be equal in size as much as possible.

12. When is a good time to conduct a needs assessment?

13. How often do I need to do a needs assessment?

14. I don't have the funds to do a formal mail out; what are some creative ways to conduct a learning needs assessment?

15. What is a good strategy for documentation of the needs assessment?

16. What time frame should be allocated for the needs assessment?

17. How can I get a good return on the needs assessment?

18. How can focus groups be used for needs assessment?

12. Most individuals will do a needs assessment prior to the beginning of the fiscal year. The data then assists the individual in planning activities for the fiscal year. Some individuals do a mini-needs assessment with each educational activity during the fiscal year, and analyze and prioritize data to plan future, upcoming activities.

13. How frequently you do a needs assessment depends on the institution and resources. Generally, an annual needs assessment should be done.

14. A formal mail out or survey is not necessarily needed to collect data. Other methods to gather assessment data are focus groups, clinical rounds, nursing reports, management meetings, planned changes or updates to the institution, observations, record reviews, satisfaction surveys, task forces, and consultations. These can provide current information.

15. The data from the needs assessment needs to be compiled in an easy, readable format. Data are usually reported in numbers and percentages. For example, 100 surveys were returned; 52 (52%) would attend a program on communication, 2 (2%) might attend a program on communication, 40 (40%) would not attend, and 6 (6%) have already attended a program on communication.

16. You want to give individuals sufficient time to complete the survey/questionnaire, but not so much time that they lose it. Usually one week is sufficient when mailing out questionnaires. When gathering information from some of the other methods, give sufficient time, but generally no more than one week.

17. To get a good return on a survey/questionnaires, offer some incentive to return the completed form. A discount on a future program is one way. I have attached a $5 coupon to the needs survey for the individual to use at a future offering. Offer a free registration to an upcoming program—have a place for a phone number on the questionnaire, select one questionnaire, call the individual, and offer a free registration.

18. A focus group should consist of individuals who are the stakeholders of continuing education or will make up the target audience. The group should include from 6 to 12 participants and be small enough to have a structured yet informal discussion. The group should have some directed questions; leave time for some brainstorming or discussion of what is needed. The group can focus on needs, potential target audience, program topics, presenters, marketing, or generating ideas to improve the overall continuing education program.

19. What about management meetings as a needs assessment methodology?

19. The management meetings could work just like a focus group. However, thc management team may have a specific goal or outcome in mind and not offer too many suggestions. A management meeting can provide information on planning programs. An example—a new specialty unit is being planned to open in six months. Nursing and support staff are going to need education for the new unit. The management team can provide information on the types of patients, philosophy of the unit, and care issues. This information is essential needs assessment data to plan the program.

20. How should the needs assessment results be analyzed?

20. Results should be analyzed so that the data are understood. The data can be analyzed by hand or by computer. The data analysis method should have been selected during the planning phase of the needs assessment. The data analysis should include a summary and interpretation of results.

21. How should the results be prioritized?

21. Data should be prioritized according to what is needed the most or what is essential to the organization. Priorities can be set by administration or the planner. Not all needs/programs can be implemented; the programs to be implemented depend on the resources available and the goals of the institution/department.

22. How do I validate a need for a given activity?

22. An activity will often be validated by the needs assessment. Many times, though, management mandates a program to be implemented. The program planner will need to validate the need/purpose of the activity with administration and with the staff by using one of the other methods such as focus groups or incident reporting.

23. My agency wants me to do a program, but it is not on the needs assessment. What do I do?

23. When administration mandates a program, the planner needs to meet with administration and gather information on the perceived need. Are there some underlying regulations or circumstances that have influenced the decision? Is it an educational deficit or a performance deficit? Sometimes, it is just easier to provide the program than disagree with administration. Just be clear on the intended outcome.

24. What do I do if needs change while I am planning?

24. Information gathered during the needs assessment allows the planner to have data to plan programs. If needs change, most times a planner can regroup and still present the program. Sometimes a need is identified and planning begins, and then someone else in the community puts on the same program. Three choices are to continue the program and hope there will be sufficient participants OR change the program and target a different audience OR cancel the program.

25. We have competence based performance standards. How can I use the competency model to assess learning needs?

25. Competence based performance standards can give a lot of information to the program planner. Competency is defined as a statement which describes an aspect of care that a healthcare professional must develop and demonstrate. These competencies may be skills, procedures, knowledge, or behaviors and should include all domains of performance—cognitive, psychomotor, and affective. Chemotherapy administration is one competence that must be validated annually. The program planner needs to then develop, implement, and evaluate staff's competence to safely administration chemotherapy in the clinical setting.

REFERENCES

Austin, E. K. (1981). *Guidelines for the development of continuing education offerings for nurses.* New York: Appleton-Century-Crofts.

Goody, A. E., & Kozoll, C. E. (1995). *Program development in continuing education.* Malabar, FL: Krieger Publishing.

Kelly Thomas, K. J. (1998). *Clinical and nursing staff development: Current competence, future focus* (2nd ed.). Philadelphia: Lippincott.

Puetz, B. E. (1987). *Contemporary strategies for continuing education in nursing.* Rockville, MD: Aspen.

Queeney, D. S. (1995). *An essential tool for quality improvement: Assessing needs in continuing education.* San Francisco: Jossey-Bass.

Swansburg, R. C. (1995). *Nursing staff development: A component of human resource development.* Boston: Jones & Bartlett.

Chapter 16: *Writing Objectives*

1. Are objectives really necessary?

1. The obvious answer is *yes!* Writing objectives is the basis for any learning activity, whether it is a 20-minute inservice class or a formal course. Objectives provide a framework for choosing what to teach and help the instructor to stay within the scope of the program. Objectives also assist in selection of appropriate teaching strategies and materials. Objectives serve as a basis for evaluation, in terms of learner outcomes and instruction. Most importantly objectives enhance communication between adult learners and adult instructors by establishing clear expectations for both.

2. What is the difference between a goal and an objective?

2. It is easy to confuse goals and objectives. The distinction is that goals are used to describe in broad terms the knowledge, skills, or attitudes that you want the learner to attain. The goal is the end product you want to achieve. In and of itself, a goal is not measurable. An example of a program goal would be *"to understand the process of pain management."* This is not directly measurable but specific objectives, if done in proper order, can be developed to achieve the overall goal.

3. How and where do I start?

3. The best place to start is by analyzing the results of a needs assessment to help answer the questions:

"What is the goal or goals of the activity?"

"Why do we need this content?"

"How much does the target audience know about the topic?"

"At what point do I start and conclude?"

The next and perhaps most difficult step is to define specifically what the learner needs to be able to do after the unit of instruction. Taking time to clearly identify these behaviors or tasks to achieve the program goals or outcomes will make the rest of the process simple and logical. The specific content, methodology, and evaluation measures all flow from these expected outcomes. Ask yourself—bottom line—what change in the learner is absolutely necessary to meet the identified need? Don't worry about the structure of the objective at this point; just identify what you want the learner to be able to do and make a list. If you are not the subject matter expert then develop this list with that person. This list will give you the springboard for writing clear objectives and developing a program to help the learner achieve them.

4. How many objectives do I need?

4. There is no magic formula! If you have decided on the goal(s) of the activity, and you have identified the critical behaviors to achieve the goal(s), you should have a well-defined list. If you train to requirements or to identified needs then you automatically will have scrubbed the list of "nice to knows" versus "must knows." Other factors may affect the number of objectives you can realistically expect to accomplish. These factors include who is going to teach the program, what the learners know about the topic, the physical facilities and resources, and time allotted. Common sense dictates that an inservice class is usually narrowly focused and the number of objectives will be minimal. Ask yourself, "What can be taught in a 30-minute time frame"? Conversely, when teaching complex topics or procedures, a longer time period must be projected. Generally, for continuing education programs three to six objectives, depending on the length of the program, will be enough.

5. How detailed does an objective need to be?

5. The objective should be written in general enough terms to describe to the learner the expected behaviors that will demonstrate achievement of the intended program outcomes. Objectives should reflect the performance domain; for example, demonstrate a skill or acquisition of new knowledge. Try to focus objectives on general behaviors, avoid minutia or trivial steps. I like to think of an objective in terms of a performance or competency checklist. The objective should reflect the overall purpose of the checklist and the steps of the checklist are actually teaching points that support the objective.

6. Should objectives be broadly stated or narrowly focused?

6. This truly depends on your goals for the program. For example, if the program presents new information, concepts, or theories, you may do well with a few meaningful, broadly stated objectives, often called general objectives or terminal learning objectives. General objectives usually state only the behavior to be achieved and the knowledge context within which it is to occur. Because the conditions and evaluation strategies are not written into the objective, it allows flexibility in the teaching and learning process. Specific or narrowly focused objectives are closed-ended and include all the contingencies of the learning situation.

These are usually used for learning activities that require sequential or linear presentation in a step-by-step manner to achieve an overall skill set or body of knowledge. Often called sub-objectives or enabling objectives, specific objectives help describe actions needed to accomplish the broadly stated or terminal learning.

7. Why does an objective need to be measurable?

7. An objective is a word picture of what we expect learners to do if they have learned the material. Measurable objectives alert the learner to focus on what is important in the program activity. If written in measurable terms, the objective provides a standard or acts as a yardstick to ascertain if achievement of intended outcomes has occurred. Keep in mind if evaluation is subjective then you don't truly have an objective!

8. How do I make an objective measurable?

8. Always use an "action" verb. The most common mistake in writing objectives is using verbs that indicate cognitive actions. This is fine for a goal statement, NOT for an objective. Verbs such as "understand, appreciate, know" are not directly measurable. I can't tell if someone "knows" or "understands" unless I get feedback that tells me they do. By using behavioral, observable terms such as "state, explain, demonstrate" you can then evaluate level of attainment.

9. What do I need to develop first, content or objectives?

9. Think of an objective as a "horse" and the content as the "cart." You never would put a cart before a horse, would you? Without objectives how would you know what to put into your cart? If you develop content first, then you are faced with developing objectives to fit the material. Objectives should be designed to meet the needs of the learner and serve as a guide for developing and organizing the content. The objectives should be arranged from the known and progress to the unknown. This helps you to develop the content or teaching sessions to move the learner through the material to achieve the objectives and overall goal(s) of the program.

10. How do I keep objectives "learner focused"?

10. The key is to identify the target audience in the body of the objective. Concentrating on the target audience (e.g., nurse, attendee, unit secretary) automatically leads you to describe "what the learner will do" NOT "what the teacher will do." If you describe, "what the teacher will do" you are referring to the *educational process* of the activity. If you describe what the learner will do you are actually talking about *learner outcomes*.

11. What are the essential components of a good objective?

11. The best description I have found relates to the acronym "**ABCD**." The "**A**" stands for the *audience* and identifies the learner as the focus of the objective. The "**B**" relates to the *behavior* or actions that indicate that learning has occurred. The "**C**" refers to the *condition*, and describes the condition(s) or circumstance(s) under which the learner is expected to perform and be evaluated. Finally, the "**D**" represents the *degree of attainment*, or standard, and describes how well or to what degree you expect the learner to perform. For example:

"Given a trauma care scenario and using the human patient simulator, trauma team members will perform a trauma nursing assessment in accordance with a performance checklist"

> **Audience:** "Trauma team members"
>
> **Behavior:** " perform a trauma assessment"
>
> **Conditions:** "using a human patient simulator and given a trauma scenario"
>
> **Degree of attainment**: "in accordance with a performance checklist"

12. Why should I include the "condition(s)" of performance in an objective?

12. The *condition* is an optional feature. I include conditions when I want to give the learner very specific information on what will be provided or denied them during evaluation of performance. Conditions are often included when the program is designed to test specific skills or knowledge. For example: "Using the human patient simulator, perform endotracheal suctioning, in accordance with the performance checklist." The first clause is the condition. Another example is "Without the use of a calculator, determine the drip rate for…." Again, the first clause provides the condition in which the learner is expected to perform.

13. How do I choose the right "behavioral" verbs to describe desired outcomes of the activity?

13. Adults are action oriented and, although measurable, verbs such as list, state, and define reflect the lowest levels of learning information. This may be an important first step, but generally adults appreciate actions that relate most closely to their job performance. Consider how the learners will use what they learn from the program. I start off by asking myself what domain of learning is the intended outcome? The three domains of learning are cognitive, psychomotor, and affective. I then ask myself at what level do I want the learners to achieve? Is it merely information or the application of the information? Thanks to a number of cognitive psychologists, sample verb lists are available for each domain. These can help you select, or guide you to the appropriate verb within each domain (see Table 1). When I choose verbs, I also ask is this something I can realistically measure, given the time and resources available?

14. *Why is it a good idea to include the "degree of attainment" within the body of an objective?*

14. Generally, the degree statement defines for the learners the standard of performance expected of them. This can be expressed in many ways. For example, the standard could be in terms of time frames (e.g., within 30 seconds); accuracy (e.g., 80% accuracy or zero discrepancy); in accordance with specific guidelines (e.g., hospital policy or another authority); or quantity (e.g., perform three venipunctures). If a degree of attainment is not specified, then degree of attainment is assumed at 100% accuracy. Although optional, including this component in the body of the objective establishes the expectation that the learner will be evaluated accordingly. Usually objectives are written as clauses in one sentence; however, if the sentence is overly long, it is acceptable to add the degree of attainment or standard in a separate sentence.

15. *What is the difference between a simple objective and a complex objective?*

15. A simple objective includes only the audience ("A") and the behavioral statement ("B"). Depending on the goal of the program this may suffice. However, if it is important to measure specific aspects of the performance, then a complex objective will be helpful. A complex objective includes the "ABCD": the audience, a behavioral statement, a condition statement, and the degree of attainment.

16. *How do I choose the right domain of learning to reflect the desired outcomes?*

16. Think about program outcomes in terms of what knowledge, skills or attitudes you want the learner to attain (the three domains of learning). **The cognitive domain** reflects *"ways of knowing."* This domain relies on facts, data, and theory, and is most frequently used when information is to be delivered. Traditional lectures, discussions, and written tests are usually the result of cognitive objectives. **The affective domain** reflects on *"ways of feeling."* This domain commonly addresses more abstract concepts that relate to "values," "attitudes" and "feelings." Programs in this domain are characterized by exploration of values and emotions and often encourage self-examination of feelings. **The psychomotor domain** reflects on *"ways of doing."* Programs that are based in the psychomotor domain generally provide step-by-step instruction to learn a new basic to advanced skill or procedure. It is certainly possible, in fact encouraged, to have objectives in two or all three domains depending on the scope and depth of the activity.

17. What strategy can I use to increase the level of objectives?

17. A common mistake is to write *all* objectives at the lowest level of learning. Objectives should be written at the level appropriate for the expected outcome. Ask yourself, how will the information and skills be used in the learner's practice setting? What level of learning will optimize the learner's ability to transfer the learning to the workplace situation? The goal is to provide educational activities that help the learner achieve a specific level of the domain. The domains of learning are written in increasing levels of complexity (or stages), with one level preparing the learner for learning at the next level. Again, these have been categorized according to the cognitive, psychomotor, and affective domains (see Table 1). Referred to as taxonomies, these are organized in such a way to act as a guide for developing objectives. Evaluation during and after the program is needed to determine if the objective and its associated level of learning is reasonable for that target audience. Also keep in mind that the more complex the level of learning, the more you must allow for a corresponding increase in learning time.

18. How do I develop objectives in the cognitive domain?

18. Think of cognitive activities as "mental skills." Decide which mental activity will provide a reliable indicator that the learner has attained the desired knowledge level. Learning within the cognitive domain includes an understanding of concepts, principles, and theories. Higher levels of intellectual skills revolve around critical thinking, problem solving, decision making, and evaluation. Again, use the classification framework found in the cognitive domain; choose verbs based on the level of learning you expect the learners to achieve; and also think about how you can evaluate attainment of the objective. Once you develop objectives and identify how you will evaluate them, then you can build content to help the learner achieve the objectives.

19. How do I develop objectives in the psychomotor domain?

19. Think of psychomotor activities as "manual or physical skills." Decide what verbs are best to describe how well the learner can perform the skill, task, or procedure. The classification framework found in the psychomotor domain provides guide words to help you develop objectives. You may find it easier to develop a terminal learning objective first that describes the skill in its entirety. Then, as you identify the sub-skills or tasks that need to be accomplished successively you are also building a list of teaching points for the content. Again, consider how you are going to evaluate performance as you select verbs and develop your objective(s).

20. How do I develop objectives in the affective domain?

20. Think of affective objectives as actions that demonstrate attitude. The affective domain relates to values and feelings. Affective skills reflect moral reasoning and the development of a value system that guides ethical and moral decision making. Indirect measures of values are "value indicators" which include moral reasoning, attitudes, and ethics. Once more, refer to the classification framework found in the affective domain. These guide words can help you build objective(s) and also help you determine the most effective way to involve the learners in activities to master the objective.

21. How can I determine if an objective is met?

21. If you include all the essential components in objectives you have an excellent guide for evaluation. You will have described the expected performance or behavior for the intended audience, the environment in which the performance is accomplished (what will be provided or restricted in the performance), and how well the learner is to perform. As noted previously, the method of evaluation should be determined at the same time you develop objective(s). The action verb indicates how you will evaluate the program. If you are using "outcome" objectives with behavioral verbs such as "perform, demonstrate, and construct" then the evaluation method should provide a means for the learner to do so; often a performance checklist may be helpful. If behaviors indicate a cognitive skill, such as "define, describe" then a written test or verbal method (e.g., discussion, games) of evaluation can be used. However, most continuing education programs focus on process objectives, with typical verbs such as explore or discuss. If this is the case then the end-of-program evaluation or critique that rates attainment of each stated objective is appropriate for adult learners.

22. How do I use objectives to develop tests and performance measures?

22. All objectives should be adequately evaluated. If you are evaluating psychomotor objectives, a checklist helps objectively rate the performance. If you are evaluating cognitive objectives you may choose between written testing and other evaluation measures such as discussion, role-playing, or games. If you choose written test items, be careful to match the appropriate item to the behavior stated in the objective (see Table 2). The most common mistake is a mismatch between the action indicated in the objective and the method of evaluation. For instance the objective may state, "perform a well baby physical examination" and the method of evaluation is a written test. The obvious flaw is that according to the objective, the learner should actually perform the assessment on either a real or simulated patient. However, if you have written sub or enabling objectives that provide cognitive content, then certainly a test item may measure that piece of knowledge. Conversely, you may infer that the learner has attained the knowledge content if he/she performs the action accurately. In this case, a written test is not necessary.

23. How do I use objectives to implement competency-based activities?

23. The hallmark of any competency assessment program is the identification of competency areas, usually written as competency statements. Development of *competency statements* and *associated performance criteria* follows essentially the same process as writing *terminal learning objectives* and *enabling objectives*. The competency statement contains a description of the general behavior in measurable and observable terms and should be validated by a subject matter expert. The competency statement is focused on "what the employee is expected to do" to fulfill the job requirements. It mirrors the *terminal learning objective* in that it includes the same components and is general enough to allow flexibility in the teaching/learning or assessment process. For each competency statement, performance criteria can be written. Much like *enabling or sub-objectives,* performance criteria represent measurable evidence of competency. Performance criteria describe a single employee behavior that is measurable and observable, the condition(s) imposed on performance, and a performance standard. These criteria also serve as "teaching points" for educational activities that may accompany competency development or verification programs. Sound familiar? If you follow the rules of good objective writing and use the domains of learning to guide you, you can write performance criteria that facilitate objective evaluation of employee performance.

24. How can I use objectives to market a program?

24. Well-stated objectives can serve many purposes. To the consumer it is considered a contract. When you advertise programs, the objectives should define the focus of the program and a program plan that is consistent with the objectives must be presented to the target audience. Provide enough detail in the marketing brochures or flyers to allow the learners to decide if the program meets their needs. The objectives should describe the benefits and outcomes of the program and the level of learning expected. An important consideration is the concept of "truth in advertising." The objectives should be reflective of the program. If the program is intended for advanced beginners, then the content should be reflective of that level. Good program marketing will build credibility with potential attendees.

25. What are some common errors in objective writing?

25. The following are few of the most common errors in objective writing. You may recognize them as you read through the list.

- Objectives that describe a "false condition" for example: *"Given that the nurse has completed the skills performance checklist."* This does not describe what the learner will be provided, denied, or the environment in which performance is evaluated.

- Objectives that contain more than one outcome, performance, or behavior: The learner may attain one performance but not the other. For example if you change *"describes and develops a patient discharge plan"* to *"develops a comprehensive discharge plan,"* you can infer that cognitive knowledge is subsumed within the learner's performance; therefore, a verbal description is unnecessary.

- Objectives that focus on "what the instructor will do," instead of "what the learner will do." For example: *"The instructor will help the student recognize the natural consequences of behavior."* A better way to describe the outcome is *"the student will identify the natural consequences of behavior."*

- Objectives that indicate a false or non-measurable performance such as *"have a thorough understanding of blood glucose monitoring."* This could be improved by inserting an action verb that is observable and measurable such as *"perform blood glucose measurement on an actual patient."*

- Objectives that include "false standard or degree of attainment" such as *"must be able to make 80 percent on a multiple choice test."* This does not describe a learning outcome; it merely describes how the learner will be evaluated. You can convert this into a realistic standard such *as "learner performs [a specific action] with 80% accuracy."*

- Objectives that are too specific and actually specify the evaluation method. For example, *"Learner will select from a list of variables"*; this is better described as *"identify key variables."*

26. What other issues should I be aware of?

26. Other related issues or pitfalls to avoid:

- Listing objectives without corresponding content, often called orphan objectives

- Using objectives that reflect a level of learning that is inappropriate for the target audience

- Using test items that do not relate to the objectives

These problems can happen for a number of reasons. Often they occur inadvertently during revision of an established program, or when mixing and matching objectives and content from multiple programs, or developing content or test measures without using objectives as the blueprint or guide.

RESOURCES

Alspach, J. G. (1996). *Designing competency assessment programs: A handbook for nursing and health-related professions.* Pensacola, FL: National Nursing Staff Development Organization.

Dyche, J. (1988). *Educational program development for employees in health care agencies: A handbook for managers, supervisors, nurses* (2nd ed.). Murfreesboro, TN: Tri-Oak.

Ferguson, L. M. (1998). Writing learning objectives. *Journal of Nursing Staff Development, 14*(2), 87–94.

National Nursing Staff Development Organization. (1994). *Getting started in nursing staff development.* Pensacola, FL: Author.

Reilly, D., & Oermann, M. (1990). *Behavioral objectives: Evaluation in nursing* (3rd ed.). New York: National League for Nursing.

Table 1. *Examples of Behavioral Objectives*

COGNITIVE DOMAIN OF LEARNING	
Level of Domain	*Behavioral Objectives*
Knowledge	Define, List, State
Comprehension	Describe, Identify, Locate, Explain
Application	Demonstrate, Apply Schedule, Use
Analysis	Diagram, Categorize, Examine, Differentiate
Synthesis	Design, Organize, Propose, Summarize
Evaluation	Compare, Evaluate, Assess, Rate
AFFECTIVE DOMAIN OF LEARNING	
Level of Domain	*Behavioral Objectives*
Receiving	Recognize, Acknowledge, Accept
Responding	Comply With, Practice, Perform
Valuing	Examine, Prefer, Value
Organization	Formulate, Relate, Identify Characteristics
Characterization	Change, Revise Judgment, Develop, Influence
PSYCHOMOTOR DOMAIN OF LEARNING	
Level of Domain	*Behavioral Objectives*
Imitation	Follow Directions, Initiate
Manipulation	Follow Written Instructions
Precision	Perform (with a degree of skill)
Articulation	Perform With Limited Errors
Naturalization	Use Action as Needed, Perform Efficiently

Pollard, M., & Green, P. H. (1995). Domains of learning. In A. E. Avillion (Ed.), *Core Curriculum for Nursing Staff Development* (p. 31). Pensacola, FL: National Nursing Staff Development Organization. Reprinted with permission of NNSDO.

Table 2. *Matching Test Items to Objectives*

Behavior	Implications	Test Item Type	Additional Comments
List	Simple memorization, no discussion or judgment needed	Listing	Before making a list, determine if it is important
State, name, define	Learner is expected to provide an answer to a problem or statement, instead of selecting from choices	Completion	Allow for synonyms, unless it is critical to use a particular word
Describe, compare, contrast, explain	Learner is expected to organize material, decide what is important, then describe it without given choices to select from	Essay	Predetermine which answers receive full credit, partial credit, or none at all. Don't let writing style influence you unless writing style is a behavior you are testing
Solve, calculate, compute	Learner is expected to solve problems, usually mathematical in nature	Computation	State whether the formula is to be given, whether the learner must select the correct formula from several formulas. Also, state the degree of accuracy desired
Select, choose, identify, match	Learner is expected to answer a question, or complete a statement when given a list of possible answers	Matching, Multiple-choice	These items can be written at any level from very low to very high
Calibrate, adjust, construct, measure, demonstrate	Learner is expected to perform a task or demonstrate a skill which involves performance as well as knowledge	Performance	You need to have a well constructed checklist for evaluating performance. Be certain the test adheres to conditions and standards stated in the objective. Also, build in time for each learner to perform the task or demonstrate the skill

Chapter 17: *Planning*

1. *Why is planning so important? Couldn't I just stand up and teach what I know?*

1. Effective educational activities are based on learning needs for a specific target audience. Taking time to plan appropriate objectives, content, and teaching methods can ensure satisfaction and achievement of outcomes. If you teach what you know, you can easily miss the mark by being redundant or over the heads of the learners. Being an expert doesn't make you a teacher. Being a planner can help you teach nearly anything.

2. *What can happen if planning doesn't occur?*

2. I remember being part of a successful continuing education department and being directed to plan an available-for-purchase activity entitled "Staff Nurse by Choice, Not Chance." It was planned for a good day and location. No one registered. You see, this hospital had a wonderfully happy nursing department with lots of satisfied staff nurses. (This was a few years ago, but still a valid example.) No one registered because there was no identified learning need nor target audience. All activities should go through a full planning process and not just be purchased or scheduled.

3. *How many people do I need to get involved in the planning process?*

3. It depends on what you are planning. A ten-minute inservice class can be successful with just you and the product representative doing the planning, or someone on staff who can describe for you the necessary outcome. Planning a CPR class can be done alone once you are sure of learners' availability to attend and there are limitations to how you can modify the program.

A new activity or a conference is best planned with at least four people: you, as the education expert, the staff expert (CNS) since this person knows everything about the topic, the manager since this person thinks she knows what the staff need to know, and a staff nurse since he knows what he knows and doesn't know. With this group you can validate topics well. A five-day conference, however, may take a few more people so that each area is well represented.

4. *How long should the planning process take?*

4. The planning process can take anywhere from 5 minutes to 2 days depending on the effectiveness of the group and the complexity of the outcome. This does not include content preparation time. Yet it has been my experience that with a good facilitator the lengthiest activity can be planned in just hours.

5. What happens if the planners do not agree?

5. A skillful facilitator should be able to bring planners back to the foundation of good continuing education. Does it meet the learners' needs? Effective meeting techniques such as reclarifying goals or resuming at a later time may help. In any case, learning needs rule. When planners start to represent personal interests, they can be reminded of their role to represent a constituency.

6. What is an effective planning process?

6. An effective planning process is one in which the goal is reached in the allowed time frame. All the planners feel invested in the outcome and are prepared to sell it to others. Starting with a blank slate is effective; use nominal group process to prioritize brainstormed topics. Maintaining flexibility while matching time slots, faculty, and topics may be necessary. Allowing creativity to enter into thinking is helpful. Be clear if you are to address scope and objectives or get down to details of who is handling name tags.

7. How can I evaluate that good planning has occurred?

7. I use the **3D Approach**—

Distance: Will they come to the setting to hear the message?

Domain: Is it the right topic for the group to present credibly?

Dollars: Is it worth spending money (or time) to attend?

8. What should be the outcome of the planning process?

8. The outcome should be known before you begin planning. A reasonable outcome is that "All staff will be able to operate the new blood glucose monitoring device." Or it could be "Transplant coordinators will come together to share expertise and improve the care of transplant patients." As you finish the planning phase, check the product against the expected outcome. During activity evaluation, be sure to address achievement of the outcome.

9. How detailed should the planning become?

9. This depends on your support systems. You do not need to start writing the script while planning. However, you may want to be clear about when you'll meet to discuss onsite coordination or a dress rehearsal. Even content outlines for American Nurses Credentialing Center (ANCC) approved activities don't need every word planned out; this is why experienced faculty are used. Using a process, documenting on forms, and checking the timetable along the way can help avoid missing any details.

10. What about negotiating details of onsite coordination during the planning process?

11. How can I negotiate co-providership or other relationships effectively and fairly?

12. What about programs that are so simple that planning doesn't seem necessary?

13. When should I give up planning to the professional meeting planners?

14. What are some important points to consider when I'm planning a schedule?

10. Co-providership is like a marriage with shared responsibilities that can be performed by either partner. However, when following ANCC criteria, the ANCC provider of the activity must be responsible for:

- determination of objectives/content
- selection of presenters/content specialists
- awarding of contact hours
- record keeping
- evaluation

It is best when sharing responsibilities to avoid confusion and create an assigned list of tasks for each partner. Sometimes the negotiation of the assignment will be based on financial contributions; other times it may be based on intrinsic value of the relationship.

11. If using a financial model, then looking at contributions and profit sharing percentages may guide the division of duties. If one partner really needs the other (for promotional purposes), then the needy partner may be willing to do more. Signing the task list can avoid confusion or misunderstanding.

12. Some planning is necessary for all programs so that the learners' needs are met and the desired outcomes are achieved. Often managers think that education will solve the problem, when in fact it is a systems or enforcement issue. Planning will help avoid teaching those who already know how but can't or won't do it.

13. Professional planners are very good at traffic flow, catering, and entertainment. However, their expertise is not in educational objectives, as is yours. So until you are expert at room negotiation, travel arrangements, obtaining permission to use popular music, and other supporting activities, let the professional planners handle those aspects. The organization will need to be clear on the desired outcome: learning, the "wow effect," or both.

14. Adequate breaks for water, exercise, fresh air, and renewal should be included. We tend to think adults can sit longer than children, and while that may be true, it isn't sensible. Consider start and end times. Nurses are hard workers and are comfortable with 7:00 a.m. starts and 6:00 p.m. endings. Yet, this is too much information for one day. Offering shorter days or an afternoon off can make learning more effective and fun. Consideration should be given to competitive concurrent sessions, speaker availability, and a logical sequence of learning.

15. *If last year's program was successful, do I have to change anything to run it again this year?*

15. Not necessarily; however, sound planning principles suggest that learners' needs and objectives are reviewed. Regardless of ANCC's approval process, being sure that the activity is still appropriate is necessary for success. Looking at last year's participant feedback can provide valuable information. It is never wise to repeat an activity without evaluation. Following formulas can result in dwindling enrollment and an intangible dissatisfaction.

16. *What should I consider if I'm planning a course that will run multiple times in several locations?*

16. When planning an activity that will be delivered several times in many locations, setting up a sensible evaluation plan and modification schedule is needed. It is impractical to make radical revisions for each delivery, yet tweaking may be realistic and vital for success. Developing adequate reporting systems, periodic review, and logical record keeping will help. In planning, geography and population density are considered for locations, while life-styles of the participants are considered for scheduling dates.

17. *When should you abort the planning process?*

17. Stopping the planning process abruptly may be necessary when there is a significant change to organizational or financial structure. When there is a major shift in initiatives, hard decisions need to be made. Making the decision to cease planning may be financial: stopping before expenses are incurred. If there is a philosophical shift as in an ownership change, the activity being planned may no longer align with the organizational mission.

18. *What happens if what you planned isn't what is delivered?*

18. The brochure becomes a contract with the learner. Any correspondence with the faculty serves as a contract with the teacher. Although as the planner you have clearly communicated the same information to both the learners and the faculty, there occasionally is a discrepancy. More often this occurs with the faculty. When this has happened, I have discussed this with the faculty during a break. If no adjustment can be or is made, then I have reduced the payment to the faculty. Other responses include providing supplemental materials after the activity, giving learners a certificate to attend another activity, not rehiring the faculty, or planning a follow-up activity.

If the problem is with the learner, after attempts to clarify the information in the promotional materials, then if the organization can afford it, a refund may be offered to pacify the customer.

19. How does the planning team fit into the evaluation process?

19. If the evaluation plan incorporates the input of the planners, it would be important to get their feedback. The planners knew their intent and are in a good position to acknowledge if their intent was met. A quick meeting mid- and post-activity provides a good checkpoint. Submitting feedback is sufficient without necessarily attending an evaluation meeting. Ideally, the planners should be the evaluators but this may not always be practical.

20. What happens if you think the program has failed despite good planning?

20. Really look at what may have contributed to the failure. Was there a change in weather, public sentiment, or some disaster that contributed? No one can predict a hurricane's path, an explosion, or a recession. Being aware of current events may save you some needless blame or guilt.

21. What happens when you have planned a successful program?

21. A successful program deserves the same attention to contributing factors as a failure, so the same factors can be capitalized on in the future. Be sure to take a moment to relish your success and congratulate yourself on a job well done.

RESOURCES

American Nurses Credentialing Center. (2001). *Manual for accreditation as a provider of continuing nursing education*. Washington, DC: Author. **www.nursingworld.org/ancc**

Aucoin, J. (1998). *101 tips to better conferences*. Pensacola, FL: National Nursing Staff Development Organization.

Chapter 18: *Implementing*

1. What creative strategies do you suggest for increasing implementation effectiveness?

1. In order to increase effectiveness, make the distinction between "awareness," "training," and "education." What are you trying to achieve? Are you trying to convey information, develop specific skills, or develop knowledge and skills for transfer to other contexts? The education methodologies you select will be contingent on the desired outcome. Use the hottest topic around with dynamic speakers at a low cost; advertise ahead of time; get supervisory commitment.

Creative methodologies include the following:

- Convey information—wallet size cards with information in a concise, easy to read format.

- Specific skills—Have hands on toys and equipment available to work with.

- Development knowledge—Guided Note Taking—fill in the blank examples; scenario with solution to be written by attendee.

In marketing training, advertise that food will be served; use a gaming strategy with prizes; advertise on bulletin boards; use colorful handouts; and try e-mail as a reminder. Strategies have to be changed regularly or they become predictable.

2. How many times should I deliver the same activity?

2. This depends on a number of variables. The number of times you present depends on size of possible audience, shifts, services involved, room size, amount of interaction desired, outcomes, staff available, and financial support available. If training is mandated, then it should be delivered until all of the targeted audience has completed it. If not, the number of times should be driven by the need for the program and the data from the evaluations (e.g., do people feel comfortable with the material, is it received well). The key issue to remember is the "shelf-life" of the material being presented.

3. How should I manage breaks?

3. As a general rule, take a 10-minute break for every hour of presentation. Audiences get restless if you do not allow them to stretch or go to the restroom. In addition, it is difficult for audience members to intently focus on a presentation for an extended period of time. By planning systematic breaks, you enable the audience to

focus their attention on you. Here are some planning tips for breaks:

- Plan breaks at strategic points. While it is important to take a break every hour or so, don't stop midway through a key presentation point to take a break. Make sure you finish a point or topic and then take a break.

- Don't tell the audience how long a break is. Instead, give them a specific time to return. This avoids any speculation.

- Vary the lengths of breaks. Consider, for example, offering a 5-minute break after the first hour of a lengthy presentation. This allows the audience to get a drink of water and go to the restroom. Because the presentation has just begun, their "needs" should be minimal. Give them 15 minutes for the second break. This allows the audience to take care of more time-consuming items. When you allow the audience time to take care of their "outside" needs, they can be more attentive and focused when they return.

- Ask for their input. If you are unsure of the participants' needs, ask them how much time they will need. In coming to a consensus about the break, you establish a psychological agreement with them to return on time. It really does work!

4. *How do I manage disasters (natural and traumatic) during an activity?*

4. Humor! Humor! Humor! You will be able to create a calm and directive environment. Everybody understands disasters; be honest and up front and let people know what's happened. There are usually enough natural leaders in the audience to initiate immediate assistance; they know who to call, how to transport, and so on. Give the whole group a disaster break.

5. *What are the best ways to ensure you have an audience?*

5. The key to ensuring you have an audience is to follow the "P" factors (product, promotion, premium, presentation, and price). You can create a successful marketing campaign even for the less- than-desirable programs (e.g., mandatory topics) by using varied promotion techniques (e.g., posters, costumes, and pictures). Actually, I have found that when I am convinced that what I am teaching is important, I can usually convince my audience. Lots of planning and practice help as well. These two things will create a "culture" of trust. People come because they don't believe that I would waste their time.

6. *How do I create a learning environment for all participants?*

6. Let's face it; presenting is all about tailoring it to the audience. To create a winning presentation, you need to know how to tailor it for the audience—and then how to present it effectively. The first step is to decide on content. Basically, all presentations should follow this structure:

1. Attention-getting opener

2. Brief overview of the topic

3. Describe what the audience needs (i.e., the problem)

4. Explain how your solution meets that need

5. Tell how the audience can implement your solution —that is, action steps

6. Brief summary and conclusion

Of course, in order to describe what the audience needs, you need to research the audience. A cardinal rule of presenting is to find out as much as you can about the audience before you create the presentation. In a worst-case scenario when no information is available in advance, chat with participants as they enter the room to learn as much as you can—and adjust your presentation on the fly. In order to explain to participants how you can meet their needs, you have to know the topic thoroughly. Then, leave most of what you know about the topic out and include only the most important points. People can only comprehend and remember a few points in one sitting. By using this six-step process, you can ensure a logical flow that the audience can easily follow.

You're not finished yet! Now you need to add visual elements that pack a punch. Research has shown that high-quality visual aids add to the effectiveness and influence of the presentation. Visual impact contains three elements and they are all important: color, graphic images, and layout.

Participants have their own motivation for attending. Tell the participants what you would like them to learn at the beginning of the program and at the end save time to discuss what they did learn. Saving time for feedback serves a two-fold purpose: the instructor learns what points registered with the audience and the audience 'realizes' some learning actually took place.

7. How do I establish a friendly and informal atmosphere?

7. Follow these tips to set a friendly, informal atmosphere:

- Come early; stay late.

- Stand as people enter the room—greet them and shake hands. It's good to know people by name.

- Begin the class on time with a positive opening (a pep talk about the program and the day's events).

- Establish the expectation that learners will take major responsibility for meeting their learning needs.

- Review housekeeping details (e.g., location of rest rooms, coffee, breaks, smoking/nonsmoking).

- Encourage participants to refill their coffee any time.

- Do not sit or stand behind a table. Perch on the corner of the table or stand beside it.

- Make eye contact with participants throughout the room.

- Let participants know how you like to handle questions—at the end or as they come to mind.

- Give participants the freedom to make mistakes. You can model this by admitting your own errors as you go along.

- Acknowledge your nervousness—transfer the energy you spend on hiding your nervousness into managing your session more effectively.

- Be yourself. Be sincere in everything you do and say.

Finally, by knowing the material, believing it, and being totally consumed by it you will create a highly effective learning environment.

8. Should I maintain control of the program at all times?

8. Yes, someone has to guide and direct the program; generally, the speaker has the most control, but expectations should be met. Encourage timeliness; if the speaker is going to run over, ask the audience first.

9. What are the best methods of encouraging active participation by all of the participants?

9. By establishing relationships with them, sincerely talking with them, watching them carefully, learning from what they say, and acknowledging them in every possible way. People define participation in different ways. I consider participation active if attendees maintain eye contact with speaker, nod their heads, smile, and laugh. There are those who will speak up at any and all programs. They have a need to process out loud. Some listen, take notes, and process information in their heads. Some combine these activities. If participation is a goal, make it non-threatening, voluntary, brief, and fun.

10. How do I ensure that the participant leaves the program with new ideas/information?

10. The rule of thumb is: (1) Tell them what you're going to tell them, (2) Tell them, and (3) Tell them what you told them. And, while you're telling them, tell them over and over again. Certainly, you don't want to repeat the same thing over and over again. But you can make an important point and use several different illustrations to drive that point home.

Why do you have to be so repetitive? Simple . . . if you want the audience to remember the important points in your message, you have to make each point in 3–6 different ways. According to research, if you make a point only one time, at the end of your presentation, just 10% of the audience will remember it. If you repeat a point six times, retention jumps to 90%. Without repetition, 40% of your audience will forget virtually everything you said within 20 minutes of the conclusion. Within 24 hours, 70% of the audience will forget almost 100% of your message.

You can validate learning occurred at the close of the program informally or formally as part of the evaluation: "List at least one new idea/piece of information you have learned as a result of attending this program."

11. What can I do to ensure that the speakers have the energy needed for a successful program?

11. Be an example; enter the room with high energy, expectations, and accountability. I also validate that the speaker will be a good match for the target audience when I call and discuss the program. You can detect the commitment and energy speakers have for the topic. During your conversation, they ask the right questions. They have an effective track record. They submit paperwork in a timely manner. During the program, they provide enough breaks to keep attendees refreshed.

12. What do I do with a person who dominates the program?

12. Be kind. You can use the direct approach, and say "thank you for your comments; we need to move on, but we can discuss this further at the end of the program. Does anyone else have a comment on this topic?" Or if you are uncomfortable with the direct approach you can approach that person at break. If you don't, some of the other learners will be turned off.

13. How do I control disruptive/hostile audience?

13. As a presenter, you may find yourself facing a hostile questioner. Your skill at disarming verbal attacks will reflect on your credibility with the audience and the impression they have of both you and your presentation. The following approach works well to diffuse the hostile questioner:

- Let the person say whatever he/she wants to say. You just listen.

- Paraphrase what he/she has just said and acknowledge the feelings in the message without being condescending.

- Ask probing questions to try to find out the real issues.

- Say one of the following statements:

  "I know what the issues are, now let me respond."

  "Let's problem solve together to work this out."

  "Let's look into this after this presentation has concluded."

By using this approach you have indicated that you value the thoughts and feelings of the questioner. The audience will respect you, and you will diffuse the hostility at the same time.

When the presentation is over, and the questions have stopped, or time is up, it's time to conclude. Don't make the mistake of giving a simple "thank you" and leaving the podium. Return to the central theme, revert to your closing statement, or talk about next steps. The closing should not be lengthy, but it should wrap things up neatly.

14. How do you promote attendance when individuals do not perceive a learning need?

14. You can win over any audience by using these persuasive presentation tips:

- Narrow the focus. Practice the speech by reducing your goal to one sentence. It should summarize the single idea you want to plant in everyone's mind. Avoid overloading remarks with too many requests, proposals, or alternatives.

- Add humanness. Weave anecdotes and experiences into the talk. This helps listeners relate to your point and accept you as the messenger. The best stories make the audience see you as one of them, rather than as an aloof, canned speaker.

- Plant seeds. Use the introduction to present the theme of your speech in a creative way. *Examples:* Pose a brainteaser that you promise to solve by the end or reveal startling facts or statistics.

15. *How can I control the physical environment?*

15. Arrange for classes to be in the best physical environment possible. Scout the area ahead of time. Check the area ahead of time for noise factors (e.g., carts rolling down a hallway, construction). Many times these factors are out of your control. Just do your best; you cannot control everything. Be frank with the participants. If they know that you know and are trying to do something about an environmental problem, they will cooperate.

16. *What factors should I consider when implementing a program?*

16. In my experience, training implementation efforts fail for a number of reasons:

- no prior assessment

- scope of program too broad

- content not presented in a logical fashion

- time frame unrealistic

- education methodology inappropriate

- no participant feedback on exercises

- poor faculty selection

- too much time lapse between training and application

- training not evaluated

- no follow-up to determine impact of training

17. *Is program implementation different for classroom programs versus online programs?*

17. Yes! For classroom programs, all the physical factors and time factors must be considered; online programs are much more flexible. In preparing an online program it is very important to assess the computer skill experience of the audience. Provide very clear, really fool proof directions for use. It's good to have a help page for reference, and it's even better to show a tutorial of how to run the program and take the test. Have a credible and knowledgeable facilitator available.

Turning a well-written presentation into an online presentation takes effort. The key principle in slide preparation is that "less is usually more." The hardest shift for authors and designers to make in their transition to network delivery is the size of their projects. As instructors, we are accustomed to producing long sequenced courses. But in building online programs you need to build shorter and much more modular courses. These may be presented as a course of study, but the modules will have to stand on their own and be compatible with short bursts of learning.

18. When implementing an online PowerPoint program are there standards to follow?

18. Some Web delivery PowerPoint standards that I have found effective include:

- Animation—Don't get carried away with the animation or movement of text. Save the animation for making an important point, not on every slide. The same goes for slide transition; if you do use slide transition, use the same transition throughout the presentation.

- Content—Unlike when you do a presentation with PowerPoint, using the slides as bulleted bits of information, and filling in the rest with speech, a presentation for the Web has to stand alone. This means that when learners read through the presentation, they need to get all the information. When you complete the presentation have someone read through it, to see if it is missing any important information. When you create a presentation with information you know quite well, it is easy for your mind to fill in the information that is missing, but learners may not be able to do the same thing.

- Clip art—Clip art and pictures should be used to enhance the text, not take away from it. They should add to the message on the slide. Do not put a picture or clip art on every slide. If you need any additional clipart or pictures for your presentation, contact your local media support for assistance.

- Footer—The footer will include the date the presentation was completed, in the lower left corner, and the author or title in the lower right corner, in a 10-pt. font. These are added in the Slide Master view only. Do not add these to each slide individually.

- Goals & Objectives—Each training presentation should have a slide stating the goal of the course, and one stating the objective of the course. These should be the second and third slides of the presentation. There should be a minimum of one stated goal and three objectives.

- Slides—The presentation should be a maximum of 50–70 slides. If you are planning more than this number, check the presentation and see if it can be divided into a couple of presentation modules. The slide should not have more than three bullets. If you only have one statement on a slide you do not need a bullet. Save the bullets for slides with several points or statements.

- Slide Master—Use the slide master. If you are not familiar with this feature, contact instructional support staff for instructions on how to use it. You can make changes here that will affect the entire presentation. If you want to add a picture or background to all slides, add it on the slide master. It will appear on all the slides. Changing the font type or size of titles or text is also done on the slide master.

- Target Audience—To whom is the presentation aimed and how long you think the presentation and test will take to complete should be included.

- Type—The only type fonts that should be used are listed below. The problem with designing presentations in fonts other than these is that if they are not loaded on the PC the presentation is being viewed on, the PC will substitute a font that is close; this may change the look of presentation. These fonts are also easy to read. You should not use more than two type fonts or three font sizes on a page.

This is a test of this font. – (Arial)

This is a test of this font. – (Verdana)

This is a test of this font. – (Times New Roman)

This is a test of this font. – (Georgia)

This is a test of this font. – (Comic Sans)

The size of font should be as follows:

  Title —44 pt. font

  Text and first bullet—32 pt. font

  Subtext and additional bullets—28 pt. font

- Test—Test questions should be written to accurately reflect the goals and objectives of the course. All questions should be multiple choice, preferably with four possible answers. The test questions should be done in Word, not PowerPoint.

All wrong answers will have a brief explanation as to why the answer is wrong. Avoid using responses like "Wrong, try again." By providing feedback on the incorrect answer, the person will actually receive some additional information. This occurs through responses such as "This is not correct because . . ."

Try not to use true and false questions; this type of question tends to be too easy to guess and requires less thinking on the staff's part.

A 30-minute presentation should have a minimum of 10 questions, and a 60-minute presentation should have a minimum of 15.

19. What education tools work best for transferring information into a practice setting?

19. Use a variety of education tools if you want to transfer information to adults. For example, use videos, demonstration, and return demonstration on actual equipment to be used, practice sessions, volunteer subjects, posttests, videotape return demos, supervision in the clinical setting, and competency forms for evaluation and proof of mastery. Stimulate as many of the 'recording' senses as possible; ask a question to guide a discussion aimed at tracking the learning process. Modular learning helps present large amounts of information.

20. What is the role of preceptor in implementation?

20. The preceptor needs to be motivated to teach, guide, and encourage, as well as to be there to answer questions. The preceptor needs to be clear on the learning objectives. The preceptee needs a desire to learn. This is basic to an effective relationship. The preceptor functions as a role model, encourages, supervises, socializes, plans, evaluates, problem solves, makes decisions, sets priorities, delegates work, organizes work, communicates, uses psychomotor skills, uses reflective listening, uses open ended questions, verifies understanding, and works to cultivate the relationship.

21. What are the tricks of the trade in implementing a program within budget and time constraints?

21. Use facilities that are low cost; use cost-effective speakers; use your own staff when possible; plan ahead. Use good presenters who are—themselves— knowledgeable about the program . . . don't rely totally on technology. Then, presenters can do without technology if needed. Make an outline of what needs to be done; delegate if there is someone to delegate to; and advertise as early and often as possible by whatever means you have.

22. *What works best for transferring information into a practice setting?*

22. Learn the material well initially! The participant must see the meaning or purpose for that information to be able to interpret and transfer it to a practice setting. At best, an adult learning situation should be self-directed. If attendees can walk away with clear, concise, brief information that they can implement right away they will, particularly if they have the support and encouragement of management. The resources of preceptors, buddies, and mentors all facilitate the adult learning process.

23. *How do you maintain consistency and reliability of programs when multiple trainers are involved in the delivery of the same program?*

23. Observe and make sure that the correct objectives are taught. You will always have different approaches, different war stories. Make concise objectives and a program outline of what needs to be communicated; review the communication with the faculty at one time, if possible. Have a facilitator in the class to keep speakers on track. Have backups in the wings. Have self-learning modules as a final backup strategy. Evaluations will indicate problem areas or target a weakness in a program/setting for learning.

24. *What strategies are most effective to ensure that participants arrive on time?*

24. When you are dealing with adults, probably none. I try setting an example by being prompt in beginning each session. Build 15 minutes into the start for an introduction, so that you can start late and still meet your time goals; don't delay programs waiting for people to arrive. You do have the right to not admit people after a certain time frame. Also, contact hours should be withheld or modified based on time and attendance.

25. *How do I ensure that speakers end their presentation on time?*

25. Talk to them ahead of time; lay out expectations VERY CLEARLY. If this doesn't work, tell them that they have a shorter amount of time to speak than they really do. Have the facilitator do the "T" signal in the back 5 or 10 minutes before completion time. Have that plan set with the speaker. If the speaker is within a minute of ending time, do the "throat slash" routine. If the speaker still does not pay attention, interrupt. Your time and the time of the audience are valuable (e.g., they have family responsibilities, other commitments).

26. *A presentation is a presentation right? Does it matter whether you are speaking to 5 or 500 people?*

26. Size Does Matter! One of the most commonly overlooked details of giving a presentation is the size of the audience. It is true that the content of the presentation doesn't have to change because of the size of the audience, but the way it's communicated should be quite different!

	Small Group (up to 6)	Interactive Group (up to 12)	Structured Group (up to 25)	Big Room Groups (25+)
Focus	Audience centered	Content centered	Content/Speaker centered	Speaker centered
Visuals	Handwritten	Unlimited	Targeted	Limited
Visual Topics	Customer-Relevant	Content-Specific	Application	Simple

Small Group (Client Presentation, Work Groups)

When delivering to a group of this size, all efforts should be focused on the individuals in the audience. Presentation style, pace, visuals, and group interaction are dictated by the audience. Given the size of this intimate group, it is imperative that you manage the audience in a way in which you maintain direction and control of your presentation while allowing a high level of interaction.

Interactive Group (Training Class, Department Meetings)

With a growing audience, the level of involvement with the audience diminishes. While audience interaction is important, a high level of audience interaction is not possible. Instead, focus on communicating the content of the presentation as clearly as possible. Make sure visuals are clear, concise and help the audience better understand the content of the presentation.

Structured Group (Committee Meetings)

The key to the presentation in this group size is effectively communicating your message as a speaker with delivery and visuals. Speaking on a more formal level, credibility and delivery are the keys to a successful presentation. All visuals should be specifically targeted to the main message in the presentation.

Big Room Groups (Keynote Speakers, Luncheon Meetings)

With large audiences, people are there to hear you speak. While the content of the presentation is important, you are part of the reason why they are there. It is extremely important that your delivery be dynamic, simple-to-follow and credible. Visuals should be simple so that regardless of where participants are sitting they can see and understand the visuals.

27. Is room layout important?

27. Room layout affects all aspects of a presentation. Just the physical arrangement of chairs can create a feeling of intimacy and cooperation or authority and hierarchy. Select the layout that works best for you, depending upon audience size, presentation content, and visuals. Some common room layouts are:

1. Theater style—This layout is primarily used for large audiences. The larger the audience, the more aisles needed in the layout. Be sure that the audience can see you and the visuals from all areas of the room.

2. Classroom Style/U-shaped Style—If the audience needs to take notes or participate in group exercises, these layouts tend to be the most effective. Classroom style is used for larger audiences while the U-shaped style is preferred for more intimate training classes.

3. Meeting Style—The most popular room layout for small groups is meeting style. The layout allows the presenter to be as formal or informal as he/she wants. In addition, the presenter has a high degree of interaction with the audience.

Preview the room—You can avoid most pitfalls with room layout if you visit the venue in advance of your presentation. If possible, speak with the venue staff to make sure that the space is adequate and they can accommodate all of your presentation needs.

Be sure to plan for visuals—When planning the room layout, make sure you accommodate for visuals and visual equipment. Leave adequate room to maneuver around all equipment.

RESOURCES

Alspach, J. (1995). *The educational process in nursing staff development.* St. Louis: Mosby.

Fuszard, B. (1995). *Innovative teaching strategies in nursing.* Gaithersburg, MD: Aspen.

Siberman, M. (2001). *The 2001 training and performance source book.* New York: McGraw Hill.

Siberman, M. (1995). *101 ways to make training active.* San Francisco: Jossey-Bass.

Chapter 19: *Teaching Strategies*

1. *What do you do when people refuse to participate in class?*

1. There are two general approaches I take: one is to engage people through participation; the other is to encourage disagreement.

   - Incorporate a small group or partner activity.

   - Encourage people to think about how they would apply this content in their setting.

   - Ask participants to disagree with the content presented.

     "What would be difficult about using this in your department?"

     "There must be at least one person who is thinking that this won't work; what are the barriers?"

2. *How can I meet multiple learning style needs of a group?*

2. When you have a group of learners you will have multiple learning styles. The best way to address this is to use a variety of teaching strategies, incorporating right and left brain approaches, and methods that appeal to auditory, visual, and kinesthetic learners.

Left Brain Approaches	*Right Brain Approaches*
Content outlines	Games
Written procedures	Music
Statistics	Color
Details	Multi-sensory activities

© 2001, Training for *Impact*®. Milwaukee, WI. Reprinted with permission.

Auditory:

Learn through hearing. Use lecture, discussions, audiotapes, and debates.

Visual:

Learn through seeing. Use demonstrations, videos, reading assignments, crossword puzzles, and activities that involve drawing or coloring.

Kinesthetic:

Learn through direct involvement or activity. Use "hands

on" activities, return demonstrations, props that can be touched/handled, and skills practice.

3. How can I meet individual learning needs in a mixed group (novice to expert)?

3. This certainly is a challenge. If possible, have separate sessions for novice and advanced, and clearly title the programs so the staff can appropriately self select. If this is not possible, separate participants in the session and give the basic case studies to the novices and the complex case studies to the experts. A next step is to buddy a novice with an expert and have the expert act as a coach or mentor both during and after the session.

4. How can I perk up my overheads?

4.
- Use color, be sure that the text and background have good contrast

- Insert clip art

- Use unusual pointers—pointing finger pointer, stirring sticks, plastic arrows

- Use small objects on overhead (e.g., small blocks, string, cut out shapes)

5. How can I use creative teaching strategies without people thinking that it is silly?

5. Start with matter of fact, straightforward presentation of content, including data, charts, and graphs for the first 5–20 minutes of the presentation. Then move to more interactive methods. A good technique for bridging to a more interactive method is to state, "The true test of content is its application to real problems. Therefore, let's apply this information to a realistic situation." You can then move to discussion or case study.

6. What's a good icebreaker for people who hate icebreakers?

6. I have two suggestions. One is in the approach you use. Give people the option to not participate in the icebreaker. If you can use humor with the group, you can say, "Now of course no one is going to *make* you do this, but the rest of us are going to have a fun-filled two minutes and I would not want you to miss out."

Second, here's a specific icebreaker that works well with a resistant group. Ask them to find one person in the group that they do not know. Introduce themselves, and state one objective they have for this session. Keep this to 3–5 minutes. When you bring them back together as a large group ask for 5–6 people to share their objective for the session and write these on a flip chart or overhead. The entire activity should take 10 minutes. At the close of the session you can ask the group to review, and check if these objectives were met.

7. How can I create new approaches for content when there is no time for development?

7.
- Network—"borrow" ideas from colleagues
- Take note of approaches you see others use
- Keep an ongoing file of ideas you like "For Future Use"
- Use the Internet to access ideas and to network with others
- Use published ideas, there are lots of books available with training activities
- Have participants develop posters or overheads. At the end of a session ask participants to develop an overhead or poster of key elements from the content. Then save and "recycle" these for future sessions.

8. How can I get money for teaching materials when money is tight?

8. The recommended strategy is the cost per learner analysis. First review several products and prices. Then calculate the cost per learner of the product(s) you would like to purchase. For example, a $500.00 video that 1000 employees would see as part of a safety training program would be 50¢ per learner. Present this information when requesting the dollars. If there has been an urgent learning need identified, clearly articulate how this product will help meet the learning need in a cost effective manner.

9. How can I spruce up the room I use for teaching?

9. Small touches can do a lot in setting a comfortable and informal atmosphere. Try:
- Plants
- Cut flowers (perhaps from your own garden)
- Posters—both educational and inspirational posters
- Flip chart sheets with fun quotes
- Balloons
- Upbeat music playing when participants arrive and during breaks

10. How can I get other people involved as learning resources instead of it always having to be me?

10. Solicit assistance from others—especially those who have identified the learning need (e.g., managers).
- "Who would be a good resource on this topic?"
- "Can you select a staff person to plan this program? I can be a resource to him/her and assist in coordinating the program."
- "Who is an internal expert in this area?"

11. What else can I do with a video—instead of just showing it?

11. Find ways for participants to interact with the video.

- "As you watch the video, identify four key concepts."

- "After watching the video, you will be asked to share three critical elements with a partner."

- Provide a worksheet with questions for them to answer as they watch the video.

- Ask them to find an error in the video if there is one.

- Inform them that they will be asked to give a demonstration of the equipment featured in the video.

12. How can I get people involved in more complex application, not just simple case studies?

12. Develop or recruit others to develop more complex case studies. Ask them to think of some of their toughest situations. Capture the ideas they identify and write them into formal case studies.

Of course maintain confidentiality but create case studies based on information in incident reports or performance improvement audits.

13. How can I use multiple audiovisuals without having the equipment become a hassle?

13. Be familiar with the equipment *before* the session. If you are comfortable with the equipment it will show. Check the functioning of equipment (focus and volume) and adjust immediately before the session. If equipment needs to be moved (e.g., moving an overhead projector before showing a video), ask a participant to help move it. You can also ask a participant to turn down lights. Avoid having the equipment become the focus of attention, and avoid bouncing back from one piece to another piece.

Have a back up plan if equipment fails. Humor can help. If you need to make small adjustments with the equipment you might have a line you use like, "Just talk among yourselves for a moment . . ."

14. What do I do if I don't know the answer to a participant's question?

14. Acknowledge that you do not know the answer. Ask other participants for their ideas and suggestions. Tell the person you will check and get back with the answer . . . and be sure to follow up.

15. What is your favorite teaching strategy?

15. Although I aim for variety, if I picked one favorite it would be games. Homemade bingo, board games, and trivia games bring out the fun in most people. Games are a great way to review content and energize the group. Candy or small prizes are appreciated too!

16. Why could your favorite teaching strategy be the least effective?

16. Any teaching strategy that is overused and excludes other methods will be ineffective. To meet a variety of learning needs, a variety of teaching methods should be used.

17. Which teaching strategy is the most expensive?

17. The strategy that is *the least effective is the most expensive.* If learning outcomes are not met, time and resources are wasted. If learning outcomes are repeatedly not met, the credibility of the educator may come into question. It is important to track and articulate the impact of meeting defined learning outcomes.

18. How can I learn new teaching methods?

18.
- Network
- Watch others—get ideas of new approaches from what works, get ideas of how to modify what does not work
- Professional journals—*JNSD* (*Journal for Nurses in Staff Development*), *Training*, *The Training & Development Journal*
- Resources on creative teaching and accelerated learning

19. How should teaching methods match my objectives?

19. Learning methods and learning objectives should be congruent. First, determine the learning domain of the objective (cognitive, psychomotor, or affective). The teaching methods should correlate. For example, if the learning outcome is competence in using a piece of equipment (psychomotor domain), teaching methods may include demonstration and return demonstration of the equipment.

20. What's wrong with good old lecture?

20. Nothing is inherently wrong with lecture. Lecture is a good method for covering a lot of content in a limited amount of time. However, use of lecture without other methods will not meet the learning styles of many learners, and, therefore, will not meet the learning outcomes. Short lectures combined with discussion, case studies, or skills practice will be more effective than lecture alone.

21. With all this Internet education, do I need to teach at all?

21. The short answer is yes. The longer answer is that other methods can be used in conjunction with the Internet. Classroom, workshop, or grand rounds sessions can enhance the content people receive on the Internet. The resources on the Internet may be great, but the application to your setting must be addressed. Coaching, mentoring, brainstorming, and problem solving in a facilitated approach can enhance achievement of learning outcomes.

RESOURCES

Lowenstein, A., & Bradshaw, M. (2001). *Fuszard's innovative teaching strategies in nursing.* Rockville, MD: Aspen.

Rose, C., & Nicholl, M. L. (1997). *Accelerated learning for the 21st century.* New York: Dell.

Russell, L. (1999). *The accelerated learning field book.* San Francisco: Jossey-Bass.

Chapter 20: *Evaluating*

1. Why do I need to evaluate educational activities?

1. Educational activities are evaluated to:
   - Determine if participants' needs were met
   - Provide speakers with feedback relative to their presentations
   - Provide a basis for maintaining and revising educational activities
   - Provide a basis for planning and providing new educational activities
   - Validate effectiveness and quality

2. Why do I need to evaluate the overall educational program?

2. The overall program is evaluated in order to:
   - Check alignment with organizational goals and mission.
   - Examine intended outcomes versus achieved outcomes
   - Analyze performance as a productive department.
   - Set direction for the next year.

3. Who should be involved in developing evaluation plans for educational activities?

3. At minimum, I try to involve the following individuals in developing evaluation plans:
   - Speakers/faculty (because they are involved in writing objectives and are evaluated on their presentations)
   - Planning committee members/staff development personnel (at least one of these individuals is generally a content expert; one is also knowledgeable about accreditation criteria/process if the activity is awarding continuing education credit)
   - Individual representing the target audience
   - Representative from co-sponsoring agency (if applicable)
   - Audiovisual media personnel

4. How can I ensure that participants complete educational activity evaluations?

4. At the start of the activity, I talk to the participants and stress the importance of completing the evaluation tool. I tell them their input is used to improve and/or plan future activities and try to give them specific examples of how information from past evaluations has been used in this way. I also tell them that their signed attendance certifications will be given to them when they turn in a completed evaluation tool at the end of the activity.

5. What is the role of the participant feedback tool in evaluation?

5. I use participant feedback (1) to evaluate a specific educational activity in terms of the

- degree to which activity objectives were or were not met

- degree to which the learner's personal objective(s) was met

- degree to which activity objectives related to activity content

- contextual considerations such as physical facility, audiovisual aids, handouts; speakers' effectiveness, teaching/learning strategies, cost

and (2) to plan and improve future activities by requesting

- suggestions for future topics

- preferred days/time of programs

- open-ended comments

- suggestions for improvement

- suggestions for speakers

6. What types of evaluation strategies other than questionnaires can I use?

6. The type of evaluation tool I use depends upon the objectives of the activity. If I want to measure knowledge, for example, I use a pre-test/posttest, essay test, role-play, case study analysis, or pre/post audit as an evaluation tool. If I want to evaluate psychomotor skills, observation, return demonstrations, skill demonstration stations, and interactive simulators are appropriate. A final test of transfer of learning is implementation into practice.

7. What constitutes an effective evaluation plan?

7. I consider an effective evaluation plan to be one that evaluates all elements of an educational activity from process to content to outcome to follow-up. When evaluating an activity, I try to answer questions such as

- To what degree were the objectives of the activity accomplished?

- To what degree were the participants' personal objectives met?

- Were the participants satisfied with the contextual elements of the program?

- Did the activity produce the desired outcome?

- Is information gleaned from educational activity evaluation used to improve future programs?

- If continuing education credit was awarded, were accreditation criteria met?

- Was the activity cost effective?

- Did the organization achieve the intended outcome?

8. What type of evidence can document that evaluation data have been used to increase the effectiveness of future educational activities?

8. I like to summarize evaluation data and compare the data to established criteria (outcomes) as well as to previous evaluation data. The use of tables, graphs, and bar graphs are effective as visual representations of written material. A table similar to the following is also a good way to depict the way in which evaluation data are used to revise or improve effectiveness.

Source of Data	Problem Identified	Action(s) Taken	Outcome

9. How does the evaluation of educational activities provided via distance learning differ from evaluation of education activities provided "on site"?

9. Educational activities provided via distance learning technologies require additional evaluation data. Additional data needs to be gathered on the

- quality of the video/audio

- degree of interaction/rapport with the speaker(s) and other participants

- degree to which the methodology enhanced or detracted from the program

- effectiveness of the site facilitator

- comparison of the experience to a live, onsite presentation

- likelihood of participating in another activity via distance technology

10. What type of information should be included when I evaluate an educational activity?

10. I examine the outcomes of the educational activity as well as the context in which the educational activity occurred. Under outcomes, I evaluate the degree to which the activity objectives were met, the degree to which the participants' personal objectives were met, and the degree to which the objectives were consistent with the content. When evaluating the context in which the activity occurred, I evaluate the speaker (i.e., knowledge, delivery, audiovisual aids, handouts, teaching/learning methodologies), the physical facility (e.g., comfort, parking, accessibility), and registration fees. In addition, I ask open-ended questions about the participants' preferred days and times for program, suggestions for improving the program if it were repeated, and topics and speakers for future programs.

11. Should both quantitative and qualitative data be included in evaluation?

11. Yes. Using both types of data will give you a more complete evaluation picture because you get subjective as well as objective data. I generally want information that cannot be obtained through the compilation of only one type of data.

12. What are some specific example of quantitative and qualitative data?

12. Examples of quantitative data include data obtained from a:

- Likert-type scale to measure the degree to which objectives were met

- Forced-choice option to evaluate the cost of a program

- Question about the preferred days/times for a program

Examples of qualitative data include data obtained from the:

- Open comments section—read these carefully to discern meaning

- Suggestions for improving the program

- Compilation of comments about the comparison of experiencing a program live, onsite as opposed to experiencing the program via distance technology

13. Can I use the same evaluation tool for all educational activities?

13. You can use a template to devise a similar evaluation tool for all educational activities. First *decide* what you want to evaluate for *every* activity; develop a template; and then add specifics for each activity. For example, you know you will always evaluate every activity's objectives and speaker(s), so you will individualize the template by including the specific objectives and names of the speakers for a specific activity. A template will also enable you to add additional evaluation areas that may apply only to a specific activity.

14. *What type of evaluation tools other than questionnaires can I use?*

14. The type of tool you choose depends upon what you want to evaluate (for example, do you want to evaluate knowledge acquisition? an attitude? a change in behavior? a psychomotor skill? a combination of any of these?). Other types of evaluation tools that can be used include:

- pretest, posttest tools (knowledge)

- return demonstrations (knowledge and psychomotor skill)

- open-ended questions (knowledge; attitude)

- audit pre and post program (knowledge; change in behavior)

- observation; peer evaluation (knowledge, change in behavior, psychomotor skill)

15. *How much time should I allow for participant evaluation?*

15. In part, this depends upon the type and length of educational activity provided as well as the type of evaluation tool you are using. A one or two page questionnaire with forced choice or Likert-type scale for a one-day program can probably be completed in 10–15 minutes. On the other hand, you can expect that a long evaluation tool that uses open ended questions or a lengthy posttest can require up to 30–45 minutes to complete. Nevertheless, time needs to be allotted so that evaluation has demonstrated importance.

16. *How do I analyze and interpret data?*

16. Analysis of data depends, in part, upon the type of data you have collected—is it quantitative or qualitative data? If you are analyzing quantitative data, you can measure your results against a predetermined standard or criterion. For example, let's say you use a Likert scale from 1–5 (with 1 being "poor" and 5 being "excellent") to evaluate the degree to which each educational objective was met. You might have set a predetermined standard that each objective would receive an average rating of 3.75 or higher; you would then compare each objective's average with the pre-set standard.

If you are analyzing qualitative data, look for trends, patterns, and similarities in comments. You might also give examples of specific comments such as, "Overheads were too small to be seen from the back of the room" or "Too many slides for such a short presentation." However, counting the comments is not necessary.

Interpret the data by drawing a conclusion based on that data. Was the predetermined standard met? Are you satisfied with the patterns or trends identified in the qualitative data? Based on the answers to these questions, you can decide what actions, if any, need to be taken for improvement.

17. When should the evaluation plan for an educational activity be implemented?

17. The evaluation plan for an activity should begin with the first planning meeting for that activity. At that point, you can begin to formulate specific areas to be evaluated and can make sure that the planning process is evaluated and that all areas required for accreditation purposes (if applicable) can be included in the plan.

18. Who is accountable for performing evaluation of educational activities?

18. The answer to this question depends, in part, upon the organizational structure. Although the planning committee for each education activity is generally responsible for performing evaluations, the Chair of the activity planning committee, or the Nurse Planner for an American Nurses Credentialing Center (ANCC) provider unit, or the Director of the Staff Development or Continuing Education Department is ultimately accountable for activity evaluation.

19. To whom should evaluation results be reported?

19. Again, this depends upon the organizational structure. Results should certainly be reported to your immediate supervisor and administrator, to planning committee members, to other members of an education department, to any co-sponsoring agencies, and to the speaker(s) involved in an activity. In addition, evaluation data may need to be shared with accrediting bodies via required reports or self-studies. Results may be used as part of performance based funding decisions.

20. Who is responsible for taking action to improve results?

20. Again, this depends, in part, upon the organizational structure. Although the Director of a Staff Development Department or the Nurse Planner of an ANCC-approved provider unit is responsible, all members of the department and/or activity planning committee should take part in reviewing evaluation data and in making recommendations based on that data.

21. Is there a time that evaluation isn't necessary?

21. Every activity deserves some attention to evaluation so that you can make decisions about continuing this type of activity or re-inviting this particular speaker. It's the degree of evaluation that varies, not whether you do it or not.

RESOURCES

Abruzzese, R. (1996). *Nursing staff development: Strategies for success* (2nd ed.). St. Louis: Mosby.

International Association of Continuing Education and Training. (1991). *A practical handbook for assessing learning outcomes in continuing education and training.* Washington, DC: Author.

Kelly Thomas, K. J. (1998). *Clinical and nursing staff development: Current competence, future focus* (2nd ed.). Philadelphia: Lippincott.

Quinn, R., & Humphreys, J. (Eds.). (1998). *Continuing professional development in nursing: A guide for practitioners and educators.* Philadelphia: Trans-Atlantic Publications.

Section 5:

Accreditation/Approval of Staff Development and Continuing Education Activities

Based on the setting, you may be familiar with the Joint Commission on Accreditation of Healthcare Organizations, the accreditation agency for healthcare organizations, and the National League for Nursing Accrediting Commission or the Commission on Collegiate Nursing Education, the accrediting bodies for schools of nursing. This voluntary process for recognition of meeting a standard is available for non-academic nursing education as well. These standards are modified periodically and are intended to guide development of activities in a systematic manner that enables quality improvement. Using the American Nurses Credentialing Center accreditation process is optional and frequently is a specialized function within larger education departments. Regardless of job responsibilities, knowledge of accreditation processes is a helpful adjunct to program planning and a component tested on the Nursing Professional Development certification exam.

21. Accreditation/Approval Criteria
Pamela S. Dickerson, PhD, RN,C

22. Continuing Education Provider Unit
RoAnne Dahlen-Hartfield, DNSc, RN

23. Continuing Education Approver Unit
Marlette Buckner, MN, RN,C

Chapter 21: *Accreditation/Approval Criteria*

1. What is accreditation?

1. Accreditation is recognition of an organization's ability to provide or approve continuing nursing education over an extended period of time. Accreditation is a voluntary process involving an in-depth analysis through self study and a site visit by appraisers representing the American Nurses Credentialing Center's Commission on Accreditation (ANCC COA). This organization, a subsidiary of the American Nurses Association, is responsible for the development and implementation of the ANCC system for accrediting providers and approvers of continuing nursing education.

Accreditation criteria and operational requirements for providers and approvers are based on the American Nurses Association publication, *Scope and Standards for Nursing Professional Development*. Manuals for providers and approvers were recently revised in 2001.

2. What is the difference between accreditation and approval?

2. *Accreditation*, as noted above, is the recognition of an organization's ability to provide or approve continuing nursing education. Within the accreditation system, there is a mechanism for accredited approvers to grant *approval* to continuing nursing education activities and/ or providers when these applicants verify that they are able to uphold the criteria and operational requirements specified by the accredited approver in providing continuing education activities. Accreditation is for a six-year period; approval is for three years.

3. What's the difference between an accredited approver and an accredited provider?

3. The accredited *approver* is granted authority by the ANCC COA to approve continuing nursing education events and/or providers if they demonstrate that they can provide quality continuing education. The accredited *provider* is authorized by ANCC COA to provide continuing nursing education events within its own system and with the direct involvement of the provider unit's nurse planner(s). Although often requested, the provider is not authorized to approve another organization's activities or activities developed within its own organization.

4. What is the difference between approval as a provider and approval of an educational activity?

4. An organization that offers numerous continuing education activities can apply to an accredited approver for approval as a provider of continuing nursing education. The applicant must submit evidence indicating that the organization has a track record of planning and

implementing approved activities and has a process in place to operate an approved provider unit according to ANCC COA criteria and operating requirements.

An organization desiring to offer a continuing education activity for which contact hours will be awarded can apply to an accredited approver for approval to grant continuing education contact hours. The application process includes verification that all criteria and operating requirements will be followed for the planned continuing nursing education activity.

5. What are the advantages of accreditation?

5. Accreditation validates to the organization and to its consumers that the organization has met rigorous criteria demonstrating evidence of its ability to provide quality continuing nursing education over time. Accreditation status in some organizations is helpful in obtaining funding and resources. Accreditation is a powerful marketing tool, because it helps potential learners to recognize providers that have proven track records in continuing education. Also, nurses who are certified by the American Nurses Credentialing Center's Commission on Certification are required to earn 50% of their contact hours for recertification from one of several types of organizations. One of these is an organization operating under the ANCC accreditation system.

6. Where do I get information about accreditation?

6. You can call the American Nurses Credentialing Center's Commission on Accreditation at 1(800)–284–2378, extension 7263, or visit the American Nurses Association Web site at **www.nursingworld.org/ancc** and click on "accreditation."

7. How do I know if my organization is eligible to apply for accreditation?

7. Eligibility criteria are specified in the ANCC COA accreditation manuals for both approvers and providers. Accreditation manuals can be ordered from the accreditation office at the phone number listed above. Three types of organizations are eligible to apply for accreditation as approvers: constituent member associations of ANA, specialty nursing organizations, and federal nursing services. Any organization may apply for accreditation as a provider as long as it meets criteria specified in the ANCC COA Provider Manual. Applicants for accreditation as either approvers or providers must have established approver and/or provider units and be able to demonstrate through self-

study and a site visit that processes are in place to carry out all of the responsibilities of an accredited unit.

8. Why is the process so rigorous?

8. The application process for accreditation involves both a self-study and a site visit. The process is designed to demonstrate that the organization seeking accreditation has the administrative support, operational structure, and resources to carry out accreditation activities during a six-year period of accreditation. An evaluation component provides evidence that the organization is continually reviewing and revising its operations in order to enhance its work and provide outcomes consistent with its goals and the accreditation criteria. These responsibilities are taken very seriously by accredited organizations. The rigor of the process protects both accredited organizations and nurses who participate in learning activities offered through these organizations.

9. How are decisions made about accreditation?

9. The nine-member ANCC Commission on Accreditation makes decisions about accreditation. Decisions are based on the self-study submitted by the applicant as well as a site visit report submitted by the appraisers who visit the organization.

10. How long does it take to get accreditation?

10. In order to be eligible to apply for accreditation as an approver or provider of continuing nursing education, an organization must have an established approver or provider unit and must have been operational for a minimum of six months. The organization completes a self-study, which typically takes from several weeks to several months. Applications are accepted by ANCC COA twice a year, in February and in August. The self-study is submitted as part of the application package. February applications are completed by the following August; August applications are completed by the following February. The actual time required to obtain accreditation varies with each organization. However, for the organization applying for accreditation for the first time, the process would take a minimum of one year (six months of operation to establish eligibility and write the self-study, and six months for the actual application review process).

11. My organization is interested in seeking accreditation. What steps are involved in the process?

11. First, contact ANCC COA at 1(800) 284–2378, ext. 7263, or visit the ANA Web site at **www.nursingworld.org/ancc** and click on "accreditation." Obtain information about eligibility criteria and the accreditation process. Then, in sequence:

a. Review operations of your organization to determine whether it meets the eligibility criteria, including operation for a minimum of six months using the ANCC COA criteria and operational requirements.

b. If it does, review and initiate processes for the self study.

c. If it does not, take steps to move the organization toward eligibility, then proceed.

d. While finalizing the self-study, notify ANCC COA of your intent to apply for accreditation in the next cycle (February or August)—the "intent to apply" form can be downloaded from the ANCC Web site (**www.nursingworld.org/ancc**).

e. Submit the self-study by February 1 or August 1. At this time, you will be asked to select several possible dates for a site visit.

f. Approve the site visit date and team based on information provided to you by the accreditation staff.

g. Participate in the site visit process.

h. Wait for word from ANCC COA after its spring or fall meeting!

12. What goes on during a site visit?

12. Before the site visit, you will receive a phone call or e-mail from the appraisal team leader. This person will review the site visit process with you, discuss a proposed agenda, and answer any questions you may have. You have the opportunity to communicate with the team leader before the site visit if additional questions arise. If you are applying for accreditation as a provider or an approver, the site visit will be one day in length. If you are applying for accreditation as both an approver and provider, the site visit will be two days in length.

The two appraisers (team leader and team member) who will be conducting the site visit will arrive in your community the day before the visit. That evening, they will meet together to review the self-study and finalize their plans for the conduct of the visit.

The purpose of the site visit is to verify, clarify, and amplify information in the self-study. The site visit gives the appraisers the opportunity to visualize resources, records, and other materials vital to operation of the approver or provider unit; to speak personally with those involved in the functions of the unit; and to clarify issues regarding the accreditation criteria and operational requirements.

A typical visit involves a brief tour of the facility, discussion with the leadership of the organization, thorough review of the processes by which the approver or provider unit operates, and interviews with personnel involved with the unit. These interviews typically include staff, volunteers, faculty, and consumers. Others may be involved at the discretion of the site visit team and the applicant organization.

The visit includes time for the appraisers to review records of previous approver or provider unit activities to determine adherence to record-keeping requirements. Appraisers also hold one or more executive sessions throughout the day to discuss their findings.

At the conclusion of the site visit, an oral report is given to representatives of the applicant organization. Appraisers then send a written report to the ANCC staff for use by the ANCC COA in making an accreditation decision.

13. When will I have the results of the application?

13. After a site visit, the Commission on Accreditation receives information from the appraisers and then acts to make an accreditation decision. For those who applied on February 1, the decision is made by the time of the August COA meeting. For those who applied on August 1, the decision is made by the time of the February COA meeting. Results are communicated to the applicant organization by ANCC COA staff by mail.

14. Once the organization is accredited, what are my responsibilities?

14. Once an organization has achieved accreditation as an approver or provider of continuing nursing education, the organization must continue to adhere to all ANCC COA criteria and operational requirements throughout the period of accreditation. Should there be changes to accreditation criteria, the corresponding changes must be made in the accredited organization's operations according to the timeline specified by ANCC COA. Accredited organizations receive periodic newsletters informing them of relevant information about accreditation and the activities of the COA.

There are two specific requirements of accredited

organizations. First, annual reports and fees must be submitted as required by COA. Information about the content of these reports is provided to accredited organizations. Second, if there is a change in organizational structure or key personnel or if there is a decision to terminate accreditation activities, this information must be forwarded to the ANCC COA office within 30 days.

15. I've developed a learning activity and I'd like to provide contact hours. What do I do next?

15. Contact the appropriate accredited approver for an application for activity approval. Accredited approvers are constituent member associations of ANA, specialty nursing organizations, and the federal nursing services. A list of accredited approvers can be found on the Web site (**www.nursingworld.org/ancc**). Some accredited approvers may have limited approval authority. For example, federal nursing service approvers can only approve activities within their own organizations.

If you are working in an organization that holds accreditation as a provider, contact the designated nurse planner for the provider unit BEFORE you develop the learning activity. Accreditation criteria require that a designated provider unit nurse planner be involved in the planning of the learning activity.

If you are working in an organization that holds accreditation as an approver but not as a provider, your organization cannot develop and present its own activities and award contact hours for them. You must submit the activity to another appropriate approver for review.

16. I've just been hired as a nurse planner for our accredited provider unit. What do I do now?

16. First, find and read the current accreditation manual, which should be available in your organization. Second, find and read the most recent self-study submitted to ANCC COA by the organization, as well as any feedback received from the Commission at the time accreditation was granted. Review any progress reports, annual reports, or other documents submitted to the Commission subsequent to the most recent accreditation. If possible, talk with the person who held the position before you to learn any tips or suggestions regarding implementation of criteria and operational requirements within the organization. Talk with members of planning committee(s), faculty, and learners to get a sense of the scope of the provider unit's activities and the perception of its strengths and needs. If you have questions about implementation of the criteria and operational requirements, call ANCC COA staff for guidance [1(800) 284–2378, ext. 7263]. Please remember to notify staff within 30 days that you are the new nurse planner for the provider unit, and send a copy of your biographical data showing that you meet the criteria for this position (i.e., graduate degree in nursing or related specialty; if the graduate degree is in a related discipline, the baccalaureate must be in nursing).

17. Are there other resources available for continuing education approval besides the ANCC System?

17. The National League for Nursing (NLN) is approved as a continuing education provider by the International Association for Continuing Education and Training (IACET). NLN has a mechanism in place for approval of continuing education programs. Contact the National League for Nursing at (212) 363–5555, ext. 266, or visit its Web site at **www.nln.org** and click on "continuing education."

IACET has a mechanism for applicants to become providers of the CEU. This involves a self-study and a site visit as well. The American Association of Critical-Care Nurses Certification Corporation (AACN) has a mechanism for application for continuing education credits for critical care activities. Although this is patterned off the ANCC guidelines, it appears that this is a stand-alone venture.

The choice of which organization to affiliate with will depend on the organization's mission and goals.

RESOURCES

American Nurses Association. (2000). *Scope and standards of practice for nursing professional development.* Washington, DC: American Nurses Publishing.

American Nurses Credentialing Center's Commission on Accreditation. (2001). *Manual for accreditation as an approver of continuing nursing education.* Washington, DC: American Nurses Credentialing Center.

American Nurses Credentialing Center's Commission on Accreditation. (2001). *Manual for accreditation as a provider of continuing nursing education.* Washington, DC: American Nurses Credentialing Center.

www.nursingworld.org/ancc

www.nln.org

www.iacet.org

www.nflpn.org

www.aacn.org

Chapter 22: *Continuing Education Provider Unit*

1. What is the relationship between the American Nurses Association (ANA) and the American Nurses Credentialing Center (ANCC)?

1. The American Nurses Association, the national professional association of registered nurses, throughout its history has been concerned about the professional growth of the registered nurses. Historically, the authority for accreditation of continuing education by the American Nurses Credentialing Center (ANCC) derives from the formal action of the 1974 ANA House of Delegates. That year, ANA established a system for accreditation and approval of continuing education in nursing. The system continues today as a voluntary peer review recognition system. Over the years, the structure of the accreditation system evolved.

In 1991, ANA's Center for Credentialing Services became the ANCC, a separately incorporated subsidiary, and the Board of Accreditation became the Commission on Accreditation (COA), which continues to be the accrediting body today. ANA's standards continue to guide ANCC COA and its program (ANA, 2000).

2. As of 2001, how many Constituent Member Associations (CMAs), organizations, and other associations are accredited as providers of continuing nursing education by ANCC COA?

2. As of December 2001, there are currently 27 CMAs and 200 other organizations and associations accredited by ANCC COA as providers of continuing education in nursing.

3. What is an example of a Provider Unit's current mission and focus?

3. The ANA Provider Unit believes it is responsible for assisting and supporting professional nurses as they pursue different opportunities for lifelong learning directed toward maintaining and increasing competence within their own areas of nursing practice. Continuing professional nursing competence is essential to the provision of safe quality health care to all members of society. The staff of the Provider Unit incorporate the roles of educator, facilitator, change agent, consultant, leader, and researcher as it creates all of the learning activities that provide direct support to professional nurses throughout their careers and to the profession of nursing.

4. What are some of the strategies for managing record keeping for the Provider Unit?

4. With limited staff and resources, the job of managing record keeping, according to ANCC COA's guidelines, for an increased number and types of programs on the CE schedule/calendar is one of the most challenging responsibilities for the Provider Unit. Each Provider Unit must decide where record keeping fits in its priorities for planning, implementing, and evaluating each CE activity and its other responsibilities related to supporting the mission, goals, and core issues of the association.

Most Provider Units develop a file folder maintenance checklist that lists the information required by ANCC COA. This checklist is stapled on the file folder for each CE activity. On a quarterly basis, the file folders for all completed CE activities are assessed, the attempt is made to locate and produce missing information, and the file folder maintenance checklist and file are finalized.

5. What type of information does the Provider Unit require for record keeping?

5. The Provider Unit should follow the guidelines set forth in the Manual for Accreditation. These were revised most recently in August 2001.

6. How long does the Provider Unit maintain the record for each CE activity?

6. The records for each activity must be maintained for five years in a secure and confidential manner. Because of the space limitations, the Provider Unit generally keeps the most recent records of the CE activity that have been provided/co-provided at the Provider Unit. The records for those CE activities provided four or five years ago are usually stored in off site storage and available upon request. An index of the records that are in storage is kept in the office.

7. Has the Provider Unit ever had to retrieve information from off site?

7. It is rare that a Provider Unit would need to retrieve records unless a customer needed recertification records. Site visitors usually request information from only the last three years.

8. If a person loses his/her nursing continuing education contact hour/ attendance certificate, how does the registrant get another copy of it?

8. The registrant is asked to request in writing, present in person with identification, or log in to a secure Web site. The Provider Unit will then attempt to retrieve the record from available information.

9. *What information do you include in the program planning minutes?*

9. With permission of members present, the planning committee meetings/conference calls are tape-recorded. The actual written minutes contain essential information of date, time, place, final decisions, next assigned tasks, person responsible, and projected date of completion.

10. *Can you describe how to pilot test a learner directed activity?*

10. While pilot testing is no longer specifically required by ANCC, it is a useful process. Pilot testing can serve to validate content and to estimate length of time to complete in order to assign contact hours.

11. *What roles do the grant funder, the faculty, and the Provider Unit planner have in the development of an activity?*

11. ANA has strict " Guidelines for Commercial Support of Nursing Continuing Education" approved by its Board of Directors. The faculty sign a Vested Interest Disclosure Form.

The provider unit must ensure that the CE content of the activity is clearly, objectively, and correctly presented. No product or device is endorsed. Often, if the grant funder is a federal agency, it will have specific data and program information that it wants to have included as part of the activity. This information is carefully reviewed by the author, provider unit, and grants director to determine its relevance for inclusion.

12. *How do the test and measurement expert reviewers help in development of the multiple choice posttest generally used in a learner directed activity?*

12. The evaluation of the multiple choice posttest questions and options addresses:

- Style and Format: concerns such as use of consistent vocabulary, correct grammar, punctuation, capitalization, and spelling; complexity minimized; and format of presentation style consistently followed.

- Content: concerns such as bases the question on something important; measures activity's purpose and objectives; avoids cuing registrants to the correct answer; avoids opinion based and trick questions; and maintains independence of other questions.

- Writing the Stem: concerns include clearly presents directions in the stem regarding the problem to be solved; includes the central idea and most of the phrasing in the stem; avoids excessive verbiage/ extraneous information; words stem positively and avoids negative phrasing such as not, except; places words in the stem rather than repeats wording in each option; avoids use of key words which gives clues to correct answer and avoids grammatical clues to the correct answer.

- Writing the Answer, Choices/Options: clearly only one correct answer; assigns correct answer randomly to a position among the alternative options; places choices in logical or numerical descending or ascending order; ensures each option is independent of each other; develops the options to be independent of each other, similar in length, detail, and complexity; uses consistent grammar; avoids use of such phrases as all or none of the above, sometimes, always, or never or not; and samples the same domain of knowledge (Haladyna, 1997; Oermann & Gaberson, 1998).

13. *What is the process used to create a learner directed activity from a workshop or education session which has been audio or videotaped?*

13. Generally if there is enough interest demonstrated in the workshop or education session, the Provider Unit will:

- Discuss with the speakers their interest in assisting in development of their education session into a learner directed activity.

- Determine the best format: audio or videotape of the education session or conversion into written format for placement on the Web site.

- Determine contact hours in a logical and defensible manner.

14. *How is copyright law applied to your activities?*

14. The Provider Unit retains the copyright of the material on its Web site and in its print materials. However, the Provider Unit:

- Considers the Web-based activities to be within the public domain.

- Allows the registrant to download and print the activity from the site.

- Suggests the user share the information with student nurses, nurses, and other health professionals.

- Requires the user to cite the source of the material.

15. *What methods have providers used to enable the user/learner to have contact with the author(s) of a learner directed activities?*

15. The author of the online activity can use several techniques:

- Set up a chat room for limited selected dates and times.

- Schedule dates and times for call-in conference calls with the author.

16. **What factors determine whether an activity is updated, revised, or removed?**

16.
- How many people completed the activity within its initial period prior to the deadline?

- Is the topic still being identified by the organization's strategic plan?

- Does the topic relate to the organization's mission and current core issues?

- Have there been new discoveries or advances made related to the topic that would be important to nurses in a variety of clinical practice areas?

- Is there a potential grant funder available to support the revision of the activity?

- Is the original author interested in completing the revision of the activity or will it necessitate locating a different expert author?

- Are there staff and resources available to support this undertaking?

17. **How does a provider of a learner directed activity verify that the individual nurse who has registered for the activity successfully passed the nursing posttest and earned the Provider Unit's nursing continuing education contact hour certificate is really the person he/she says they are?**

17. Passwords, registration information, and the answers to the posttest can be shared. At this point, the Provider Unit must rely solely on the honesty of the individual nurse and assumes the individual abides by the Code of Ethics for Nurses which states " the nurse owes the same duties to self as to others, including the responsibility to preserve integrity and safety, to maintain competence, and to continue personal and professional growth (ANA, 2001).

18. **How does the nurse planner participate in the development/planning, implementation and evaluation of multiple conferences, workshops, or conventions?**

18. ANCC criteria require that a nurse planner trained to use ANCC criteria be involved in planning.

The nurse planner becomes involved in the meetings of the Program Planning Committee throughout the planning process either in person or electronically.

19. How does the nurse planner put together a program schedule?

19. There are software packages available to assist in the scheduling of the education sessions and finalization of the CE program. However, the majority of associations still use the basic schedule table board format. Scheduling of education sessions within a concurrent time period should:

- Offer a variety of topics (e.g., clinical practice, ethical/legal, professional practice, advocacy, collective bargaining).

- Be directed toward different audiences (e.g., staff nurse, nurse administrator, nurse educator/researcher, and advanced practice nurse).

- Allow for the repeating of the critical important sessions on the same day.

- Permit a speaker who has had more than one education session accepted to present at different time periods.

- Schedule exciting and lively sessions immediately after meals.

- Allow at least 5–10 minutes for the registrant to move between education sessions scheduled in different classrooms.

- Schedule frequent 15-minute breaks, adequate time for lunch, and free time to tour, network, or have fun throughout the entire program.

20. What are the advantages and disadvantages of using tracks and learner leveling in scheduling the education sessions?

20. Since 1994, the ANA has used the designation of tracks such as staff nurse, nurse administrator, nurse educator/researcher, nurse consultant/entrepreneur, and advanced practice nurses in the scheduling of its education sessions. The speaker/faculty identifies the tracks for their specific education session. This designated track(s) is reconfirmed by the Program Planning Committee. It is possible for an education session to be assigned more than one track.

The symbols of each track are labeled and defined within the program book. The appropriate track symbol(s) is placed by the title of each education session. A schedule page of the education sessions for each track is also in the program book. The program book also clearly states that the registrants do not have to remain within their track, but are free to attend all of the education sessions.

The advantages of the tracks are:

- The registrants can easily locate those education sessions of most interest to them in their current and future professional nursing career.

- Registrants who stay within their role track more quickly begin to introduce themselves and network with each other.

The disadvantage of using tracks is that registrants may fail to carefully read the program or understand the announcement and not realize they are free to attend all education sessions. They may unknowingly limit themselves as to what they are able to learn and experience within the conference.

In considering the use of terms such as basic, intermediate, and advanced levels, the Program Planning Committees have reaffirmed the Association's position of not using these terms to identify the level of knowledge that the registrant must bring to the session and, thus, the results from attending the session. This type of labeling is too restrictive and often in error. The definition of the levels varies from individual to individual.

21. *How can the nurse planner assist in the implementation phase of these CE activities?*

21. The role of the Nurse Planner in the implementation phase of the CE activity is dependent upon staffing, resources, and scheduling. The Provider Unit:

- Prepares the CE Guidelines Program Book, Personal Verification Form, and Education Session and Total Program Evaluation Form and ensures sufficient numbers are produced.

- Orients appropriate staff to the forms and the process/ procedure for distribution, collection, and return to the Provider Unit.

When on-site:

- Staffs the Speaker Ready room and assists speakers and handles problems as needed.

- Attends part of each education session in the schedule.

- Obtains feedback from the registrants within the education session.

- Networks with speakers, registrants, and others as time permits.

22. What types of evaluation can the provider unit conduct for its provider directed CE program activities?

22. In collaboration with the Program Planning Committee:

- Reaffirms the continued use of the Likert Scale format of the responses 1 = low/poor to 5 = high/excellent to each question.
- Determines the core questions that it wishes to ask related to the evaluation of the education session.
- Develops the basic education session evaluation form which is used for all provider directed CE.
- Allows faculty/speaker to add questions if they wish.
- Determines the core questions which it wishes to ask related to the Total Program Evaluation Form.
- Collaborates with the Program Planning Committee to identify additional questions it wishes to add to the Total Program Evaluation.
- Enters the data obtained from the registrants' completed Education Session Evaluation forms and Total Program Evaluation forms into the Survey Pro Software Program which computes the average score for each question posed.
- Analyzes the data and written comments made by the registrants on the evaluation forms.
- Generates a Total Program Evaluation Report and an evaluation report for each individual education session.

23. With whom should these evaluation reports be shared?

23. The Provider Unit identifies the appropriate audiences to receive these reports:

- Members of the Program Planning Committee, the Association's Board of Directors, Executive Staff, and others as appropriate.
- Individual speakers/faculty receive a thank you letter, the Total Program Evaluation report, and the report of their individual education session. The ratings of the other speakers within their specific session are kept confidential. Each speaker should be informed on his/ her rating only.

24. How can an annual conference planning committee most effectively use the findings of last year's conference evaluation report(s)?

24. The annual conference planning committee should review and discuss last year's conference evaluation report. If the format and scheduling of this conference remains unchanged from year to year, it would be important to review the evaluation reports of the previous 2–3 years. This will enable trends to be easily identified as to what should be kept the same or discarded. Conferences need to be exciting to continue to attract new attendees and retain attendees who faithfully attend each year.

25. Why should I maintain provider unit status?

25. The accreditation of the provider unit by ANCC COA ensures:

The continuing education activities are of high quality and meet specific standards established by the American Nurses Association as the only general professional association representing all nurses, and the requirements of the major general continuing education accrediting body of nursing which is ANCC.

26. What is the correct statement that a provider unit should use with each of its CE program activities that will enable a nurse to tell if a CE program is being provided by an ANCC COA accredited provider?

26. The following entire statement should appear on the program and marketing materials: "The _____ (name) is accredited as a provider of continuing nursing education by the American Nurses Credentialing Center's Commission on Accreditation." It is important to note ANCC COA does not assign an accreditation number to accredited provider units.

27. Whom should a nurse call to determine if a CE program is being or was provided by an ANCC COA accredited provider, especially since ANCC certified nurses must obtain 50% of their continuing education credits from ANCC accredited or approved providers?

27. It is suggested the nurse confirm this status of the association or organization providing the CE activity before paying the money to register and attend the activity. Certification and licensing boards and employers generally want their required CE activities to be provided by an accredited provider. They may not accept the CE credits/contact hours issued by a non-accredited provider.

The nurse can confirm this status by accessing the Directory of ANCC COA accredited providers on ANA's Web site, **www.nursingworld.org**, or call directly at (202) 651–7263 or 7753.

28. What criteria does your provider unit use to determine if you want to co-provide a CE program activity with another nursing specialty organization/association or for profit CE Provider?

28. The areas to be explored are:

- Agreement as to the goals, audiences, location, and dates of the CE activity.

- Ownership/copyright of the audio or videotapes of the education sessions within the conference.

- Agreement as to specific responsibilities of each party related to meeting services, site location/contract, travel and transportation arrangements.

- Division of expenses related to booking/hotel room confirmation; food, beverages, meals, exhibits; speaker expenses (e.g., travel, hotel, per diem, honorarium, handouts, audio visual equipment; marketing; registration services, operations/staffing; program planning committee meeting/conference calls).

- Division of revenues, setting of registration fee.

29. What are the differences between co-providership and co-sponsorship?

29. Co-providership is generally much more complex and requires a formalized signed letter of agreement which clearly outlines that the Provider Unit is responsible for: determination of objectives and content, selection of presenters/content specialists, awarding of contact hours, record keeping, and evaluation.

Co-sponsorship is generally handled by sending a formal letter to the Executive Offices describing the planned CE activity and requesting the Association to provide an expert speaker, sponsor a reception, have an exhibit, make a financial contribution, or just lend its name and logo.

ANCC doesn't use the term "co-sponsorship." It's a formal term for a relationship that is not co-providership.

30. What can a co-sponsor expect in return for giving permission to another Provider for use of its name and logo and a listing as a co-sponsor for the CE program?

30. The Provider might agree to:

- Have the co-sponsor appoint a member to the program planning committee.

- Pay the designated speaker's total expenses to speak at the conference.

- Use the co-sponsor's name and logo in the format as requested on the marketing and program materials.

- Provide free conference registration for 1–2 members of the co-sponsor association.

- Provide free exhibit space, provided the co-sponsor is responsible for the mailing and packing up of exhibit materials and appropriate staffing of the exhibit.

31. What is the Provider Unit's response when any health organization or nursing specialty organization asks it to approve their organization's CE program activity?

31. The Provider Unit:

- Explains the differences between an ANCC accredited approver and provider and confirms that it is not an approver.

- Asks the theme and location of the conference and the organizations' headquarters office.

- Refers the organization to the appropriate Constituent Member Association which is accredited as an approver by ANCC COA or specialty nursing organization.

RESOURCES

American Nurses Association. (2001). *Code of ethics for nurses with interpretive statements.* Washington, DC: American Nurses Publishing.

American Nurses Association. (2000). *Scope and standards of practice for nursing professional development.* Washington, DC: American Nurses Publishing.

American Nurses Credentialing Center's Commission on Accreditation. (2001). *Manual for accreditation as a provider of continuing nursing education.* Washington, DC: American Nurses Credentialing Center.

American Nurses Credentialing Center. (1996). *Manual for accreditation as a provider of continuing education in nursing.* Washington, DC: American Nurses Credentialing Center.

Haladya, T. M. (1997). *Writing test items to evaluate higher order thinking.* Needham Hcights, MA: Llyn & Brown.

Macklin, N. R., & Mathews, J. H. (1998). Ensuring quality in continuing education. *American Journal of Nursing, 98*(4), 60–62.

Oermann, M. H., & Gaberson, K. B. (1998). *Evaluation and testing in nursing education.* New York: Springer.

White, G. (2001). Issues update: The code of ethics for nurses. *American Journal of Nursing, 101*(10), 73–75.

Chapter 23: *Continuing Education Approver Unit*

1. Who is responsible for accrediting the Approver Unit?

1. The American Nurses Credentialing Center's Commission on Accreditation (ANCC COA) is the only accrediting body for Approver Units. ANCC is a separate, yet cooperative, subsidiary of the American Nurses Association (ANA).

2. Why would an organization want to become an Approver Unit?

2. I think the best reason would be to demonstrate a belief in the importance of continuing education and professional development for the Registered Nurse. Other reasons include providing a way for nurses and organizations to obtain approval as providers and/or offer individual activities for continuing education credit.

3. Can any organization become an Approver Unit?

3. Only those organizations that meet criteria in one of the categories of Approvers identified by the ANCC COA are eligible to be accredited as an Approver Unit. The three main categories are:

1. CMA—Constituent Member Association, formerly State Nurses Association (SNA) (e.g., GA Nurses Association)
2. FNS—Federal Nursing Service (e.g., Veterans Affairs Medical Centers)
3. SNO—Specialty Nursing Organization (e.g., Oncology Nursing Society, American Association of Critical-Care Nurses, Academy of Medical-Surgical Nurses)

CMAs and FNSs can approve providers and individual activities. SNOs can only approve individual activities.

4. How can my employing organization become an Approver Unit?

4. First of all, make sure you meet criteria for one of the categories of approvers. If so, then you will need to obtain a copy of the ANCC COA *Manual for Accreditation as an Approver of Continuing Nursing Education.* In the *Manual,* the Accreditation process will be described in detail along with the necessary forms, documentation, and fees to submit with the application. Once the application has been reviewed by the ANCC COA and is determined to meet eligibility criteria, a site visit will be scheduled. The ANCC COA meets in February and August of each year to discuss each application and make the accreditation decisions.

The ANCC COA Accreditation Manuals can be downloaded from the ANCC Web site: **http://www.nursingworld.org/ancc/** or you can request a copy by mail by calling: (202) 651–7265 or 1(800) 284–2378.

5. How often must an organization reapply to be an Approver Unit?

5. Full accreditation by the ANCC COA as an Approver Unit is granted for a period of six years. The Approver Unit is notified by the ANCC COA when renewal is imminent and the Approver Unit must reapply prior to that expiration date.

6. How does the Approver Unit set fees for the provider and individual activity applications?

6. Everyone always wants to know why the fees seem so high. I assure you that the Approver Unit is not a money-making business. Because there is no mandated universal fee schedule for the provider and activity applications, each Approver Unit is free to determine what its fees will be. This decision is based on costs involved in the ANCC COA Approver Unit application process, a market survey of other Approver Units fees, and the amount of effort and time required to operate the Approver Unit. The mission of the organization can also influence setting fees, based on the financial versus customer service orientation.

7. Can one Constituent Member Association (CMA) approve another state's activities or provider applications?

7. A CMA that has been accredited by the ANCC COA as an Approver Unit must determine whether or not it is going to accept applications for providership and activities outside of the state boundaries. If so, the CMA can only approve providers and activities for those states in which the CMA is not already an Accredited Approver Unit. If a CMA is an Accredited Approver, all provider and activity applications from that state must be submitted through that CMA.

8. Why do some states (Constituent Member Associations) choose not to become Approver Units?

8. While I can't speak for all states, I do know that in some of the states that require continuing education for nursing license renewal, ANCC COA approved continuing education hours are not automatically accepted. The continuing education activities must first be approved by the State Board of Nursing. Also, states that do not mandate continuing education for registered nurses may not feel the need to provide this service to nurses, especially since it is costly, requires staff, and is time-consuming.

9. Can an Approver Unit approve an application for providership where several organizations have applied together on one application as a "Consortium"?

9. This is a situation I have actually experienced. I was part of a multi-facility consortium that belonged to the same parent corporation. We applied to be a Provider Unit under one application. The application was approved because the main purpose of forming the consortium was not to obtain providership, but to serve as a support network for sharing between the facilities. So, the answer to this question depends on why the organizations formed a Consortium. If the common purpose and mission of forming a Consortium wasn't solely related to the providership application (such as several healthcare facility sites belonging to the same healthcare system), then yes. If the Providership Approval was the reason for the consortium formation, then no.

10. *How often must a Provider Unit reapply to an Approver Unit for approval?*

10. A Provider can be *approved* by an Approver Unit for a period of two years. This is different from a Provider Unit, which is *accredited* by the ANCC COA for a period of six years and involves a more in-depth process, including a site visit.

11. *What kind of records must an Approver Unit maintain?*

11. Here is a word of advice—don't throw anything away! Always remember the phrase "If you didn't document it, then you didn't do it." All provider applications and individual activity applications approved by the Approver Unit must be kept in their entirety for a period of six years. This includes *all* documentation regarding the review and approval process.

12. *Can an Approver Unit provide activities?*

12. No, there must be a freestanding Provider Unit. Any activities that are provided or co-provided by the Approver Unit may not be approved by that Approver Unit. If an Approver Unit also wishes to provide activities, it must apply to be an **Accredited Provider** directly through the ΛNCC COΛ or an **Approved Provider** through another ANCC COA Approver Unit. If an entity has both an Approver Unit and a Provider Unit, then separate records must be maintained for each unit.

13. *Why must activities be submitted to the Approver Unit at least "30 days prior to the activity" in order to obtain contact hours?*

13. Before I became a reviewer, this was a question I often wondered about. I soon found out that the 30 day time frame gives the Approver Unit reviewer(s) time to evaluate the activity using the established ANCC COA criteria and give feedback to the applicant prior to the activity. This is especially important in situations where the applicant is required to submit further documentation in order to obtain activity approval for contact hours.

14. *How does the Approver Unit review the provider and program applications?*

14. Each Approver Unit must establish its own process for reviewing the applications. This process will be evaluated and approved by the ANCC COA during the Approver Unit application process. Options include, but are not limited to, hiring qualified staff specifically to review the applications or forming ad hoc review committees composed of either paid or volunteer reviewers.

15. What are the qualifications of the reviewers?

15. According to the ANCC COA guidelines, a reviewer must be a registered nurse holding a baccalaureate or higher degree in nursing. Other criteria regarding selection of the reviewers is left up to each Approver Unit. Regardless of the method of selecting the reviewer(s), the goal should be to provide the applicant with qualified, competent, objective nurse reviewers. Generally, reviewers have had experience with the application process.

16. How are the reviewers trained to be reviewers?

16. That was one of the first things I asked when I was chosen to be a reviewer. I found out there is no mandated way to train the reviewers. The procedure for training is determined by the Approver Unit. You must remember that it is important to prepare the reviewer to consistently and objectively apply the ANCC COA criteria when reviewing applications. Helpful items to include in the training process are orientation manuals, ANCC COA review guidelines for provider and individual activity applications, as well as assigning preceptors and mentors.

17. How does the Approver Unit ensure a fair review for the provider applications?

17. In addition to providing trained reviewers, the Approver Unit must have an appeals process in place. If the applicant disagrees with the results of the review, the applicant can follow the Appeals Process. The ANCC COA requires that the Appeals Process be separate from the review process.

18. How does the Approver Unit handle provider and individual activity applications that don't meet ANCC COA criteria?

18. Provider and individual activity applications that don't meet the criteria for approval are provided recommendations in writing to assist them in obtaining approval. These recommendations may include revising the application, submitting additional documents, or participating in the consultation process.

19. How much revision to a Provider Unit application is allowed?

19. As a reviewer, I have seen minor revisions and major revisions. There is no limit to revisions. A provider applicant is allowed to revise and resubmit an application for approval as many times as desired. When a provider applicant shows evidence of being severely deficient in meeting the criteria for approval, the applicant will be given the opportunity to participate in a consultation with the Approver Unit. However, no application will be approved until it meets ANCC COA criteria for approval.

20. When is it determined that a Provider Unit applicant needs consultation?

20. Once again, each Approver Unit sets its own criteria for consultations. Consultations are usually required when the Provider Unit applicant has demonstrated deficiencies in meeting the ANCC COA criteria that clearly require verbal explanations or instructions prior to revising the application. A consultation may be via phone conversation or in person—it depends on the preference of the reviewer(s) and the severity of the deficiencies. The goal of consultation is to enable the provider applicant to successfully revise and submit an application that meets the criteria.

21. Can an organization be turned down for an Approved Provider Unit?

21. Yes, if the organization fails to meet eligibility requirements or fails to comply with the recommendations made by the Approver Unit by the allotted deadline. A new provider application along with the applicable fees can be resubmitted for approval in the future as desired.

22. What qualifies an activity as continuing education in nursing?

22. This is one of the most frequently asked questions by applicants. Continuing education in nursing is defined as that which builds upon RNs' education and experience as well as enriches their contribution to health care. Inservice education and orientation processes are not eligible for continuing education credit because they are specific to the facility and/or employer. You can find out more detail regarding what constitutes continuing education in nursing by consulting the *Scope and Standards of Practice for Nursing Professional Development* (ANA, 2000).

23. How does an Approver Unit ensure that providers are maintaining the ANCC COA standards on the activities they are providing?

23. Each Provider Unit is required to submit three current activities that represent the ability to provide activities along with the Provider Unit renewal application to the Approver Unit every two years. In addition to that, the Approver Unit has the right to conduct audits of Provider Unit records randomly or if there is a reason to believe that the provider is no longer meeting the ANCC COA criteria for continuing education. Violations of ANCC COA standards could result in revoking the Provider Unit's approval.

24. Can the Approver Unit or Provider Unit accreditation be transferred with mergers or acquisitions of organizations?

24. There is no exact answer to this question. In some cases, accreditation may be transferred, while in others it may not. The **Accredited Approver** and the **Accredited Provider** must notify the ANCC COA regarding the changes and obtain direction for what must be resubmitted for continued accreditation. If the Provider

Unit status was obtained from an **Accredited Approver** instead of the ANCC COA, the Provider must submit the changes to that Approver Unit. The Approver Unit will decide whether or not to grant transfer of the approval.

RESOURCES

American Nurses Association. (2000). *Scope and standards of practice for nursing professional development.* Washington, DC: American Nurses Publishing.

American Nurses Credentialing Center's Commission of Accreditation. (2001). *Manual for accreditation as an approver of continuing nursing education.* Washington, DC: American Nurses Credentialing Center.

American Nurses Credentialing Center's Commission of Accreditation. (2001). *Manual for accreditation as a provider of continuing nursing education.* Washington, DC: American Nurses Credentialing Center.

Section 6:
Approaches to Learning

This section encompasses a variety of concepts that will contribute to your success. Each topic is developed from a wealth of literature to support the contributors' summaries and recommendations. Attention to each of these components is difficult to handle at once for the novice educator; however, the more expert Nursing Professional Development specialist will be able to integrate attention to learning styles, critical thinking strategies, cultural competence, humor, performance improvement, and development of others in each planned activity. These aren't the extras to consider, but are important concepts that will make a difference in learner satisfaction and eventually patient outcomes.

Chapter 24: *Cultural Diversity*

1. What is culturally competent nursing education (CCNE)?

1. CCNE relates to a celebration of all the similarities and differences within an employee pool. CCNE includes competent, efficient, and effective delivery of teaching programs to all staff, regardless of background, learning style, language ability, experience, disability, age, gender, or any other cultural diversity attribute. Diversity among healthcare providers is increasing and can be obvious or hidden. Confusion, misunderstanding, and client harm are direct results of culturally incompetent nursing education.

2. Why is learning to teach to a diverse workforce so important?

2. Diversity is real. Within healthcare organizations, diversity is an ever-growing social and demographic influence. The growing numbers of culturally diverse caregivers and clients has made CCNE an important skill and commitment. Integrated, interactive, individualized outcome based teaching/learning is essential because education requirements for healthcare employees are also increasing.

3. How much workforce diversity can I expect?

3. Diversity includes gender, culture, age, education, sexual orientation, religion, seniority, education, job title, economic and geographic environment, language, and more. Here are some important statistics. According to US Health Resources and Services Administration there are 2,696,540 licensed RNs in the US with nearly 82% employed as nurses. The average licensed RN is 45 years old; about 32.5% are under age forty and 4.4% are over age 64. For new RNs, the average age upon graduation is nearly 31 (compared to about 24 years old for new graduates in 1985). Nearly 43% of RNs hold baccalaureate or higher degrees. Nearly 6% of employed nurses are male and 12.3% self-report as members of racial or ethnic minority groups. Importantly, 86.4% of RNs with minority backgrounds are working as nurses (compare this with the 81% of Caucasian RNs). Additionally, minority RNs are more likely than non-minority RNs to be full-time employees (86% report full-time employment compared to 70% of Caucasian RNs). Of all employed nurses, 59% work in hospitals. Thus, the nurses in the classroom and on clinical units are older, better educated, and more ethnically diverse. Furthermore, because of a growing nursing shortage, ever-greater numbers of foreign born and foreign educated nurses are employed by US facilities.

Non-RN healthcare workers are younger and more diverse. Currently, over 27% of Americans between 18-64 report minority status and by 2050 this number will increase to 50%. In 1998, 73% of working age minorities were under 45 (compared with 62% of Caucasians).

4. What do I need to know about teaching to a diverse workforce?

4. Healthcare workforce diversity increases daily. First, please understand that each employee-learner is both an individual and a member of one or more distinct social groups. Members of minority groups are often afraid to ask questions and admit lack of knowledge, skill, or understanding. Culturally diverse staff may be unaware of differences in perceived roles and duties.

5. What is my responsibility in addressing a diverse learning population?

5. The burden is on you to assess learning needs and implement CCNE. Initially, it will be important to fully understand the facility's diversity climate. You will need to compare the demographics of professional and non-professional staff with that of the community and client population served. Assess staff perspectives and perceptions and how these perceptions differ from the facility's stated policies, mission, and strategies.

6. As I prepare to learn culturally competent teaching skills, what must I do first?

6. First, you need to learn about yourself. Sit quietly and consider these questions. Who am I? What are my own values, beliefs, and attitudes, as a socialized, cultural person? What is my ethnic heritage; what are my ethnic beliefs regarding health, illness, teaching, learning? How comfortable (and why) am I about and with members of diverse groups? How much (and of what type) contact have I had with diverse groups? Do I seek out formal and informal diversity learning opportunities?

Most of us have grown up "ethno-centric." Our traditions and core beliefs have been largely assumed and unexamined. Thus, we tend to believe that our world view is best; yet, these core values and learning styles are a mere reflection of family and culture. Thus, we first need to know and then question the very basis of what makes us human. Second, we need to question and constantly evaluate what and how we teach and learn.

7. What specific cultural competence techniques should I use?

7. CCNE means using a diverse repertoire of teaching/learning strategies within each teaching/learning encounter. CCNE is highly flexible and balanced in order to take full advantage of diverse relational and learning styles. According to Marchesani and Adams (1992), CCNE includes:

- Collaborative and cooperative goals vs. individual competition

- Visual and auditory demonstrations vs. verbal or written materials

- Group, peer, cross-age learning projects vs. individual questions/answers

- Study groups, group projects based on peer relationships vs. solo study

    - When requiring group work, it is best to randomly assign group membership (self-segregation may harm the teaching/learning process and marginalize minority group members). With prior explanation, random group assignments are well received by all and learners believe they are fairly treated.

    - Tell groups that you assume disagreement

- Active learning projects, simulations, role play vs. passive lecture/listen classes

CCNE integrates alternative perspectives and methods.

Staff demonstrating obvious stress during teaching/ learning sessions need to be queried in private. Learners may not automatically disclose problems, however. That is, look carefully at nonverbal cues that may suggest questions, concerns, or confusion. When learners are approached in private regarding possible uncertainty, they are more likely to disclose a lack of understanding. Do not expect culturally diverse learners to overtly seek answers to their questions.

8. What is the difference between cultural competence and cultural sensitivity?

8. Cultural sensitivity is a kind of cultural empathy that includes understanding and appreciating others. Cultural competence (CC) goes beyond sensitive interactions. Cultural competence is a continuous process of cultural awareness, knowledge, skill, interaction, and sensitivity. Culturally competent caregivers constantly seek skills, practices, and attitudes that help them transform interventions into positive health outcomes (Smith, 1998). By enhancing the potential and effectiveness of every single healthcare worker, the overall goal of CC is improved client health outcomes and improved quality of work life for all staff members.

9. *How can I incorporate cultural competence into teaching-learning plans?*

9. How you teach is just as important as what you teach. Most of us teach the way we have been taught, reusing tradition and unproven strategies. By teaching to the majority, learning needs and expectations of diverse employees are threatened. We often expect workers to be assertive, independent, and competitive yet those expectations may create tremendous conflict with cultural norms. Staff development goals also need to address the older nurse. The best advice—vary instruction content and approach to accommodate multiple learning styles and needs.

10. *Which Internet Web sites might be most beneficial as I implement culturally competent staff development?*

10. **www.diversityrx.org** is a Web site that promotes language and cultural competence so that health care to minority, immigrant, and culturally diverse groups and communities can be improved.

A resource to help you and the facility locate and mentor minority management staff is **www.diversityconnection.com**

www.inform.umd.edu/diversityweb/ was developed by the Association of American Colleges and Universities.

The White House Initiative on Race Web site addresses the challenge of living and working together in the 21st century. The site: **http://clinton4.nara.gov/initiatives/oneamerica/america_onrace.html**

One of my favorite sites is **www.yforum.com**, which is an international interactive diversity forum.

For a great list of Internet resource links including education, human/ethnic resources, government, and healthcare go to **www.nadm.org/**

11. *What do I need to know about educating and developing an aging workforce?*

11. The licensed healthcare workforce is aging. Therefore, CCNE must include consideration of the older learner. Effective teaching/learning strategies for mature learners are more important than ever. The first step is to recognize the tremendous facility-wide value increased age and experience brings. Yet aging workers are more likely to work part-time, experience health insults, and require time off to care for elder parents and grandchildren. Aging workers are also more likely to have visual and hearing impairments and they may not be as sure-footed or as quick to learn as their younger counterparts. Thus, teaching/learning strategies must include:

- Greater allotments of time to learn new skills and behaviors

- Plenty of visual and audio reinforcement

- Speaking clearly (never shout), with eye contact and plenty of gestures and enthusiasm

- Ongoing knowledge checks as well as final skill evaluations

- Good light, minimal visual/audio distraction, plenty of take-home materials

- Focus groups of older workers to identify learning needs, concerns, suggested strategies

- Heavy doses of respect and group work integration

- Variable times and dates for offerings

- Collaboration with management regarding workplace ergonomics

- Reevaluation of personal stereotypes, biases, and prejudices for and about the older worker

12. What do I need to do if staff members are not fluent in English?

12. Regardless of the preferred language, effective training is essential. For millions of healthcare workers, English is a poorly understood second language. Workplace function and safety depend on clear standards of operation. The driving force behind hiring non-English speakers is their availability.

13. Should I prepare translations of teaching materials?

13. Yes, but you will still need to evaluate staff members for language literacy, even if they are non-English speakers. For certain non-English groups, native language literacy rates are low. Just as with English literacy rates, there are many levels of language literacy among foreign-born US residents. When needed, written materials should be multilingual. Training sessions could be conducted in two languages either simultaneously or consecutively. Additionally, you will want to:

- Use photos, drawings, symbols, and charts to make key points

- Use easily understood analogies, metaphors, and examples

- Distribute a side-by-side translation of key points whenever possible

- Use volunteers to mentor non-English speakers

- Facilitate English conversation classes through the facility, local community college, or immigrant resource center

14. What do I need to know about teaching and developing the staff member who is disabled?

14. Always consider the disabled class member as a capable participant in the teaching/learning process. The Americans with Disabilities Act (ADA) had as its goal the integration of persons with disabilities into U. S. social and workplace environments. What accommodations you make will depend on the disability. Mostly, you will find that teaching disabled staff requires only a few modifications. Guide dogs, interpreters, and wheelchair access may be classroom additions. The Center for Teaching and Learning (1998) suggests that you:

- Use appropriate terminology— visually impaired vs. blind, mobility restricted vs. wheelchair confined.

- Treat each employee as an individual, not a disability; focus on learner needs and interests.

- Teach to the person, never to the disability.

- Inform staff of all training requirements (written and oral). Do this at the beginning of each class session.

- Make modifications as needed; plan alternatives ahead of time.

- Make sure learners fully participate in class and group work.

- Query about special needs ahead of time, never during class. State, "Please give me a few suggestions on how we can make this class easier and more meaningful…."

  - How do you take notes?

  - What will improve access to class information?

  - What are the problems you expect to face in this class/training?

15. What if the learner is hard of hearing?

15. • Determine what can easily be heard; position the person close to speakers.

- Look directly at learners when speaking (tell peers to do the same); don't turn your back or cover your mouth.

- Speak slowly and directly to the learner, not to the interpreter.

220

- Make sure room has good lighting; minimize noise/distractions.

- Place class participants in a circle when possible.

- Use PowerPoint presentations with handouts or write key terms on overheads or flipcharts.

- Point to questioner and repeat all questions before answering.

- Remember, video tapes are usually full of helpful, visually displayed information.

16. What if the learner is visually impaired?

16.
- Keep classrooms consistent.

- Comfortably accommodate learner and guide dog
  - Explain to the class that guide dogs are workers, not pets.

- Place visually impaired learners close to the action.

- Minimize extraneous stimuli (noise, distractions).

- Describe all written information verbally, especially regarding charts, graphs, or photos when Braille translation might be unavailable or inadequate.

- Accommodate audio taping and Braille or computer note-taking devices.

- Clearly, carefully announce all training requirements ahead of time.

- Provide audio tapes of important materials whenever possible.

- Remember, sound and dialogue on video tapes are great teaching/learning tools.

17. How do I assess learner literacy?

17. Here are some ways to assess learner literacy levels:

- Use open-ended questions: Instead of asking, "Do you understand this new policy?" Ask, "What will you do differently…?"

- Look for cues. Staff with low literacy levels often ask peers to read and interpret complex documents.

- Use formal literacy screening tests.

18. What do I need to do if the staff member functions at less than the 7th grade level in reading, writing, and mathematics?

18. All printed materials must be developed at or below the employee's literacy level (most workplace materials are written at or above the 9th grade level). Although few US residents are totally illiterate, nearly 44 million adults (about 22%) cannot read well enough to fill out an employment application or read a food label (National

Institute for Literacy [NIFL], 1998) and most Americans read three or more grade levels below their education attainment. For a good summary and evaluation of readability formulas see the text by Zakaluk and Samuels (1988). In the absence of a formal literacy assessment, ask staff members to interpret a short document or news item. You may also use powerful software programs such as Microsoft® Word to evaluate readability levels of materials you write.

Prior to beginning any teaching/learning project, perform an employee skill level assessment (reading, writing, math) with subsequent, appropriate class placement. Many times, these assessments are completed prior to employment. Use tutoring and mentoring services, learning laboratories, or career guidance to translate nonspecific learning goals into organized study programs. Here are some additional steps to follow (Smith, in press):

- Use teaching tapes as needed. These resources allow staff members to use and reuse materials until competence is achieved. For example, if teaching a new spill cleaning procedure, have the facility tape the demonstration and discussion.

- Use teaching/learning software that provides self-paced learning. This software often uses pictorial descriptions and simple commands that return learners to previous screens if questions are missed.

- Use audiotapes. Audiotapes are small, inexpensive, and mobile. Tape discussions; have staff members repeat the instructions; then give them the tape to keep for further review.

- Keep teaching/learning sessions short.

- Use short words, sentences, paragraphs; keep instruction brief, clear, specific; break tasks into short, basic, easily digested segments.

- Write handouts at the 5th grade reading level, limiting information to basic essentials, and peppering key concepts with illustrations. Use font size no smaller than 12 point (Times-Roman), upper/lowercase presentation, and understandable terms. If using MS Word 2000 software (or equivalent) readability charts are available immediately after performing a spell check. These statistics include number of words, sentences, paragraphs; number of sentences/paragraph, words/sentence, characters/word along with the Flesch-Kincaid grade level equivalent. This chapter was written at the 10.8[th] grade level.

- Repeat important information.

- Express yourself with plenty of paralanguage, gestures, expression.

- Teach with and by example.

- Ask often: "What are your questions? Explain in your own words what you have just learned. Show me how to …."

- Document all your teaching efforts as well as employee responses/behaviors.

19. What should I consider in preparation of case studies?

19. Integrating case studies into teaching plans is a perfect way to emphasize the growing prevalence of chronic illness and disability, an aging population, a growing emphasis on community-based long-term healthcare delivery systems, and most importantly of all, culturally competent care. Case studies gently guide learners into concepts of case management, which shorten hospital stays and increase effectiveness and efficiency by organizing care using teamwork and collaboration.

20. How do I teach culturally competent care (CCC)?

20. CCC is a learned skill! It can be learned and evaluated. CCC begins with the perception that all persons have equal access to healthcare resources and services and all groups within a service area compare equally regarding healthcare outcomes. CCC includes an organization-wide commitment to improve the service links among client needs, expectations, and health outcomes. CCC is a total commitment, not just a single project or mandate. Thus, you will be able to teach CCC by being a culturally competent nurse educator.

21. How do I improve diversity at voluntary CE program offerings?

21. Staff development is people improvement. In conjunction with a local university or community college, conduct a community-wide needs assessment of the target population via ground or e-mail delivery. Until you do this, you will only "think" you know their wishes and needs. Those assumptions will damage your ability to attract and keep diverse CE participants. Broaden your concept of staff development (beyond a sit-and-get mentality) to include programs with growth-promoting processes such as study groups, action research, and peer mentoring. To attract a diverse audience, you should provide a spectrum of CE programs that meet the needs of all local and regional nurses. Broaden the program format and timeframe to include teleconferences, forums, custom workshops, and online course delivery.

22. As I teach and develop a diverse staff, what must I never do? Never —

22.

- Interpret culturally influenced behaviors as stupidity, lack of motivation or preparation.

- Lower your standards.

- Expect one member of a group to speak for and on behalf of the entire group.

- Ignore or single out any one student based on diverse group membership.

- Allow classmates to create an uncomfortable learning environment by ignoring offensive behavior or remarks. You should take issue with off-color jokes or statements and when possible, challenge stereotypic remarks with valid data. If necessary, explain harassment policies.

- Reinforce stereotypes with ethnocentric course materials.

23. How do I evaluate my own cultural competence in the classroom and clinical settings?

23. So often, we teach what and who we are without evaluation. However, our perspective may seem offensive and obtrusive to a diverse audience. Branch out; examine covert course assumptions and balance these with learner input via qualitative and quantitative report tools. Remember, staff may be very reluctant to contact you with questions or concerns. Therefore, seek each person individually; stay receptive and open to change. You could schedule regular informal sessions prior to or immediately following each teaching/learning session and give all staff your phone and e-mail contact numbers. Using focus group techniques, ask all learners to contact you two weeks following any major training sessions. With their permission, record these sessions, transcribe them, and learn from them. Whenever possible, ask a trusted culturally competent nurse educator to sit in on your teaching sessions. One very inexpensive yet effective method is to videotape yourself, create a checklist, and self-evaluate what you see and hear.

While watching this tape, ask yourself: Did I . . .

- make eye contact, give feedback, and temper criticism with praise?

- give learners plenty of time to ask and answer questions (ethnic minorities need triple time to consider both)?

- recognize all learners equally; address learners by name?

- facilitate discussion (do not patronize); assign collaborative learning activities?

- send identical messages to all class members?

- engage even non-assertive learners; stop offensive behavior and remarks?

- convey to learners in word and deed that cultural competence with peers and clients is essential? Did I walk the talk of CCNE?

- encourage learner contact (through word and deed) with me?

- clearly state learner objectives, outcomes, criteria, and ongoing evaluation processes?

- follow all teaching with personal contacts?

- use unbiased language and course materials? Remember, CCNE includes the ability to identify bias in written, audio, and visual materials.

RESOURCES

Center for Teaching and Learning. (1998). Chapter 13: Students with special physical or medical needs. In *Diversity in the college classroom*. Retrieved July 8, 2001, from the University of North Carolina at Chapel Hill Web site: **http://www.unc.edu/depts/ctl/tfi13.html**

Health Resources and Services Administration [HRSA]. (2001, February). *The registered nurse population: National sample survey of registered nurses*. Retrieved May 1, 2001, from **http://phpr.hrsa.gov/**

Marchesani, L. S., & Adams, M. (1992). Dynamics of diversity in the teaching-learning process: A faculty development model for analysis and action. *New Directions for Teaching and Learning, 52*, 9–20.

National Institute for Literacy [NIFL]. (1998, May 28). *Frequently asked questions*. Retrieved April 2, 2000, from **http://novel.nifl.gov/nifl/faqs.html**

Population Reference Bureau. (1999). America's racial and ethnic minorities. *Population Bulletin, 54*(3). Retrieved March 10, 2001, from **http://www.prb.org/pubs/population_bulletin/bu54–3/part3.htm**

Smith, L. S. (1998). Concept analysis: Cultural competence. *Journal of Cultural Diversity, 5*(1), 4–10.

Smith, L. S. (in press). Help! My client's illiterate. *Nursing2002*.

Zakaluk, B. L., & Samuels, S. J. (1988). *Readability: Its past, present, and future*. Newark, DE: International Reading Association.

Chapter 25: *Learning Styles*

1. *What is meant by "learning style?"*

1. A learning style is the individualized process a person prefers for learning. It has nothing to do with a person's intelligence, but rather how a person takes in and processes information. Just as no two people are alike, individual differences also occur in terms of learning styles.

When you can offer educational material in alignment to the learning style that a person prefers, it is analogous to traveling by fast car on a highway. Conversely, if you are trying to teach in a way that is difficult for a learner, the journey will feel like you are walking uphill on a bumpy, gravel road.

2. *Why are learning styles important to the nurse educator?*

2. Learning styles can be helpful to the nurse educator because they help to explain some learner behavior. In addition, they can guide the nurse educator's attempts to improve learning outcomes for a particular individual. Caution is in order though as learning styles have the potential to be detrimental and limiting if they are used to stereotype individuals or force fit them into "pigeon holes."

Multiple authors have espoused differing explanations for learning styles. This can be confusing, but each model makes its own unique contributions to understanding learners and how they learn. For that reason, it is worthwhile to take a look at some of them in this chapter. However, it is also important to note that no single theory of learning styles is in itself sufficient to explain all learner behavior because people are complex. An individual may shift to a different learning style depending on the subject matter, the work involved, and the context in which it all takes place.

3. *Does personality influence learning style?*

3. Personality traits do influence personal preferences, including those involving learning. As one example, our personalities might influence how much we like to participate in group work versus working independently on an educational project.

One of the best known tools for understanding personality traits is the "Myers-Briggs Type Indicator." Called the "MBTI," this tool is not an inventory of learning styles, but rather an analysis of personality traits that can be helpful in knowing how people might approach a learning situation. It is based on the earlier work of Carl Jung. The model presents four dimensions, each one being a continuum of characteristics from one extreme to the other:

1. Mode of relating to others: introversion versus extroversion. Introversion is manifested by an interest in one's own inner thoughts and preference for solitude in study. Extroversion equates with interest in others; extroverted people prefer interaction in learning situations.

2. Preferred way of judging: thinking versus feeling. Thinkers judge based on objective rules or criteria while feelers judge based on emotions, values, and interpersonal concerns. People who are feelers appreciate social support.

3. Preferred way of perceiving: intuition versus sensing. Intuitive learners like to see things as a whole, to theorize and conceptualize in order to learn. Learners who prefer sensing are more comfortable gathering practical data from the use of their five senses. They are drawn to facts and concrete events.

4. Preferred mode of decision-making: judging versus perceiving. Judging learners like to systematically plan and organize information, while perceivers prefer open and unstructured learning approaches and they like to accumulate large amounts of data.

Related learning styles that flow from the Myers-Briggs model (Silver, Strong, & Perini, 2000):

Sensing plus thinking is called the "Mastery style." This learner is practical and prefers active learning, specific expectations, and seeing outcomes. He/she learns best from repeated practice, drill, or hands-on experience.

Sensing plus feeling is called the "Interpersonal style" of learner. This type of person is highly oriented to people and prefers team learning, personal feedback, and exploring the personal impact of content and learns best from group projects, individual feedback, and sharing experiences.

Intuitive plus thinking is called the "Understanding style." This type of learner has an affinity for theory and knowledge and prefers studying, independent projects, logic, debate, and problem-solving. The understanding style learns best from lectures, reading, rational discussion, and self-chosen project work.

Intuitive plus feeling is called the "Self-expressive style" of learner. He/she prefers using creativity and imagination, real problems, and working on multiple projects. Self-expressive learners benefit most from art, stories, drama, and creative methods for learning.

4. Have other authors addressed personality and learning styles?

4. Yes, one is David Kolb (1984) who was strongly influenced by Carl Jung and the Myers Briggs typology; however, he took a somewhat simpler approach. Kolb believed that there are two separate processes important to how people learn: perception and processing. He believed that perception was either oriented toward concrete experience or abstract conceptualization. He thought that processing could either be oriented toward active experimentation or reflective observation. Kolb suggested that these two dichotomies of perception and processing form four learning modes that may be identified through the following kinds of questions:

- How does the learner best process information (active versus reflective)? Active learners learn best by doing something with the subject matter, while reflective people learn best by thinking about it.

- How does the learner prefer to perceive information (sensing versus intuiting)? Sensing learners have a decided preference for facts and data, while intuiting learners prefer theories and interpretation.

- How does the learner prefer to receive information (visual versus verbal)? Visual learners like seeing information in print, diagrams, or illustrations, while verbal learners prefer the spoken or written word.

- How does the learner develop understanding (sequential versus global)? Sequential learners like taking individual steps and making logical connections between them. In contrast, global learners need to get the "big picture" first before smaller pieces fall into place.

Kolb used the answers to these kinds of questions to point the way to four learning styles.

- **Convergent.** This learning style consists of people who are oriented to both abstract conceptualization and active experimentation. They like logic, ideas, concepts, and quantitative processes. They are good at problem solving and enjoy decision making. Kolb named them "convergent" because they are very adept at narrowing the information to converge upon a single correct answer. Such learners are pragmatic, and they prefer hands on, intuitive, action-oriented learning experiences.

- **Divergent.** The "divergent" learning style consists of people who emphasize both concrete experience and reflective observation. Imaginative and creative, they can look at a concrete situation from a number of perspectives and generate alternative implications. Divergent learners like to think, watch, and organize material. They also learn by watching another person learn. In contrast to "convergent" learners, the "divergent" person has a special gift for generating new and different ideas from review of existing information.

- **Accommodative.** This learning style is comprised of people who are oriented to both active experimentation and concrete experience. They are very good at adapting themselves to changes around them. Such learners prefer to do things, carry out plans, complete tasks, and use trial-and-error.

- **Assimilation.** The "assimilation" learning style is comprised of people who prefer abstract conceptualization and reflective observation. These learners have a capacity to observe data and extrapolate theories and generalizations that are logical and concise. They are very good at inductive reasoning and called "assimilators" because they are able forge discrete facts into coherent conceptual models.

In a mixed group of learners encompassing all four Kolb learning styles, a nurse educator could address the needs of all by presenting a learning situation that can be experienced, reflected upon, analyzed, and acted upon.

5. *Do sensory preferences influence learning style?*

5. Yes. Although this belief does have some critics, I have personally found this to be one of the most practical models for my own work in education. We all seem to have a favorite way to take in information through our senses. This makes for distinct differences in how we approach learning. The three most predominant sensory modes are:

- **Visual.** Learn best by seeing things, reading, looking at illustrations, watching videotapes, observing a procedure, or looking at lecture notes.

- **Auditory.** Learn best by listening to lectures, audiotapes, or talking it through.

- **Kinesthetic.** Learn best by touching, taking notes, return demonstration of procedures, or manipulating equipment.

Taste and smell are also possible, as are combinations of all the various senses; however, the most commonly expressed modes are visual, auditory, and kinesthetic. It is well established that people often reveal their preferred sensory mode to others in their speech patterns. For example, visual learners might say, "As you can clearly see," "I am not getting the picture," or "I am in the dark." An auditory learner might say, "that rings true," "hear me out," or "listen up." A kinesthetic learner might say, "I have a bad feeling about that," "this sits well with me," or "it is going smoothly."

Some authors (Lewis & Pucelik, 1990) believe that in addition to speech patterns, you can also identify a person's preferred sensory mode by posture, body movements, voice characteristics, listening behavior, and other observable patterns.

Once the sensory mode preferred by the learner is identified, the nurse educator can use this information to facilitate learning. When you detect a person's predominant sensory mode and choose words that match it with your own speech, you will find it easier to establish rapport and easier to work with the person. You can also tailor learning strategies to fit more directly with learners' preferred sensory mode, making their learning more efficient and effective. For example, you may allow a visual learner to read an article and have an auditory learner listen to an audiotape on the same information.

6. How do multiple intelligences factor into learning styles?

6. Multiple Intelligence theory proposes that there are eight distinct content areas or fields of knowledge. The theory does not really address how people perceive or process information, but rather the domain of knowledge involved. Based on the work of Gardner, as described in Silver and colleagues (2000), there are eight areas of intelligence, each with its own symbols, biological basis, and manner of expression within a culture:

- Verbal/linguistic—words, reading, poetry, debate, writing

- Logical/mathematical—numbers, symbols, patterns, experimentation

- Spatial—photographs, pictures, images, sculpture, location, direction

- Musical—melody, rhythm, musical expressions

- Body/kinesthetic—dexterity, athleticism, dance, acting

- Interpersonal—social, emotional, team players, relationships

- Intrapersonal—self awareness, self-understanding, independence

- Naturalist—natural sciences, attuned to environment

Gardner believed that people possess all of these intelligences and employ them in differing degrees in various settings. As this theory has become more widely embraced, the school system fell under criticism because of its heavy emphasis on just the verbal/linguistic and logical/mathematical intelligences. In response, many school systems are now working to design learning activities to address and develop students in the other areas as well.

Certain areas of content seem suited to teaching methods that can address the various areas of multiple intelligences. For example, you might augment learning about heart sounds by having the learners tap out the various patterns with their fingers instead of just listening to them with a stethoscope. Content in the affective domain might be reinforced through photographs and images in addition to just discussion of a sensitive topic or case study. I have even used song (albeit humorously) to reinforce some of the key content in advanced cardiac life support during my tenure as a clinical nurse educator. All of these give a glimpse of the potential for multiple intelligences to spawn creative teaching approaches that bring the content to life for varied learners.

7. How does hemispheric dominance influence learning style?

7. There are demonstrable differences in the style of thinking that people prefer based upon brain hemispheric dominance. Early work on this subject differentiated between the strengths of the left and right hemispheres. The left hemisphere was attributed with logic and analysis and believed to be responsible for functions such as mathematics. Conversely, the right hemisphere was identified with music, creativity, artistry, and emotions. Critics believed this simple dichotomy was not adequate to explain the complexity and differences observed among people.

The early hemispheric dominance theory and other work of that time evolved into a new model of hemispheric dominance by Ned Herrmann in the 1970s. Basically, Herrmann (1996) proposed that there are four interconnected quadrants that function together in the working human brain. These quadrants form the thinking styles that people use. Although all are present in each of us, a preference usually emerges for one quadrant and this can be identified. Herrmann provided the following specific descriptions of each quadrant:

- A or "Rational self" is the left cerebral hemisphere and is identified with logic, analysis, and quantitative and fact-based thought processes. People with preference in quadrant A like to analyze and solve problems.

- B or "Safe-keeping self" is the left limbic system and it is attributed with organization, planning, details, and sequential thought processes. People with a preference for quadrant B like to plan, administer, and organize.

- C or "Feeling self" is the right limbic system and it is associated with emotions, interpersonal understanding, kinesthetics, and feelings-based thought processes. People with a preference for quadrant C are expressive, spiritual, and social in nature.

- D of "Experimental self" is the right cerebral hemisphere and it is identified with holism, intuition, synthesis, and integrating thought processes. People with preference for quadrant D are visionary and good at conceptualizing.

It is important to note that in Herrmann's model, mental preferences do not equate with ability, meaning we can all tap into the thought processes attributed to any of the four quadrants. However, just as right-handed people use that extremity more, people usually tend to use their preferred quadrant more frequently. These preferences have been linked to the kind of work people enjoy and how they approach the process of learning.

Herrmann contends that tapping into all four of these quadrants strengthens creativity and innovation. A nurse educator can use this "whole brain" approach by ensuring that all his/her teaching methods are not oriented to just one quadrant. For example, you might present logic/theory, supporting data/facts, the interpersonal impact with a case study, and then have learners strategize how they would apply the subject matter in their practice.

8. Is there a way to recognize my own learning style?

8. Remember your nursing school days? You probably identified whether you learned best from listening to lectures, reading the book, or practicing on mannequins. You probably also quickly determined your weaknesses (e.g., "I fall asleep in lecture, but can make up for it by reading the related text."). On a practical basis, this self-assessment may be all you need to figure out your learning style preferences.

Formal assessments of learning style certainly can be done for many of the models discussed here. You will likely find that the results serve to validate what you have already discovered about yourself as a learner.

A formal "Myers-Briggs Type Indicator" test can be done through attendance at a Myers-Briggs workshop. This proprietary instrument can also be administered by some authorized psychologists and counselors. As an alternative, the Keirsey Temperament Sorter addresses similar areas with a 70-item self-assessment tool (Keirsey & Bates, 1978).

You can determine your strengths relating to the eight multiple intelligences through the "Multiple Intelligence Indicator for Adults" developed by Silver, Strong, and Associates.

Hemispheric dominance can be revealed by the Herrmann Brain Dominance Instrument.

Silver et al. developed a "Learning Styles Inventory for Adults" which is presented in sample form in Silver et al.

The Learning Style Inventory developed by Kolb has been extensively used and empirically analyzed. Like the Myers-Briggs tool, this one is also a proprietary instrument.

On the World Wide Web, you will discover a number of Web sites that offer learning style assessments. It is interesting to try them. Caution is in order, though, because you cannot always tell whether such tools have been validated by scientific research.

9. Why can't I just assume others learn the same way that I do?

9. Each person is unique. Each learner is a little different in how he/she learns. If you assume each learner is the same as you, you may be presenting material in ways that actually make it harder for the learner to learn. Conversely, reaching a learner in the way that is most efficient for him/her can truly help that person to remember and apply the information more easily.

There is no such thing as a good or bad learning style; however, difficulties can and do arise when there is a conflict between the learning style preference of a student and how the material is being conveyed by a teacher. If the person you teach looks bored, can't seem to pay attention, and does poorly on tests, it is possible this could indicate a learning style difficulty.

10. What is the easiest way to identify the learning styles of those I teach?

10. You could certainly use any of the assessment tools already mentioned. I honestly don't know too many nurse educators who routinely go to that much effort, though. I tend to take a simpler approach. I listen to conversations to identify their primary sensory mode. I ask them about their nursing school experiences and how they found it easiest to learn new material. I ask them what approaches they find most helpful when they are trying to learn. Generally by the time they are entering the clinical arena, most nurses have some self-awareness of these areas and can tell you if you simply ask them. Once you find out how they learn most readily, then you can employ that kind of approach to convey material to them.

11. When a learner is struggling, how can I tell whether learning style differences are at the root of the difficulties?

11. As the old saying goes, "when you find that you are in a rut, quit digging." If you have been presenting by only lecture and the learner is struggling, change to a different teaching approach. Try readings, videos, mannequin practice, or other methods to convey the material. If it truly is a learning style problem, converting to an approach better aligned with the learner's style will promptly resolve it. If it is not a learning style conflict, then changing teaching approaches will probably not help. I always try a change of teaching approaches first when I encounter poor learner performance and in many instances that is all that is needed to bring about improvement.

12. How can I use this information to be a more effective nurse educator?

12. I always endeavor to tailor my teaching methods so that they are aligned with what learners have told me about how they learn best. When I expect to be covering a similar subject with multiple learners over time, I appreciate the fact that they will not all learn best in the same way. For that reason, I stockpile alternative teaching materials related to that subject (e.g., articles, videos, audiotapes, slides, models, case studies) so that I can adjust my approach to learner preferences. This also allows me to quickly "shift gears" to a different method in the event that a learner is having difficulty understanding the material.

For efficiency sake, I recommend aligning with the learner's preferred style to convey the bulk of the information you wish to teach. Then if you choose, you can augment what is learned by reinforcing it with approaches that address the learner's non-dominant learning styles as well. The thinking behind that is that just like athletic training, we can develop strength by deliberately exercising learning styles that are outside of our "comfort zone."

13. What resources can help me find out more about learning styles?

13. Much has been written on this subject and work is ongoing. Vast information is available on the Internet although the quality is quite variable. The most helpful Web sites I have found are those associated with colleges and universities or those of recognized experts on this subject.

RESOURCES

Bransford, J. D., Brown, A. L., & Cocking, R. R. (Eds.). (2000). *How people learn: Brain, mind, experience and school*. Washington, DC: Committee on Developments in the Science of Learning, National Academy Press.

Herrmann, N. (1996). *The whole brain business book*. New York: McGraw-Hill.

Keirsey, D., & Bates, M. (1978). *Please understand me: Character and temperament types*. Del Mar, CA: Prometheus.

Kolb, D. A. (1984). *Experiential learning: Experience as the source of learning and development*. Englewood Cliffs, NJ: Prentice Hall.

Lewis, B. A., & Pucelik, R. F. (1990). *Magic of NLP demystified: A pragmatic guide to communication and change*. Portland, OR: Metamorphous Press.

Silver, H. F., Strong, R. W., & Perini, M. J. (2000). *So each may learn: Integrating learning styles and multiple intelligences*. Alexandria, VA: Association for Supervision and Curriculum Development.

www.keirsey.com

Chapter 26: *Critical Thinking*

1. Why is there so much emphasis on critical thinking?

1. When I began working with critical thinking almost 15 years ago, nursing faculty members were extremely interested in critical thinking (CT). They wanted to operationalize CT in curricula, enhance students' clinical judgment and document students' growth in CT. The National League for Nursing had included requirements related to CT in the accreditation process.

Today, nurses in leadership positions have recognized that CT strategies support clinical excellence, address management issues and contribute to interdisciplinary collaboration. Healthcare organizations have responded to Joint Commission on Accreditation of Healthcare Organizations (JCAHO) competency standards by validating CT skills of staff.

Whenever the Department of Labor or futurists project skills needed in the workforce, CT, or at least component skills and attitudes of CT, always figure prominently on the list.

2. What is critical thinking?

2. One CT guru, Richard Paul (1995), refers to definitions as "scaffolding for the mind." He's encouraging us to use definitions to stimulate our thinking rather than to bring our thoughts to a close.

His own definition of CT is "The art of thinking about your thinking, while you're thinking, to make it better, more clear, accurate, and defensible" (p. 9).

Paul's definition emphasizes reflection—an important component of CT. Watson and Glaser, pioneers in studying CT, identified three components of CT: knowledge, skill in application, and attitude of inquiry.

Another authority, Steven Brookfield, emphasizes the importance of recognizing and validating assumptions.

Sometimes the definitions expressed in just a few words fail to communicate fully the flavor of CT in nursing. Collier, McCash, and Bartram (1996) defined CT in nursing as . . .

> "a special way of handling information that calls upon all of one's resources—intellect, knowledge, creativity, experience, intuition and reasoning. Using these resources, the nurse generates ideas, considers alternative explanations, draws conclusions and makes accurate judgments about the client's needs

... always purposeful and goal directed ... Examples include recognizing pertinent, significant data; clarifying, verifying and validating clinical data; using appropriate resources; using an organized assessment format to obtain the necessary data base; and generating multiple diagnostic hypotheses for consideration in the diagnostic process" (p. 7).

Most research, including recent nursing research, identifies two components of CT: skills (e.g., analyzing) and attitudes, or habits of mind (e.g., flexibility). Nurse researchers Rubenfeld and Scheffer (1999) enumerated both skills and habits of mind in their recently published research:

Critical thinking in nursing is an essential component of professional accountability and quality nursing care.	
Critical thinkers in nursing exhibit these **Habits of Mind**	Critical thinkers in nursing practice the **Cognitive Skills** of ...
Confidence	Analyzing
Contextual Perspective	Applying Standards
Creativity	Discriminating
Flexibility	Information Seeking
Inquisitiveness	Logical Reasoning
Intellectual Integrity	Predicting
Intuition	Transforming Knowledge
Open-mindedness	
Perseverance	
Reflection	

CT is both a logical, left-brained process and a creative right-brained process. I like to represent CT as a light bulb (representing the creative part) that has a question mark for a filament (representing the logical part). The question mark (or Watson and Glaser's attitude of inquiry) drives the critical thinking process.

3. Isn't critical thinking just the same as nursing process or problem solving?

3. CT certainly contributes to using the nursing process expertly and solving problems well. CT skills and attitudes are important to success with both processes. However, CT goes before and beyond nursing process and problem solving. CT is a goal-directed, outcome-oriented process, BUT an important part of CT is identifying problems or those well-known "opportunities for improvement."

One of my favorite CT questions is "What's wrong with this picture?" or "What in this picture can be improved?" That's the part of CT that goes before nursing process and problem solving. CT is active in the assessment phase of nursing process—it also functions in a broader and more holistic way than we often view assessment. CT guides the effective application of nursing process and problem solving.

Sometimes we solve the wrong problem because we fail to view a problematic situation from a variety of perspectives and with all the information we can get our hands on. How many times have you put a new policy in place to solve a problem only to find that despite the new policy the distressing symptoms of the problem still remain? That's usually a result of solving the wrong problem.

We need to walk around the elephant to fully view the aspects of the problem and their interrelationships. Walking around the elephant is a metaphor taken from John Godfry Saks' parable of the blind men and the elephant. Each blind man palpated a different part of the elephant and therefore each constructed an image of the elephant that differed from the others. For example, one felt the tail and found the elephant like a rope; another, the ear and found the elephant like a fan. I like to use that metaphor not only to emphasize the importance of redefining problems, but also to highlight the idea that each of us develops perspectives based upon our own experiences (i.e., the blind man who thought the elephant was like a fan must have known something about fans). We're all unavoidably prisoners of our own perspectives. But we must both recognize and expand our own perspectives to think critically.

Beyond nursing process and problem solving lies the reflective aspect of CT. It's more than evaluating a solution or intervention—it's reflecting on your own thought process and becoming consciously aware of how your knowledge base evolved as a result of this episode of CT.

4. *Isn't critical thinking only for the RN? Some delegation guidelines direct RNs to delegate no activities that require critical thinking.*

4. If you have any exposure to school age children, you know that most schools today are teaching critical thinking strategies to children at a young age. So, if school age children can think critically, I don't believe that RNs are the only nursing care providers who exercise those skills. I believe that CNAs, UAPs, patients, and significant others use CT and that RNs need to support CT by all of these.

The difference between RNs and unlicensed nursing caregivers is the knowledge base. I certainly think that giving unlicensed nursing caregivers structure to follow promotes safety and I believe that these roles need to be clearly defined. *BUT* I also think that CNAs, for example, can think critically about issues of patient safety and infection control. True, they have procedures to follow—but we expect them to recognize "What's wrong with this picture?" on at least safety, infection control, and customer relations issues—and we can't put every eventuality on their procedural checklists.

One thing unlicensed nursing care providers need to think critically about is when they need to report something to the RN and how urgently they need to do so. Again, many circumstances are defined and described in policy. I think we need to respect the thinking experience that unlicensed caregivers have had in their lives and help them transfer the skill to the nursing practice setting.

Don't misunderstand me—I think analyzing assessment data, making the nursing diagnosis, planning, implementing, and evaluating nursing actions belong to the RN. But, as others carry out their delegated duties, situations will arise for which there is no established procedure. Unlicensed caregivers need some criteria with which to decide what to do when those situations arise. And, within the scope of their practice, making those decisions wisely is CT.

5. *What are some approaches to get interdisciplinary groups using critical thinking in their work together?*

5. I think that collaboration is an interpersonal form of CT. But unfortunately, all interdisciplinary encounters are not collaborative processes.

In true collaboration, as a first step, the parties together define, and redefine the problem. They walk around the elephant together. They take into account the needs of all stakeholders. Each party identifies the most important ingredients of a solution to a problem from his/her perspective. And, they bring forth evidence of the perspectives of those who are not present—such as patients and their families.

So, especially when interdisciplinary perspectives are involved, it's important to take the time to state and restate the problem until you achieve a precise and comprehensive understanding of the problem. This is what I mean by CT going before problem solving.

The second step in collaboration is an analytical one, to be taken by each party to the collaboration. Each party identifies the most important ingredients of an effective solution from his/her point of view. This does not mean that each party presents a solution. Instead, each party specifies what makes for an effective solution: specifications such as patient safety, a target dollar figure, a target reduction in medication errors, a time factor, or compliance with documentation guidelines.

The second step is a difficult one because representatives of the various disciplines usually come to the table with a formulated solution to advocate on behalf of the department that each represents. Sometimes each advocates vociferously for his/her preformulated solution. Francie Wolgin calls this the anti-disciplinary approach.

To effectively reach a collaborative solution, each party must exercise some critical thinking skill to identify the criteria that are truly important to his/her discipline.

In the third step, all parties put their specifications on the table.

Finally, the group honors these specifications and works together to generate solutions that fit the specifications. Then, the group selects a solution to implement, does so and evaluates the results.

The graphic on the following page represents this process.

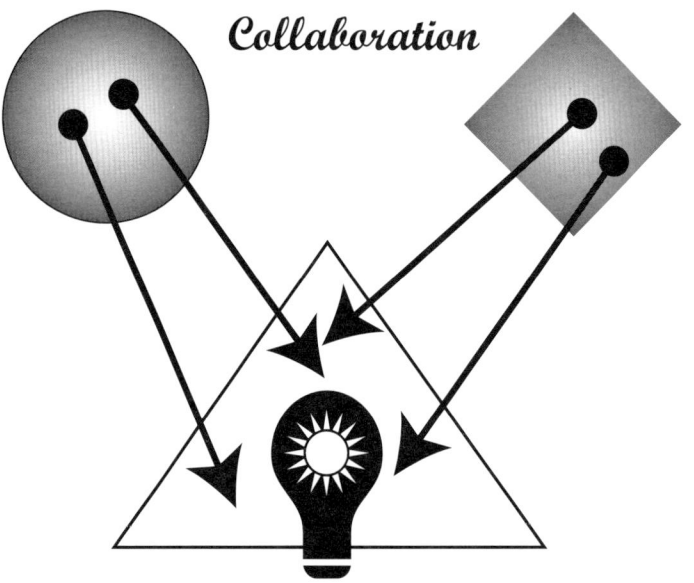

Collaboration

The circle represents one perspective, perhaps nursing, and the square represents another, perhaps pharmacy. The small circles within each represent the most important needs that an effective solution must satisfy from each perspective. The triangle represents the collection of these specifications—a decision-making platform of a slightly different shape and texture from that of either of the collaborating parties. From the collaboration, emerges a new approach, represented by the light bulb.

Did you pick up on the skills and habits of CT in this description of collaboration?

6. *What difference does critical thinking really make in an organization?*

6. When CT comes to life in an organization it facilitates professional, collaborative, outcome-oriented behavior. Because CT involves taking all perspectives into account, it also facilitates truly patient-oriented care and patient satisfaction. When leaders and staff are exercising their CT skills, they don't allow faulty assumptions to guide their behavior. Instead they validate (or invalidate) assumptions before proceeding.

Hansten and Washburn (2000) described CT in an organization as characterized by empowerment, rapid action, managers modeling CT, educators using CT strategies and evaluating their effectiveness, preceptors and mentors using CT widely, multi-disciplinary teams functioning effectively, participative management, mistakes viewed as opportunities for improvement, new ideas and risk taking supported, and a reward system for CT.

7. What does critical thinking look like in staff development practice?

7. The most important use of CT skills in staff development is to identify and align with organizational goals. This keeps the staff development department a viable, valued, and contributing member of the organization. Staff Development Specialists also use CT skills when they:

- sort out essential competencies

- present staff education after identifying what problem this new learning will solve for staff

- teach new policies and techniques by identifying and emphasizing the differences between current and new practice

- use critique as a strategy (e.g., critique plans of care, documentation, or approaches to reduce medication error, research findings)

- model CT

- develop preceptors and managers as coaches

- promote examination of perspectives and validation of assumptions

- use lots of varied strategies that help staff develop CT skills. Many of these are enumerated in Case (1998). Adult education means to always leave the class with a lingering question to promote further use of the content. It is hoped that question is not, "What the heck was that all about?"

8. What does critical thinking look like in clinical nursing practice?

8. Nurses who use their CT skills in practice demonstrate sound clinical judgment. They ask themselves, their colleagues, and their resources lots of questions, such as:

What's wrong with this picture? How do can I do this more effectively? What do I already know about this patient? Who (or what resource) is the most credible source of information? What will I ask? What will I look for? Where will I look?

What's the priority? To whom can I safely delegate this task?

9. What does critical thinking look like in management/administrative practice?

9. Managers who use CT model it. They show openness to challenge from staff. They ask questions about clinical care, how departments can improve quality, and how they can obtain resources and use resources more effectively. They experiment. They reward CT among the staff. They use inquiring techniques in the interview process, in counseling

10. How can I get nurses and other staff to think?

staff, in appraising staff performance, in conducting meetings, and in searching for ways to improve quality of care in departments.

10. Henry Ford once said, "Thinking isn't easy, which is the probable reason why so few people do it." Thinking is hard work and it's risky. Challenging long-standing policies and procedures, continually asking "What's wrong with this picture?" or looking for new alternative approaches is risky. Let's face it—few nurses will do it unless:

- Nurses are expected to think critically.

- There are consequences for thinking critically (or not) specifically in daily feedback to staff and in performance appraisal.

- The environment fosters CT.

- Leaders, colleagues, and peers model CT behavior.

Two maxims apply:

- Expect it or forget it.

- What gets measured gets produced; What gets rewarded gets produced again.

Make the question mark ubiquitous, or everywhere. Picture a big, puffy, helium inflated question mark, floating around the unit and hovering over problem situations.

Ask questions and question answers. Come up with a relevant "Question of the Week." Make it a question relevant to a specific aspect of patient care—perhaps medication safety. Ask that question on rounds. Good questions for busy nurses are targeted questions. Instead of "How can we improve patient satisfaction on the unit?" ask "What was the one thing you did so far today that patients most appreciated?" or "Which one of the patients seems least happy with his/her care today?" followed with probes to get at the sources of dissatisfaction and suggestions for fixing those dissatisfiers.

Alfaro-LeFevre (personal communication, May 17, 2002) has identified some indicators of CT which are useful in helping managers spell out expectations for CT. However, the manager must still create the connection between the behavior and the specific unit practice.

11. *Aren't there some people who just can't learn to think critically?*

11. Probably, but let's not give up without a good try. Most people of average intelligence and certainly people who have graduated from professional education programs can improve their CT skills with systematic practice, coaching, and an environment that *expects* people to think critically.

12. *The nurses say they're just too busy for this critical thinking stuff. Don't they have a good point?*

12. CT is more a *way* of doing nursing than another task to do. Applying CT to identify priorities and make a plan *before* you get overwhelmed can actually save time and aggravation. Staff, managers, and Staff Development Specialists need to be alert to threats to CT such as illness, short staffing, stress, distractions, multi-tasking, and all the attitudes that are the opposite of habits of mind stated earlier. When conditions threaten CT, we all need to recognize the threat and remain alert for the picture that has something amiss.

13. *How do you assess critical thinking in applicants for positions?*

13. You can't until you define specifically and operationally what CT looks like on the unit or in the department. When you've defined it, then ask applicants what they would do in situations that commonly occur on the unit and call for CT. The applicant won't know the policy and procedure, but that's not the purpose of your question. You want to assess the applicant's ability to think critically. What does the applicant identify as priorities? How does the applicant use prior experience and recognize the need for more information? What sources would the applicant consult?

14. *How can managers assess critical thinking in managing and appraising performance of staff?*

14. Managers must function as coaches. They must realize that unlike skill performance (where we can see errors as they occur), with CT we often see only the result. So, we have to ask staff to think-out-loud in order to offer corrective feedback. Remember that it's possible to obtain a good result or outcome totally by accident and despite some precarious errors in thinking.

Long before the first performance appraisal, when the manager orients the staff member, the manager can ask "What will I see you doing when you are demonstrating this particular item on the performance appraisal form?" The response and the manager's follow up response or questions help clarify and reach a mutual understanding of expectations.

15. How do you teach critical thinking? Most nurses I work with never had a course in critical thinking. Does it work best to design separate courses in critical thinking?

15. I think that staff and managers relate to CT strategies best in terms of the usefulness of CT strategies in solving problems that are important to them. For that reason, I think the "course" or learning activity needs to be about attacking the issues, rather than presenting an academic discourse on CT. I have done this in creating the self-study modules cited in the Resources at the end of this chapter (Case, 2000). It's not so important for staff to learn the CT jargon—it's more important that we give the strategies some practical anchors and applications.

Published accounts of success with emphasizing CT in nursing departments (Hansten & Washburn, 2000; Ulsenheimer et al., 1997) encourage the use of a model as an advance organizer and an ongoing reference point.

Below are a couple of the models that I've found quite useful. I encourage readers to explore the full description of these models in the references cited.

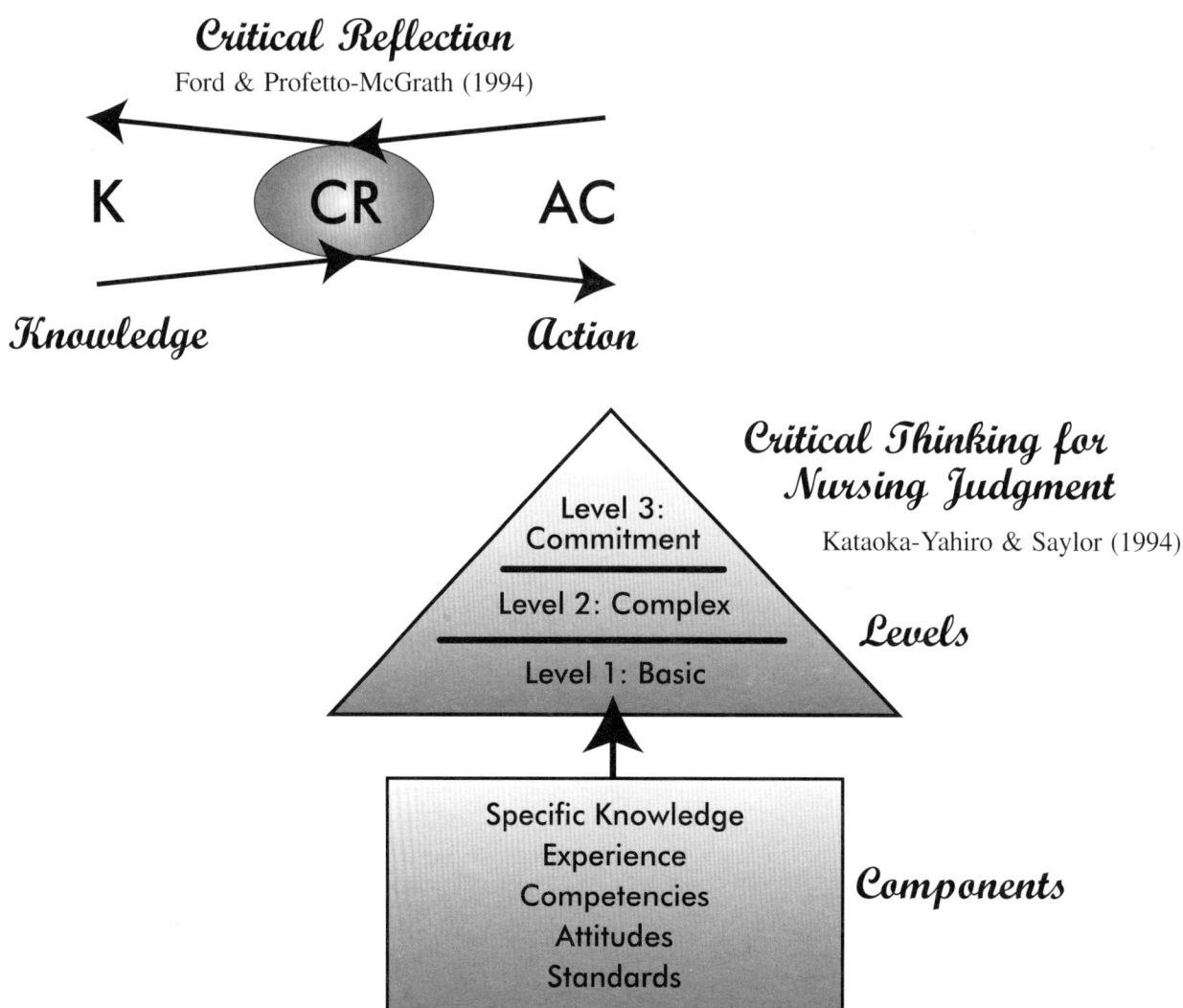

Critical Reflection
Ford & Profetto-McGrath (1994)

K   CR   AC

Knowledge   *Action*

Critical Thinking for Nursing Judgment
Kataoka-Yahiro & Saylor (1994)

Level 3: Commitment
Level 2: Complex
Level 1: Basic

Levels

Specific Knowledge
Experience
Competencies
Attitudes
Standards

Components

16. What are schools of nursing doing about critical thinking?

16. Schools of nursing are doing a lot about CT. To meet accreditation standards, they have defined CT for their curricula. They also identify CT outcomes in student performance. I encourage Staff Development Specialists and managers to give feedback to school of nursing faculty—to the faculty of local schools and faculty of the schools from which your new hires graduated. If you perceive a discrepancy between what you see in the new graduates and what you believe is a reasonable expectation of CT on the part of a new graduate, the faculty need to know this and you need to take the initiative to open the dialogue.

17. How can I prepare myself to teach and evaluate critical thinking?

17. The first step is to operationalize CT. Look at the characteristics, the models, Alfaro-LeFevre's (1999) indicators, and then identify *exactly and specifically* what CT looks like in your setting. When you have determined that, you have identified the outcomes of the education program. When you attach the measurement to your outcomes you have the means of evaluation.

I believe that the educational process is really an opportunity for learners to gather and practice the knowledge, skills, and attitudes they need to demonstrate the outcomes. So, with outcomes defined, plan learning activities that will allow learners to actively gather the knowledge they need and practice CT.

If you have trouble with what CT looks like, observe the practice of star clinical performers. Also, refer to Fonteyn's (1998) book.

Use lots of cases and situations, problems to solve, and open-ended questions. Remember that you can express a case or situation in a sentence or two and then ask the alternative-response style of question. That is, given this 2- or 3-sentence situation, were infection control practices adequate or inadequate? Or do you see an ethical issue? Or is documentation adequate or inadequate? And then, ask the learner to give evidence to support his/her answer and correct those situations that do not satisfy the criteria. Better still, ask the learners what the criteria need to be to make those decisions.

When evaluating CT it's important to triangulate. That is, to look at a number of sources of evidence, such as:

• Performance appraisal—preferably 360°—to

incorporate all those important perspectives: the manager's, the patient's, nursing colleagues, interdisciplinary colleagues, preceptees or preceptors, and other relevant persons

- Self-appraisal and self-description of patient care situations

- Patient outcomes

- Committee and other project work

- Quality improvement contributions

- Unit problem solving

- New approaches suggested

- Research findings applied

- Performance as a preceptor

Very importantly, take a large dose of courage and sense of humor. For help in that regard read Brookfield's 1993 article in the reference list.

18. How can you incorporate critical thinking into classes and still have enough time to cover the material?

18. Take every opportunity to ask rather than tell. Question the answers instead of answering the questions. Instead of telling the nurses information that they probably know anyway, ask them for examples. If they can't come up with any, then give your mini-lecture. Think *mini*-lecture and only as a default.

Use multiple-choice questions for discussion instead of lecturing. Instruct learners to think-pair-share (pair with another learner and respond to a question or come up with an example)—it only need take 2–3 minutes of precious class time. Use lots of critique strategies. Use lots of case studies and patient care situations. Ask for lots of examples.

19. How do you test critical thinking in written tests?

19. Start with those CT outcomes you defined when you planned the learning activity. The idea applies equally if you are creating a competence assessment rather than a post test. As Dorothy del Bueno said, "Few patients present nurses with four possible options to solve their health problems." So, we need to require some open-ended responses.

Present a situation and ask "What else do you need to know?" or "What is your priority?" or any of a number of questions that are germane to objectives. When you have a clear picture of what CT looks like in the practice area of concern, the questions will flow readily.

Use novel situations—that is, situations that the person being tested has not encountered previously in exactly that form. Ask trouble shooting questions, questions that require identifying missing information. The key is to ask questions that require the person being tested to demonstrate the behavior you are after—Is it validating data? Is it asking questions? Is it identifying missing information? Whichever of the CT behaviors or indicators it is, that is what your question needs to require the person being tested to answer.

20. Can you test critical thinking with objective-type test items like true/false (also known as alternative-response) and multiple-choice?

20. You can test some aspects, but not all. To fully evaluate CT you need to provide some open-ended questions. When you give alternative-response or multiple-choice you are restricting the field to two or four choices. This is a miserably small sample of all the possibilities a nurse might come up with left to his/her own devices.

21. Are there some good standardized CT tests available?

21. There are numerous tests available both to measure CT as a general construct and in nursing. I have recently worked with the National League for Nursing (NLN) on a standardized test and companion online course that the NLN is developing for nursing students who are close to graduation. But the question about any test is "good for what?" Tests are valid for a purpose and not valid in the abstract.

The results of standardized tests have not shown consistent results in correlation with clinical practice or academic measures in nursing. You can review these studies in the articles by Rane-Stoszak and Robertson (1996) and by Adams and colleagues (1999) in the Reference list.

Research purposes are different from our purposes in developing staff. I believe that the most valid tests of CT for use in staff development are carefully constructed using situations common in the practice arena of those being tested.

I've provided a list of a few published test resources. In

addition, Hansten and Washburn (2000) are researching tools for use in clinical practice.

- Watson-Glaser Critical Thinking Appraisal
  Psychological Corporation, Cleveland, OH

- Cornell Critical Thinking Skills Test Level Z
  Critical Thinking Press & Software
  P.O. Box 448
  Pacific Grove, CA 93950

- California Critical Thinking Skills Test
  California Critical Thinking Dispositions Inventory
  California Academic Press—**www.calpress.com**

- Arnett Critical Thinking Outcome Evaluation
  Critical Thinking Level Exam
  Critical Thinking Entrance Examination
  http://www.arnettdevcorp.com

- ATI Testing Critical Thinking Assessment
  http://atitesting.com/Critical Thinking.asp

- InterEd Critical Thinking Assessment for Nursing
  Education: phone (602) 894–5550

- NLN Critical Thinking Assessment:
  phone 1(800) 669–1656

- Mosby Assess Tests: phone 1(800) 633–6699

- CNET: phone (908) 469–8615

- Association of Women's Health, Obstetric and
  Neonatal Nurses (AWHONN) ACATs:
  phone 1(800) 673–8499

- Performance-Based Development System
  Performance Management Systems, Inc., Tustin, CA

22. What differentiates a test item that tests critical thinking from one that does not?

22. A critical thinking item requires the person being tested to perform one of the CT behaviors, demonstrate one of the habits of mind, or demonstrate an indicator of CT. This does not mean reciting facts and principles—even when the facts and principles are complex. Research has shown that college faculty often overestimate the cognitive level at which they are testing—that is, they are often only testing rote learning or recitation of principles and concepts (albeit complex ones) rather than requiring students to generate an original answer that shows analysis and synthesis.

Asking nurses to apply criteria to situations, or to come

up with criteria to evaluate situations is a sound CT measure. So is asking for priority nursing diagnoses. But there are many more. Think of all the ways you can answer the question, "What does CT look like in this practice area?" The answers to your questions are what you want the nurse to demonstrate.

23. What are some good products and materials for teaching critical thinking?

23. Case studies and computer-based case studies are good materials for teaching CT. Look at the nursing texts in the Resources list for some ideas and then translate them into the staff development setting. Multiple-choice questions are good discussion material too—if you require learners to think through their own answers and then present evidence to support their conclusions.

REFERENCES

Adams, M., Whitlow, J., Stover, L., & Johnson, K. (1999). Nursing education for critical thinking: An integrative review. *Journal of Nursing Education, 38*(3), 113–118.

Alfaro-LeFevre, R. (1999). *Critical thinking in nursing: A practical approach* (2nd ed.). Philadelphia: Saunders.

Brookfield, S. (1993). On impostership, cultural suicide, and other dangers: How nurses learn critical thinking. *The Journal of Continuing Education in Nursing, 24*(5), 197–205.

Case, B. (1998). Competence development: Critical thinking, clinical judgment and technical ability. In Kelly Thomas, K. J. *Clinical and nursing staff development: Current competence, future focus* (2nd ed.). Philadelphia: Lippincott.

Case, B. (2000). *Critical thinking.* San Diego: American Mobile Healthcare, Professional Development Council.

Part one: Strategies to master floating

Part two: Working with UAP

Part three: Staffing

Part four: Managing stress (2001)

Part five: Administering medications to the elderly (2001)

Part six: Identifying and preventing polypharmacy (2001)

Collier, I. C., McCash, K. E., & Bartram, J. M. (1996). *Writing nursing diagnoses: A critical thinking approach.* St. Louis: Mosby.

del Bueno, D. (1990). Evaluation: Myths, mystiques, and obsessions. *Journal of Nursing Administration, 20*(11), 6.

Fonteyn, M. E. (1998). *Thinking strategies for nursing practice.* Philadelphia: Lippincott.

Ford, J., & Profetto-McGrath, J. (1994). A model for critical thinking within the context of curriculum as praxis. *Journal of Nursing Education, 33*(8), 341–344.

Hansten, R., & Washburn, M. (2000). Facilitating critical thinking. *Journal for Nurses in Staff Development, 16*(1), 23–30.

Kataoka-Yahiro, M., & Saylor, C. (1994). A critical thinking model for nursing judgment. *Journal of Nursing Education, 33*(8), 351–356.

Paul, R. (1995). *Critical thinking: How to prepare students for a rapidly changing world.* Santa Rosa, CA: Foundation for Critical Thinking.

Rane-Stoszak, D., & Robertson, J. F. (1996). Issues in measuring critical thinking: Meeting the challenge. *Journal of Nursing Education, 35*(1), 5–18.

Rubenfeld, M. G., & Scheffer, B. K. (1999). *Critical thinking in nursing: An interactive approach.* Philadelphia: Lippincott.

Ulsenheimer, J. H., Bailey, D. W., McCullough, E. M., Thornton, S. E., & Warder, E. W. (1997). Thinking about thinking. *The Journal of Continuing Education in Nursing, 28*(4), 150–156.

RESOURCES

Case, B. (1994). Walking around the elephant: A critical thinking strategy for decision making. *The Journal of Continuing Education in Nursing, 25*(3), 101–109.

Case, B. (1995). Critical thinking: Challenging assumptions and imagining alternatives. *Dimensions in Critical Care Nursing, 14*(5), 274–279.

Case, B. (1997). *Career planning for nurses.* Albany, NY: Delmar.

Case, B. (1999). Manager as infusion pump: Facilitating continuous flow of critical thinking in the nursing department. *Advance for Nurses, 1*(17), 16–17.

Facione, N. (1997). *Critical thinking assessment in nursing education programs: An aggregate data analysis.* Millbrae, CA: California Academic Press.

Fowler, L. P. (1998). Improving critical thinking in nursing practice. *Journal for Nurses in Staff Development, 14*(4), 183–187.

Hansten, R., & Washburn, M. (2001). Intuition in professional practice: Executive and staff perceptions. *Journal of Nursing Administration, 30*(4), 185–188.

Hansten, R., & Washburn, M. (1999). Individual and organizational accountability for the development of critical thinking. *Journal of Nursing Administration, 29*(11), 39–45.

Maynard, C. A. (1996). Relationship of critical thinking ability to professional nursing competence. *Journal of Nursing Education, 35*(1), 12–18.

Miller, M. A., & Babcock, D. E. (1995). *Critical thinking applied to nursing.* St. Louis: Mosby.

Oermann, M., & Gaberson, K. (1998). *Evaluation and testing in nursing education.* New York: Springer.

Scheffer, B., & Rubenstein, G. (2000). A consensus statement on critical thinking in nursing. *Journal of Nursing Education, 39*(8), 352–359.

VonOech, R. (1983). *A whack on the side of the head.* New York: Warner Books.

Jossey-Bass Publishers, San Francisco, CA, (415) 433–1767—many critical thinking titles

Sonoma State University, The Center for Critical Thinking, (707) 664–2940—annual meeting and publications

Massachusetts Institute of Technology, The National Center for Teaching Thinking, (617) 965–4604—meetings

Critical Thinking on the Internet **http://www.criticalthinking.org**

Chapter 27: *Performance Improvement*

1. What is meant by performance improvement?

1. Performance improvement is a continuous, ongoing measurement and evaluation process with the intended outcome of quality care. The process includes those activities an organization/department/agency conducts to monitor, analyze, improve, and sustain performance. Each agency or organization must determine how it defines quality care.

2. What role does competency play in performance improvement?

2. Competency forms the basis for performance improvement. Competency assumes that a predetermined standard or level of excellence has been established as a guideline for practice and evaluation. If this level of excellence is not met, then action needs to be implemented to ensure that performance is improved and sustained and quality care assured.

3. How do I assess staff competency?

3. Staff competency must be assessed by measuring knowledge, behaviors, and/or psychomotor skills against predetermined standards known and understood by staff. Knowledge, behavior, and skills may be determined via objective tests, essay tests, computer simulation, case studies, observation, peer evaluation, nursing audits, and surveys.

4. What is the role of the staff development department in performance improvement?

4. A staff development department's role in performance improvement depends, in part, upon an agency's organizational structure. Typically, such departments may be responsible for any or all of the following:

- Assessing staff competencies
- Developing corrective action programs based upon identified staff needs
- Evaluating and monitoring effectiveness of actions to improve performance
- Communicating effectiveness to staff and administration

Staff development departments may be part of an interdisciplinary team assigned to assess performance, provide and evaluate performance improvement activities, and monitor performance for maintenance of improvement.

5. What are performance indicators and how are they established?

5. Performance indicators are predetermined standards or levels of excellence that serve as a guide for practice and/or quality. Indicators are measurement tools, and therefore must be objective, measurable, and achievable.

Indicators are established by individuals in authority positions in organizations and may be derived from professional nursing practice standards, ethical codes, accreditation and regulatory standards, and an organization's philosophy, mission, and culture.

6. What data sources can I use to identify areas for performance improvement?

6. Possible data sources include:

- Nursing audits
- Problem focused studies
- Patient surveys
- Infection rates
- Competency testing
- Performance appraisals
- Inservice program evaluations
- Continuing education program evaluations
- Staff meetings
- Committee meetings

7. The hospital has identified a quality management deficit and sent it to education for resolution. What do I do now?

7. Apply the nursing process!

- Assess: Review the deficit and your resources. Do you have all the data you need about the deficit in order to take corrective action? Do you have the resources and authority to address the deficit?

- Plan: Make a plan for taking correction action. The plan should include WHO (both who will be responsible for plan implementation as well as who will be the target population); WHAT (what specific action needs to be taken); WHEN (time schedule); WHERE (geographic location); and WHY (objectives/outcomes for correction action).

- Implement: Take the corrective action you have decided upon.

- Evaluate: Determine how and when you will evaluate the outcomes of the corrective action. One strategy is to reassess the deficit using the same assessment tool that identified the deficit.

Be sure to document and share results with appropriate individuals and continue to monitor the deficit to ensure that improved performance is sustained.

8. What role does benchmarking play in performance improvement?

8. Benchmarking allows you to measure an agency/organization's practices and services against those organizations that provide the "best practices and services." You can determine where your organization or department is on the quality scale. Your position on that scale can be used as a starting point from which you can measure progress toward higher quality.

9. Whom should I include when planning performance improvement activities?

9. Interdisciplinary teams should be involved in performance improvement activities to the degree possible. Specific individuals who may take an active part in planning performance improvement activities include:

- Staff development personnel or individuals who will assist with the corrective action

- Individuals representing areas where deficits have been identified

- CQI or TQI staff

- Nurse managers and/or representatives from nursing administration

- Vendors

- Individuals with expertise related to accrediting body, regulatory agency, or reimbursement guidelines

10. How do I set priorities?

10. Any deficit area that compromises patient safety (e.g., falls, medication errors) should receive highest priority. Routine monitoring areas that should receive priority include issues concerning:

- High risk and/or high volume procedures and processes

- Standards, accreditation, or regulatory agency compliance

- Problem prone procedures or processes

- Customer satisfaction

In setting priorities, you also need to look at the resources you have available to devote to the problem as well as the impact on quality if corrective action is taken. Those corrective actions that have the greatest impact on quality should receive the highest priority.

11. What should we teach everyone about performance improvement?

11. At the very least, everyone in the organization needs to know:

- How the organization defines performance improvement

- The goals of performance improvement

- How the organization defines quality

- The individual's role and responsibility related to performance improvement

- That performance improvement is a continuous and dynamic process essential to the organization

- How quality is measured, monitored, and evaluated

- Organizational activities implemented to improve performance

12. What is a reasonable amount of improvement to achieve?

12. Although we'd generally like to document 100% improvement after every corrective action taken, frequently this is not a realistic expectation. For example, we doubt that an organization will achieve a zero medication error rate or a 100% patient satisfaction score. Therefore, the organization or department must decide what an acceptable, achievable, and realistic degree of improvement is for any specific performance indicator of quality.

13. How often should performance be measured?

13. To determine how often performance should be measured, review guidelines established by accrediting agencies, regulatory bodies, and organizational policies and procedures. These guidelines and policies establish time frames for routine performance measurement. Annual monitoring may be sufficient for competency testing whereas monthly monitoring of patient falls may be mandated by hospital policy.

In addition, if any area has been identified as a deficit, performance needs to be measured more often than the established guideline or policy requires. Monitoring should continue until an acceptable level of performance has been achieved. Once the performance level has been achieved, monitoring can be resumed on the originally established time frame.

14. What tools/activities can be used to improve performance?

14. The most common activity to improve performance is an inservice class or other educational activity. Other methods include memos, counseling sessions, policies and procedures, bulletin boards, posters, and return demonstrations. The tool/activity used will depend on the type of information that needs to be conveyed and the outcome you want to achieve.

15. A program was implemented for an identified deficit and there was no performance improvement. What do I do now?

15. The educator and manager need to address whether or not the deficit was truly a performance deficit. If no performance improvement has occurred after implementation of corrective action, then you need to reassess. Is the deficit a process, structural, organizational, or motivational deficit? Depending on the reassessment, revision of the corrective action plan needs to occur.

16. How can I determine if a performance improvement activity was effective?

16. Observation of behavior, clinical competence, surveys, improved documentation, questionnaires, or interviews are some methods used to determined the effectiveness of a plan. One method involves using the same measurement or assessment tool that was used to discover poor or inadequate performance. Did a nursing audit discover a 20% medication error rate? If so, then repeat that audit after corrective action has been implemented. Compare medication error rates before and after corrective action. Did you achieve the desired performance level?

17. How can I measure the current status of a performance indicator or deficit?

17. Data need to be collected on the performance indicator. Data collection may take place during chart review/ audits, observation, patient/customer satisfaction surveys, patient/family complaints to patient advocate/ administration, staff complaints, accreditation surveys, utilization review, questionnaires, and peer reviews. Statistical and non-statistical tools can also be used. Statistical tools include run charts, histograms, control charts, scatter diagrams, and Pareto charts. Non-statistical tools include flow diagrams, fishbone diagrams, and cause-and-effect diagrams. The main concept is to look at performance indicators to assess for deficits.

18. How long after a performance improvement activity should outcome evaluation be performed?

18. Evaluation should not take place until staff has had enough time to improve performance; this may mean weeks or, in some cases, months. The key is to allow enough time for a change in behavior to occur. The timing of evaluation will also depend on whether the desired performance improvement is a knowledge, competency, attitude, or performance deficit. You must allow time for corrective action to be implemented, for behavior to change, and for reevaluation to occur.

19. What methods can be used to evaluate performance improvement outcomes?

19. Tools that can be used to evaluate performance improvement are the same ones used to assess and collect data on the performance indicator. After the corrective action/plan has been implemented, any of the tools can be used to evaluate whether outcomes have been met or performance improvement has occurred.

20. What is the role of leaders and managers in performance improvement? The role of the nurse? The role of the client?

20. Leaders and managers will often identify a performance deficit and include staff development in the performance improvement process. Management can give the necessary support to accomplish the corrective action/plan and identify the plan as a mandatory activity.

The nurse's role is to monitor and maintain quality care. In the performance improvement process nurses may identify the performance deficit, collect and monitor data, participate in the corrective action/plan, and evaluate and monitor performance.

The client is the internal customer of the organization. Clients are more knowledgeable about treatment choices and want more input in their care. Clients can and do make complaints and/or suggestions to improve performance and care.

RESOURCES

Huber, D. (2000). *Leadership and nursing care management* (3rd ed.). Philadelphia: W. B. Saunders.

Jeska, S. B., & Fischer, K. J. (1996). *Performance improvement in staff development: The next evolution*. Pensacola, FL: National Nursing Staff Development Organization.

Kelly Thomas, K. J. (1998). *Clinical and nursing staff development: Current competence, future focus* (2nd ed.). Philadelphia: Lippincott.

Marquis, B. L., & Huston, C. J. (2000). *Leadership roles and management functions in nursing: Theory and application* (3rd ed.). Philadelphia: Lippincott.

Yoder-Wise, P. S. (1999). *Leading and managing in nursing* (2nd ed.). St. Louis: Mosby.

Chapter 28: *Preceptor Development*

1. Why would anyone want to become a preceptor?

1. As I'm sure you are well aware, not every nurse wants to be a preceptor. Nurses who *do* want to serve in this capacity are usually those who enjoy both the professional as well as personal experiences involved with meeting new people, helping new staff feel at home / get accustomed to their unit, and providing any guidance and instruction their new colleague may need or request. Many nurses become preceptors just because they enjoy sharing their knowledge and skills with others or because they find helping to develop the next generation of nurses so satisfying. Precepting can also be edifying at times, reminding nurses of how much they do know and how skilled they are.

2. Although our facility desperately needs more preceptors, a number of nurses say that they are not interested in becoming a preceptor. How can I recruit these nurses to try this role?

2. Your potential for success here depends on the reason(s) why those nurses are refusing the invitation to join the preceptor ranks. Some of those reasons may be open to modification and others may not. If they are saying no because they lack self-confidence in their own skills or experience as a nurse when this not the case, that misperception could be readily corrected at a tripartite meeting with their manager and you. If they are saying no because they fear failure or feel inadequate as a teacher, you can assure them that all of the requisite capabilities can be developed in a preceptor development program. But if they are refusing the invitation because they simply do not want to be bothered with the added responsibilities of serving in this capacity, or because their firsthand observations suggest that nurses who volunteer to work as preceptors at that facility get too much patient care responsibility, too little staff or managerial support, and no appreciation of their efforts, then all of your recruitment attempts will most likely be in vain. Just as with all of us—they have to see "what's in it for me?" To successfully recruit new preceptors, they need to be convinced that the extra burdens imposed on them from this added role are "worth it" to them in some meaningful way.

3. I work in a 300-bed hospital where there is no preceptor development program for nurses, despite repeated requests from staff

3. The fundamental rationale for providing preceptor development programs is that the knowledge, attitudes, and skills required to function effectively as a preceptor are not the same or equivalent to those required to function effectively as a staff nurse. For example, providing direct patient care is not the same thing as

to provide this training. The "reason" that administration offers for denying our requests is that "nurses should be capable of teaching nursing to other nurses." I know that isn't the case, but am at a loss as to how to respond. Could you please reiterate the rationale (justification?) for providing training programs for preceptors?

4. We have a number of preceptors who are excellent as staff nurses, but who seem to have no facility whatsoever as preceptors, except to either "take over" clinical situations or to say something comparable to "watch me do this." What's the problem here? What can I do about this situation?

teaching and supervising others to provide that care; being responsible only for one's assigned patients is not equivalent to being responsible for your assigned patients as well as for the preceptee's assigned patients, and that preceptee's learning and development. Although serving as a role model is part of a preceptor's job, it does not encompass everything that a preceptor needs to know or be able to do. Preceptor training programs focus on developing those additional areas in which nurses need to be proficient to be effective as preceptors.

4. At least three possible causes may account for the situation you describe, so at least three avenues of response are possible. First, that nurse may never have developed the knowledge and skills needed to be an effective preceptor. This situation may be due to "grandfathering" of senior staff who had functioned as preceptors prior to initiation of a preceptor preparation program or to provision of an ineffective or poorly designed training program. The obvious solution to this situation is to provide an opportunity for the nurse to acquire and refine these skills via a thorough and quality training program. A second possible cause is that the nurse already possesses the requisite knowledge and skills needed by preceptors, but does not enjoy functioning in this capacity. Unless there is some way to build that nurse's interest, motivation, and/or level of satisfaction in precepting, there isn't much you can do about this situation. A third possible etiology is that the nurse's attitude at work is being negatively affected by circumstances unrelated to either skill in or desire to precept. The immediate cause may be anything that preoccupies the nurse's attention, diminishes the threshold and tolerance for expanded responsibilities, or interferes materially in the ability to do the job. Examples of such situations range from concerns over or caretaking burdens posed by a very ill or troubled child, spouse, parent or partner; coping with personal demons such as depression or substance abuse; or overwhelming issues related to financial problems or divorce.

5. What are the primary roles of a preceptor?

5. A preceptor has three primary roles: 1) staff nurse role model, involving emulation of how a nurse in this position is expected to perform the job; 2) socializer, who helps the new staff member integrate socially and professionally with the work group and employer; and as 3) educator, providing instructional assistance and support to the new staff members by helping them assess their orientation learning needs, plan appropriate learning experiences, implement their learning plan, and evaluate their job performance. Because the educator function spans all four phases of the instructional process, it may also be viewed as consisting of four sub-roles.

6. Is a preceptor the same as a mentor?

6. No, a preceptor and a mentor are not synonymous terms, although these roles share a number of features in common. For example, both refer to a knowledgeable, experienced, and highly skilled person assisting a less knowledgeable, experienced, and skilled colleague in developing the capabilities necessary for acquiring expertise in a particular field. Unlike the mentor, who typically works on a voluntary basis with the less experienced staff member for an extended period of time throughout career development, a preceptor's working relationship is not always voluntary in nature and typically extends only for the limited duration of that new staff member's orientation to that facility.

7. With this persisting shortage of nurses, our facility is now communicating that all RNs are expected to serve as preceptors as part of their professional responsibilities. Although this has not yet been formalized into a written policy, we are hearing intimations that our jobs will be on the line if we refuse to work in this capacity. What are the downsides to mandatory precepting?

7. Healthcare facilities that assume this posture toward the scope of an RN's job responsibilities are indicating that they are willing to sacrifice the long-term loyalties and contributions of senior staff nurses in order to achieve acute or persisting short-term staffing gains. Institutions already experiencing shortages of RNs would do well to not only avoid alienating their most precious staff resource, but rather, to add a generous set of incentives for more highly experienced RNs to work in this capacity and tangible forms of organizational appreciation for RNs who are willing to assist their employer by sharing their time, knowledge, and expertise with new employees. Unless orientation via preceptors is viewed and treated as an investment rather than as merely a task carrying a price tag, healthcare facilities that persist in using veiled threats and intimidation risk losing not only the senior staff they most need, but also the new staff members who

8. What kinds of incentives or recognitions could we award to celebrate the contributions of preceptors?

can see firsthand how professional nurses are treated at that facility.

8. Healthcare agencies have a wide variety of possible means for acknowledging the contributions of time, effort, and expertise that preceptors make. Monetary rewards include a meaningful pay differential (via a shift bonus, hourly differential, or higher base pay accorded for advancement on a career ladder). Educational incentives might include employer-paid attendance at national or regional continuing education conferences, paid educational leave days, paid membership in a professional nursing association of choice, paid subscription to a nursing journal of choice, a higher level of tuition assistance, or choice of any nursing book or audiovisual product. Other forms of recognition could include an annual luncheon or reception in preceptors' honor, preferences in regular or holiday scheduling, distinctive uniform scrub tops, distinctive name tags or lapel pins, wall plaques with names of all preceptors engraved, free garage parking space in designated area, free meal pass, and the like.

9. How can I keep preceptors motivated?

9. As you recall, motivation comes in two varieties: external and internal. As wonderful and valuable as all of the external rewards mentioned in the previous answer can be in affording preceptors some tangible indication that their efforts are acknowledged and appreciated, I truly don't know of any staff nurse who ever picked up the added responsibilities of precepting to ensure a seat at the annual chicken dinner in the hospital cafeteria or to have his/her name etched on a dusty hallway plaque. Without internal motivation, external incentives are merely tokens with minimal value. Internal motivation—derived from the satisfaction gained by helping to develop a new staff member, from the satisfaction of teaching, from the knowledge that you have made a difference in both the orientee's career and also in the quality of nursing care provided on that unit, and the like—is the primary driving force by which nurses decide whether serving as a preceptor is "worth it" to them. As an educator, you can facilitate this process by ensuring that the resources (e.g., time, patient access, teaching materials) and administrative supports (e.g., adequate staffing, ability to modify schedules or assignments when useful or necessary) that preceptors need to do their jobs well are in place. With your ongoing support, preceptors will generate their own internal motivation.

10. My employer has only offered a preceptor development program for the past few years, as the nursing shortage has worsened. During this time, we have operated largely on the "any warm body" approach to assigning staff nurses to work as preceptors. That strategy hasn't worked out very well, so we are now interested in identifying the criteria used to select preceptors. Can you mention a few of these criteria?

10. The most frequently used selection criteria for preceptors include:

- knowledge of nursing and of their specific job responsibilities as well as their employer's policies and procedures,

- effective interpersonal and communication skills, and

- clinical nursing skills and experience that enables them to provide nursing care and to troubleshoot common clinical situations in a competent and consistent manner.

In addition to the obvious need for preceptors to be clinically capable and professionally adept, other important personal attributes include:

- empathy and patience with others,

- being realistic in their expectations,

- respectful, open-minded, and mature in their manner, and

- having a healthy sense of humor.

The desire to function as a preceptor is fundamental to most of these traits.

11. Which aspect of the role is usually most problematic for preceptors and why?

11. Preceptors typically find their role as an evaluator of the orientee's clinical performance to be the most difficult aspect of their responsibilities. Unlike their functions as role model of the staff nurse position and as an assistant in socialization of the new staff member, which are familiar and comfortable to them, their role as evaluator is the least familiar and often the most daunting aspect of their job. Related sources of problems may be as follows:

- the discomfort experienced by preceptors when they need to offer feedback to correct or improve an orientee's performance,

- when they are having professional disagreements over the acceptability of an orientee's practice,

- whenever an orientee gets angry, defensive, impatient, arrogant, or condescending toward them, or

- when their appraisal delays that new staff member from independently taking on a full workload and contributing to staffing on the unit.

12. How can preceptors support the special needs of new graduate preceptees?

12. When the nurse preceptee is a new graduate, preceptors can respond to the preceptee's special needs by recalling the insights that Marlene Kramer provided regarding new nurses in the publication titled *Reality Shock.* As you recall, Kramer identified four stages of reality shock that new graduates progressively experience: honeymoon, shock, recovery, and resolution. Healthcare facilities that welcome new graduate nurses need to have preceptor development programs that include an explanation of each phase of reality shock and how to recognize it, as well as strategies that preceptors can use to assist new graduates through satisfactory resolution of each phase.

13. Preceptors often request some feedback on how well they are doing. What kind of feedback should be provided and by whom?

13. Preceptors should anticipate receiving feedback related to various aspects of their performance so that they can determine whether they are functioning at, below, or above others' expectations of them. A majority of this feedback would be based on how effectively they fulfill the duties and responsibilities delineated in the preceptor's job description. The job description for this position would, in turn, specify the preceptor's responsibilities to the orientee and distinguish preceptor duties from those of other staff who participate in the orientation program. Feedback may be sought not only from each orientee being assisted, but also from the educator or coordinator responsible for developing and supporting preceptors in their role, the nurse manager of the clinical area, and possibly, peers and other staff nurses. At some healthcare institutions, preceptors may also complete self-appraisals of their performance in this role.

14. Are there stages of expertise that a preceptor will achieve?

14. As with any other type of skilled performance, preceptors practice their craft at various levels of practice that may range from a level comparable to the Beginner to that of the Expert in Benner's Novice-to-Expert model. For example, a preceptor functioning at the Beginner level may be able to recognize a few of the principles of adult education, but not be able to consistently translate those principles into actions with preceptees. Likewise, in correcting some aspect of an orientee's practice, preceptors can vary markedly in the facility with which they identify, modify, and improve that practice so that it coincides with the facility's expectations. In contrast to preceptors who function at the Advanced Beginner or Competent levels and manage potential errors only as they are recognized and evidenced, those at the Expert level of preceptor practice have the knowledge, skills, and experience to anticipate many areas that new staff will find problematic and plan learning experiences to ensure that those performance areas are addressed.

15. What happens if a preceptor gets pulled back into staffing?

15. Two of the fundamental resources that preceptors need to do their job are sufficient time to work with the new staff member and immediate availability to the preceptee. When preceptors are yanked out of their role as preceptors to cover staffing inadequacies, they are no longer truly or immediately available to the preceptee and their professional loyalties are forcibly split between the patients they are personally assigned to and the orientee they are supposed to assist. Because patients' lives and welfare often depend on the nurse's ministrations, patient care needs virtually always and necessarily take precedence over the orientee's educational needs. The preceptor can neither be in two places at one time nor deal with competing sets of work priorities at the same time. Common outcomes of this situation include a frustrated, thwarted, and fearful preceptor who is hoping that the orientee inflicts no harm on patients and a frustrated, angry, and insecure orientee who feels that he/she cannot trust the preceptor will be available when needed and who feels "hung out to dry" to fend for herself/himself by the new employer. Either situation is potentially detrimental to patient care and plants the seeds for either or both nurses to consider finding a new employer that actually supports rather than forsakes simultaneous needs of both staffing and orientation.

16. What do I do about a preceptor who just isn't working out?

16. The most effective approach to managing this situation is via basic problem solving. First and foremost, it will be necessary for the nurse educator to identify and verify the nature and extent of the performance problem(s) as explicitly as possible. This amounts to defining what "just isn't working out" refers to. What is the specific nature of the preceptor's deficiency(ies)? In which and how many of the preceptor's roles does the problem exist? Once the nature and extent of the performance problem has been identified and validated with the preceptor, the next step is to work with the preceptor to determine the source or cause of the problem. Is the problem due to a lack of knowledge and/or skills necessary to function competently as a preceptor? Is the problem attributable to the preceptor's attitude or demeanor? Or is the problem caused by circumstances outside of the preceptor's control (e.g., that the preceptor is simultaneously assigned to serve as charge nurse for that shift or simultaneously expected to carry a heavy patient workload in addition to serving as a preceptor)? Once the source of the problem is distinguished, the remedy is usually easy to discern: if the source is a need for instruction or practice, these can be readily provided; if the source is unrealistic expectations that the nurse can function effectively in two roles simultaneously, the unit manager needs to decide which of the two competing sets of priorities (staffing, precepting) will take precedence at that time. If the etiology of the preceptor's problem is not something amenable to instruction (e.g., if the preceptor is preoccupied with some stressor such as a parent's increasing need for caregiving or if the preceptor truly dislikes serving in that role and/or lacks the temperament, patience, or interest to serve in that capacity), then a temporary or permanent lifting of preceptor duties would seem warranted.

17. What is the "Preceptor's Bill of Rights?" the "Preceptee's Bill of Rights?"

17. Each role in the preceptor-preceptee relationship has a set of rights as well as responsibilities that need to be recognized and respected. Historically, orientation programs and the preceptor's role in the program have primarily emphasized the full spectrum of preceptor's responsibilities to the orientee and have virtually neglected the reciprocal set of rights that the preceptor should be able to rely on if expected to fulfill obligations to the preceptee. The *Preceptor's Bill of Rights* (Alspach 2000a, 2000b) represents a summary of the rights that preceptors should be afforded to enable them to do their job. These rights represent forms of administrative and/or educational support that need to be in place to facilitate the preceptor's work. Similarly, the *Preceptee's Bill of Rights* (Alspach 2000a, 2000b) represents a reciprocal set of the rights that each preceptee (orientee) is owed in this relationship.

18. What is the preceptor's responsibility when the orientee is just not progressing satisfactorily?

18. When an orientee is not completing orientation in a satisfactory manner, the preceptor is a convenient and frequently used target for blame, particularly when staffing shortages are acute and pervasive. Although it is easy for other staff or managers to play this "blame game," it is rooted in the false assumption that it is the preceptor's job to get the preceptee oriented. Successful preceptorships, by contrast, are managed with the clear and mutual understanding that it is the *orientee's* responsibility to complete orientation. The preceptor's responsibility in this situation is to facilitate this process to the maximum extent possible. When progress in an orientee's performance is lagging, the preceptor works with the orientee to determine the nature and cause(s) of this situation, to determine an appropriate instructional remedy, and to verify whether performance has satisfactorily improved. If the preceptor is unable to identify or resolve whatever obstacles are limiting the orientee's progress, the preceptor's responsibility extends to securing assistance from the nurse educator or manager, as appropriate. The nurse educator who provides instructional and ongoing support to preceptors is responsible for monitoring the preceptor/preceptee relationship and for identifying and resolving any orientee performance problems attributable to an ineffective preceptor.

19. The hospital won't give us more than four hours to prepare staff to function as preceptors. How can I modify the development program to deal with this restriction?

19. Whether you are using a published program to prepare preceptors or need to design your own program for this purpose, review or develop an outline of content and learning activities as well as an estimate of time that each requires. Then reach consensus among nurse managers, educators, and experienced preceptors on which content and instructional activities are of highest priority for meeting learning needs and for completion within the time available. After the priority instructional areas have been designated for the four-hour training program, nurse educators can plan to provide instruction in the remaining areas as part of a continuing support program for preceptors.

20. In addition to just asking, how else can a preceptor determine what an orientee's learning needs are?

20. Other means for identifying a preceptee's orientation learning needs include the following:

- Encouraging the preceptee to ask questions

- Listening carefully to the nature of questions the preceptee asks

- Reviewing the preceptee's résumé

- Observing the preceptee's clinical practice

- Reviewing orientation evaluation tools with the preceptee

- Having the preceptee complete a self-appraisal of needs relative to the expected outcomes of orientation

- Having preceptee complete a battery of written tests, computer-assisted scenarios, or laboratory simulations

Of these, the most valid means of assessing preceptees' learning needs is through observation of their clinical practice.

21. As a preceptor, how do I decide where to start in orienting new staff?

21. Since preceptorships are conducted as cooperative endeavors between preceptor and preceptee, this issue can be decided by one of these participants or by a simple negotiation between the two parties. Because orientees are adult learners, they should be granted as much discretion as possible in making decisions such as these. In this context, the preceptee may have specific preferences of starting points they would like to use (e.g., starting with familiar and simple aspects of care before advancing to less familiar and more complex aspects). If the orientee either has no preferences or wishes to defer to the preceptor's guidance, possible starting points might include clinical priorities of care, a typical patient course from admission to discharge, phases of the nursing process, and the like. As long as all performance areas that need to be verified are completed, the order in which this is accomplished is generally not important.

22. Nursing has used preceptors to orient new staff for many generations, but this practice is foreign to most other hospital departments. Why are other hospital departments now training and using preceptors for this purpose?

22. Historically, nursing has been a service that has nurtured its new graduates and new employees for extended periods of orientation. I've never been convinced that nursing is the only health profession that fails to fully prepare its practitioners for the realities of its work, but we seem to be the only profession with an established tradition of lengthy forms and varieties of orientation programs. Where nursing has, perhaps, tended toward the use of protracted programs for staff orientation, departments other than nursing have, traditionally, offered little or no substantive orientation program to new staff.

Changes in that situation began when the Joint Commission extended the requirement for verification of staff competency from applying only to the nursing department to applying to all hospital services. Suddenly, managers of those departments needed to provide some form of documentation of initial and ongoing competency of staff, so the use of preceptors to provide and document staff competency has become more prevalent. As a result, many hospital educators now find it necessary to provide comparable training programs for preceptors throughout the agency. An additional contributor to this practice has been the merging of nursing education and inservice departments into staff development services now responsible for hospital- or system-wide orientation and competency verification.

23. What is a reasonable amount of experience someone should have before precepting?

23. The answer to your question is, I believe, more legitimately measured by a nurse's performance rather than by the number of months or years that the nurse has occupied a particular position. As you recall from Benner's "Novice-to-Expert" model, nurses at the two most fundamental levels of nursing practice (novice, advanced beginner) are still functioning on the basis of very general guidelines, still struggling with consistently discerning (more versus less) relevant clinical data, still stymied when clinical situations differ from what they anticipated, and still quite capable of demonstrating clinical performance that is marginal in quality. Not until a nurse is functioning at least at a competent level of practice is that nurse in any realistic position to serve as a role model to a new staff member. At the competent level of nursing practice, the RN is able to both manage and modify practice for a variety of clinical situations that deviate from textbook norms, to work in an organized and efficient manner, to interrelate effectively with patients, family, other nurses, physicians, and other departments, and to be confident in the ability to handle the great majority of clinical scenarios. As Benner pointed out, most nurses require two to three years of clinical experience with the same or comparable patient populations before they practice at a competent level, but the calendar is no guarantee that this level of practice has been either attained or maintained. Some nurses will need more time to attain that level of practice, others will need less time, and

24. What kind of ongoing support should be in place for preceptors?

24. still others may never quite maintain that level of practice on a consistent basis.

In addition to providing both educational and administrative support during the course of each preceptorship, both of these avenues of support need to be provided in an ongoing manner. Continuing educational support may consist of regularly scheduled instructional sessions that address topics relevant to preceptors' work that are not included in the preceptor development program. These topics might include in-depth coverage of cognitive styles or learning style preferences, applying Benner's model to orientation programs, or more advanced topics related to creative clinical teaching techniques. In addition to these informal instructional programs, time needs to be allotted for preceptors to ask questions and to resolve problems that may arise during preceptorship programs. Ongoing educational support for preceptors can benefit by joining preceptors from many clinical fields together to share ideas and solutions to common issues. Preceptor motivation and support are also aided by the provision of continuous administrative support in the form of adequate time to do their jobs, intermittent assignment to this role to avoid burnout, necessary relief from their customary workload, and the support of their peers. Healthcare facilities that genuinely appreciate the work of preceptors find monetary and/or other tangible ways to express that appreciation.

REFERENCES

Alspach, J. G. (2000a). *A preceptor training program for professional healthcare staff—Instructor's manual*. Aliso Viejo, CA: American Association of Critical-Care Nurses. (Related materials include *Preceptor Handbook,* color transparencies, CD-ROM of PowerPoint files of visuals.)

Alspach, J. G. (2000b). *From staff nurse to preceptor: A preceptor development program—Instructor's manual* (2ⁿᵈ ed.). Aliso Viejo, CA: American Association of Critical Care Nurses. (Related materials include *Preceptor Handbook,* color transparencies, CD-ROM of PowerPoint files of visuals.)

RESOURCES

Alspach, J. G. (1995). *The educational process in nursing staff development*. St. Louis: Mosby.

Benner, P. (1984). *From novice to expert*. Menlo Park, CA: Addison-Wesley.

Kramer, M. (1974). *Reality shock: Why nurses leave nursing*. St. Louis: Mosby.

Chapter 29: *Humor in Teaching*

1. *Can humor teach?*

1. Somewhere in time, humanity has forgotten that humor is a very powerful teaching tool. Many old world parables were written with the intent that they be funny. Scholars knew they had to capture the attention of students, and humor was the only technical device available. With the advent of television, computers, and all the other modern devices available to distract learners, we now find ourselves looking for new avenues to capture learners' attention. Humor helps to do that.

2. *What's funny?*

2. What's funny to one person may be annoying to another. Since there is no universal code of humor, it's hard to say exactly what's funny. Keep in mind that humor is highly relative. Years ago, NBC's "Saturday Night Live" aired a skit entitled "If Eleanor Roosevelt Could Fly?" The image of Eleanor Roosevelt leading Allied bombers on raids over Germany during World War II was hysterical to my eight months pregnant wife. She laughed so hard at that skit, tears flowed freely from her eyes and she could not catch her breath. The other ten people in the room watching were not even amused.

3. *What kinds of humor are there?*

3. There are three basic forms of humor: physical humor, spontaneous humor, and jokes. Physical humor involves the application of a physical movement or action. Lucille Ball performed lots of physical humor on her television show. Falling over an ottoman or a pie in the face can be funny. Spontaneous humor involves reaction. On the Carol Burnett Show, many of the skit performers broke into laughter because one or two of the performers flubbed their lines, sending others and the audience into laughter. Jokes are funny short stories or one-line questions that require a punch line.

4. *What kind of humor should I use?*

4. When trying to incorporate humor into the classroom, use the form of humor with which you are most familiar. Start small. No person expects you to entertain him/her for ninety minutes. Many of my own attempts at humor fall short of my expectations. Keep reminding yourself you are an educator. It's the class that wants to be entertained. It's your job to find the middle ground.

5. *How do I become comfortable using humor?*

5. To borrow a marketing phrase from a popular athletic shoe, "Just do it!" After a while, it will become second nature. Using humor will begin to feel natural. On the rare occasion you don't use humor, you will miss it.

6. When is humor appropriate?

6. Humor can be best used at the beginning and end of sessions. In the beginning, you want to focus attention and a humorous moment will help to accomplish that. As a closing, a humorous activity will have participants leaving with a smile. Keep in mind that spontaneous humor can happen at any moment. Looking at this question from another perspective, the content must drive the humor we use, not be driven. Use of humor at the expense or the misfortune of others is inappropriate.

7. What are the benefits of using humor?

7. When I was a young boy and would get in trouble, if I could get my parents to laugh, my punishment was usually not as severe. I tried to keep them laughing. Humor can do many things besides reduce anger. It can also reduce stress and that is one of the obstacles to learning. Humor also serves as a method to refocus attention in the classroom. When a participant's brain wanders, a funny moment will get him/her back and engaged. It also can be used when the energy of the group is waning. Humor adds energy to the group.

8. I'm no good at telling jokes; can I still use humor?

8. By all means, use humor. My mother would ruin every joke she heard. Either she remembered every fact up to but excluding the punch line, or she missed the important fact that made the joke funny, but got the punch line right. But she was a very funny person. Why? Because she found herself in some of the funniest situations imaginable. The stories that she told were hysterical because they were real and you could relate to them. Find out what you do best, and stick to it.

9. If I use humor, will I lose control of my class?

9. The possibility exists, although slim, so use humor sparingly. After all, we are educators teaching professionals or future professionals, so our primary focus is educating participants, not performing a sixty-minute monologue.

10. Will humor lessen the importance of my content?

10. No! Important content is just that. What humor will do is frame that content so that everyone knows that the content is important. The application of humor will wake participants up so that they hear the important content.

11. I don't normally think of myself as funny, so how do I become funny?

11. Your audience may already think you are funny. Now, take a deep breath. Relax, and think of one thing that happened in your life that you found funny. Not amusing, downright funny. Now share it with a friend or co-worker. Did you get a smile? Laugh? Chuckle? Don't look now, but you're funny! Now just apply humor in small doses to content and let it grow.

12. *How do I handle the audience's laughing and I haven't a clue why?*

12. Just smile, pretend like you said or did that on purpose, and go on. Don't ever ask for an explanation because the moment or situation will lose its humor. You really did want that reaction. The audience will not know differently unless you tell them.

13. *Where do I find things that will make me funny?*

13. Start looking right under your nose. Dress using a theme for the day, or use different pointers on an overhead. Exciting overheads, cartoons, and quotes are all sources of humor you can incorporate. There are numerous books available with copyright-free humor for educational purposes. Just ask about the copyrights before using. Nobody likes being visited by the copyright police in the middle of an educational session.

14. *Can I overuse humor?*

14. Yes. When humor is used too much, you cease being an educator and become a stand up comic. Students don't have a lot of money to tip well, so keep the humor fresh and in small amounts, and you will find the experience rewarding. (You still won't get many tips.)

15. *Can humor solve all my teaching problems?*

15. Well, humor hasn't cured the common cold, balanced the national budget, or eliminated terrorism, but it has kept us laughing, and when you can laugh, your problems don't seem so big.

16. *What's the most important thing to remember about using humor?*

16. There may not be a universal code on humor, but there is one thing all people do, no matter their race, creed or occupation, national origin or ethics. We all laugh. Use humor to unify your own part of the world.

Section 7:
New Approaches to Staff Development

At one point, our focus was on audiovisuals, but it is now on media and technology. Although we still teach with overhead projectors and VCRs, there is room now for computers and patient simulators. It is difficult to discern whether increased technology has fostered creative approaches to teaching or whether decreased human resources have led to increased use of technology. Nevertheless, these creative approaches are yielding good results and opening new pathways for learning. This section is intended to introduce a variety of concepts and strategies to consider in an electronic era.

Chapter 30: *Selecting Technology*

1. My supervisor suggests we use more technology. Where do I get started?

1. The first step in using technology is to determine the objectives and goals for using it. Will this new technology be used to disseminate information, make testing more efficient, provide video instruction, or a combination of all of these?

   Once you have determined what the needs are, find out more about the types of programs available by contacting vendors for demonstrations, or by polling facilities similar to yours regarding their use and opinions of equipment.

2. There is a lot of talk about the Internet. Should I consider other options such as CAI on diskettes or CD-ROM, laser discs, closed circuit TV (CCTV)?

2. All of these options play a significant role in getting information out among large populations. Although the Web-based learning program you choose may be excellent for those familiar with Internet-based functions, there will be others who are more comfortable with disc drive operations or CD-ROM, and thus, more inclined to use them. While laser discs may already be outdated, CCTV, with its ability to easily adjust program menus, may be one of the best ways to keep people abreast of current topics.

3. Can I mix different technologies?

3. Mixing different technologies is not only possible, it is preferable because it better meets the learning styles of a broader audience. As stated above, people have various preferences and comfort levels around technology, and will be more apt to use the one with which they feel the most familiar. However, caution should be used when mixing technologies to ensure the facility has the means to support the additions (e.g., network servers accommodating simultaneous users, licensing fees for large numbers of users), and to minimize redundancies within the programs that you are opting to use.

4. What should I do with the old equipment and software?

4. There are three major ways in which to dispose of old equipment.

   - **Recycle.** Probably the most efficient plan for old equipment is to recycle it within the organization. Keyboards, monitors, and even terminal parts can be used with other systems.

   - **Donate.** Donating is another great way to get the most from equipment that may be outdated for you, but not for another institution, such as the local school district.

   - **Disposal.** Dispose of equipment in an environmen-

279

tally approved fashion. Components may contain lead or other compounds and should not be deposited in landfills.

Software can also be donated or recycled, but be sure to include the original license, so that the recipient is within the copyright guidelines of the manufacturer.

5. *What is a Learning Management System (LMS)?*

5. A Learning Management System is a comprehensive approach to e-learning. These systems generally include:

- tracking capabilities

- course management tools such as roster, information access, and testing

- technology to allow for discussion threads, chat features, and video streaming

a) Why would I need an LMS?

A good LMS will assist you in maximizing resources by automating records. If you need to track training for a large number of employees or students, these systems are ideal. Learning management systems also provide the most rapid processing available. They are excellent in providing updated information to the audience in the shortest amount of time. Since the information is Web-based, bulletins, policies, and modules can be uploaded in minutes for same day viewing and interaction. A good program will also interface with other systems, providing access to information you would otherwise not have. In addition, organization analysis, quality improvement information, and course categorization can be developed using a LMS.

b) What about a tracking system for training? Is this part of a good technology purchase?

A comprehensive tracking system should be an integral part of any training program. Tracking provides necessary documentation for training and is crucial to increasing efficiency, especially in a healthcare organization where regulatory agencies influence record keeping. A good system will have components of documentation that include the following:

- ability to build a comprehensive database for staff and all training attended

- ability to electronically alert the author of use by

a specific individual (this allows for checking proficiency if there is an evaluation or testing component involved)

- ability to provide credit to the individual upon completion, and also the exact time involved in taking the test.

6. What is an Application Service Provider (ASP)? Do I need it for implementation on the Web?

6. An ASP is a somewhat recent approach to providing service to purchasers of programs. For facilities with inadequate server capacity to use a desired program, the manufacturer can base the program on its own system, and the users access it from the Internet. If you have adequate support for the program, you can access it from your own server, rather than relying on the manufacturer. The decision is ultimately one of resources and preferred service. For those institutions with a large Information Services (IS) department, service may not be an issue, but others may opt to focus on access only, and allow the manufacturer to house, service, and update the purchased program.

7. I'm a clinician at heart. How can I learn about all these educational technologies?

7. Ask to participate in distance education, clinical informa-tion system, IS, or purchasing meetings where technological decisions are made. It is to these audiences that the vendors will most likely be providing marketing and presentations. If this is not possible, ask a resource in the facility for a brief update on the direction of technology and do an Internet search of the topic. This will not only point you to explanations and definitions, but the major names in technology in the industry will become evident.

8. Once we decide on a technology, how can we choose a vendor?

8. Once the technology is decided upon, using a Web search, attending a vendor fair, or asking a similar facility about its experiences can help identify possible vendors. Vendors are also very willing to come to an institution to present their programs. It is helpful to have a core group of people, who may be invested in making a decision regarding technology, to preview several similar programs from different vendors.

One of the most important aspects in choosing technology is to determine the amount of vendor support available following the purchase. Ask a lot of questions to ascertain what the exact contractual agreement states for training. Does inservice training involve one or two sessions only, with costly charges for revisits? Are travel, lodging, and per diem costs the responsibility of the purchaser? Is there an annual support fee? If telephone support is available, what are the hours of operation, and will that benefit you should it be in distant time zones?

In addition, you will want to know about updates. How often are updates provided? Are updates for the first year free of charge? When is the next update anticipated? Depending on the needs of the facility, getting the most information possible regarding training can prevent an extremely costly (not to mention frustrating) decision should implementation fail due to lack of training and support.

9. *How can I make sure that I don't end up with obsolete technology?*

9. By adequately researching the programs that you are interested in, seeking counsel from experts, and forming a task force to help balance decision making, you can usually be assured that your technological choices will be competitive. Unfortunately, one of the hazards in choosing technology is that programs can quickly become obsolete following purchase and implementation. This is more an effect of continually improving technology rather than a weakness in the system of choice. A common mistake in choosing technology is inadequate information regarding the ability to support it once implemented. For successful long-term use of new technology, you must ensure that it will fit within the infrastructure of the institution. Both the potential vendor and the IS department can work to ensure that the fit is a good one.

10. *Courses offered by vendors are fine, but many times we have very special learning needs. What can we do to make these courses more applicable to desired learning outcomes?*

10. Here are a few options:

a) Ask the vendor to customize the inservice classes to meet special learning needs. This may require working together to educate the vendor regarding what the special needs are and why it is essential to meet them.

b) If the vendor is unable to alter the training package, supplementing the inservice session with literature that relates to the facility will help bridge the gap between the training you receive and the training needed.

c) While it may seem costly, designing specialized training using the experts in IS and clinical areas often is the best way to implement a system with the highest usage and compliance. You can negotiate with the vendor to subtract training and transportation from your costs, which will offset the cost of using staff. Ultimately, conversion may be more seamless based on the familiarity of the teachers with the institution and its needs.

d) Preview pre-packaged modules that can be loaded onto your system for use in the organization. Keep in mind licensing requirements and additional costs when choosing this option.

11. How can I convince administrators to invest enough in learning technology?

11. *Do your homework.* Sounds simple, but presenting a request for a significant purchase should always be prefaced with a comprehensive cost benefit versus risk analysis report. The best technologies available will not be cost effective if they don't fit the needs of the organization. Include projections specifically related to the organization. Why do you need this program? If the issue is risk management related to insufficient training, emphasize how the desired program will not only improve performance and staff satisfaction, but also reduce incidents and liabilities.

12. What are the most important steps in implementing a new learning technology?

12. The implementation of a new learning technology can be an exciting yet challenging endeavor. Many of the steps are equally vital to the success of the implementation. These are: analysis, planning, implementation, support and development, and transition.

13. Who should be on the implementation team?

13. Many disciplines should be represented on the implementation team. Administrators are effective with such processes because of their authority and decision-making abilities, which can be useful in propelling the project forward. Educators are proficient in need identification, developing initial and subsequent training schedules, and training evaluation. Naturally, Information Services staff need to be involved. These staff members are exceptionally knowledgeable regarding not only the newly purchased program, but the existing mainframe and collateral technology available. Vendors should be available, if not present on the team, to answer questions and receive feedback. While often excluded, it is important to include administrative support staff on the implementation team as they are often the highest users and can help train and encourage other staff in the transition.

14. How can I market new learning technologies to staff?

14. Beta testing or trials are the best ways to market to specific populations. This can be done either by setting up the program as it would be used in the area and providing vendor support, or by providing guest passwords and use through the program server. In a testing arena, comprehensive evaluation is essential to define potential problem areas. Once a program is purchased, incentives will help motivate staff to convert to the new technology. Another way to support staff is to develop user groups. These are comprised of one or two representatives from each unit. This group represents the areas converting to the new program. They meet at intervals with IS staff or the vendor to identify problems, provide feedback, and receive support to help them to better assist their co-workers.

15. We have many employees with limited computer skills. What can I do to support them?

15. Encourage practice, practice, and practice! The more online opportunities available, the faster and more proficient students will become. Vendor inservice classes are available, at least initially, and if the facility has an education and IS department, these departments should be able to provide additional inservice classes, and literature to support computer literacy. Pairing expert with novice staff may help improve the students' skills. Many programs have internal help features that can answer questions, provide short tutorials, or demonstrate various functions, as well.

16. Once a learning technology is implemented, how can I keep the momentum going?

16. A good program will ultimately catch on and maintain its own momentum, however, in the beginning, there are some things you can do to prevent staff from reverting back to familiarity. Change or continuous development is important to keep the interest of the users. For experienced staff, the same pages, modules, and information will not attract them back to the site. For a program to be effective, it must be used. This is best accomplished by continual updates of information. If the facility does not support continual training, post committee minutes, newsletters, accomplishments, interactive Q/A, or a weekly message from the CEO to keep staff interested and using the technology. This will help to keep staff experienced, comfortable, and ultimately more compliant with the process.

RESOURCES

Chapman, L. (2001). Distance learning in nursing. *Seminars in Oncology Nursing, 17*(1), 48–54.

Kaas, M. J., Block, D. E., Avery, M., Lindeke, L., Kubik, M., Duckette, L., & Vellenga, B. (2001). Enhancing traditional, televised, and videotaped courses with Web-based technologies: A comparison of student satisfaction. *Nursing Outlook, 49*(3), 132–137.

www.dailyprincetonian.com/Content/2001/12/04/news/1421.shtml

www.e-learninghub.com/Selecting_an_LMS.html

www.thejournal.com/magazine/vault/A3753.cfm

Chapter 31: *Integrating Technology Choices Into Practice*

1. *Why would I want to use media when I teach?*

1. There are several reasons why you might want to consider using media in the classroom. First and foremost, each learner has a unique style of learning. Some learn better by taking notes while others may find it easier to learn if they watch a video. As instructors, we should try to meet as many learners' learning styles as possible.

   Secondly, research has shown that when media are used in a teaching-learning activity, the learners have an easier time learning and they retain more of the information. Remember, learners remember 20% of what they hear, 50% of what they see and hear, and 80% of what they see, hear, and do.

   Keep in mind, too, that media appeal to today's visually oriented society. Some media appeal to the learners' entertainment sensibilities and many learners expect technological support in the classroom.

2. *When you talk about the use of technology in teaching, exactly what are you talking about?*

2. I usually mean just about any medium that will enhance my teaching capabilities and learners' learning abilities. In addition to the equipment itself, I also consider the way I use the equipment to teach. So, for me, the list includes simple equipment like blackboards and handouts. Not flashy enough for you? Remember, once upon a time the typewriter and the phonograph were considered the latest in technology! Today, there is much in the way of multimedia for us to use to enhance teaching including but certainly not limited to:

   - Flip charts
   - Paper and electronic handouts
   - Black and white boards
   - Overhead transparencies and projectors
   - 35 mm slides and projectors
   - Motion pictures (big screen)
   - Computer-based presentations (computer disk and CD-ROM)
   - Internet and Web-based programs including chat rooms and instant polling
   - Video cameras and tapes (live and canned)

- Audiotapes

- Television (standard and cable)

- Patient simulators

While technology has become very valuable and almost expected in the classroom, you should always choose the media that truly enhance your teaching and fit you as the presenter, as well as the learners, and the content matter.

3. How does technology change the way I teach?

3. Technology certainly does not eliminate work for you. It may move you from the forefront of the classroom to the background of the material being presented. Using technology means time looking for media to enhance content or maybe even turning out a product of your own like a video or slides.

Technology does not change the principles of adult learning but in fact underscores some of them—like self-paced learning, individual learning styles, and interactivity. The advantages of using technology in the classroom should be obvious. Technology allows content to be delivered in a variety of formats, is self-paced, and almost always allows visual learners to "see" the content. It can make the learning experience extremely interactive.

4. Will using media make teaching easier?

4. I wouldn't necessarily equate using technology with easier teaching. In fact, when you run into problems with the technology you are using, it could make your job a lot harder. Also, if not used correctly you can wind up with an awful presentation and more headaches than you bargained for.

There is quite a bit of preparation that goes into the use of media, above and beyond the normal preparation for a learning activity. It takes time and careful consideration to select the proper technology for a learning activity.

Remember to weave the media into the presentation. Introduce the technology and explain it to keep the audience focused on you and to make sure that the message you wish to convey through the technology is on target.

Having said that, I would have to admit that when everything goes right, using media in learning activities will make your job fun and will probably make learning easier for students, which in the end does make your job easier. Remember, the media are not meant to be a substitution for teaching but an enhancement. Be sure that you keep that in mind when selecting the appropriate technology for learning activities.

5. How do I choose the appropriate medium to integrate into a learning activity?

5. As with any learning activity, begin by identifying the topic, the audience, the learning objectives, and the best method for delivering the content.

Identifying the audience goes beyond whether there is a homogenous group in terms of education and experience. When choosing media you really need to think about the learners and the type of technology they are used to using in their everyday lives.

Next, you need to consider the learning objectives and decide which available technology would be the best way to enhance the content you are planning to present. For example, if you want to identify reasons teenagers smoke, then you might decide to show a video tape of teens interviewing teens who smoke.

6. How many media should I integrate into one activity?

6. The number of different media that you integrate into one learning activity depends on the information you are trying to convey to learners and the best way to convey that information to them. This being said, it is a good idea to keep it simple and not to go overboard by using too many different media in one session. If you do, you could very well wind up distracting learners. Remember that you are using the media to convey the information in the best way possible to supplement and complement content.

There is one place, however, where you should have any and all technology available to learners and that would be in a learning lab. Learners can then select a method of choice. But in an organized classroom setting, choose the minimum number of appropriate technologies to meet the needs of the majority of learners.

7. How can I become more comfortable using media in my classroom?

7. Be familiar with how the equipment works. Get comfortable with the equipment. Learn how it works, troubleshoot common problems, replace parts like bulbs and batteries, and know what all the buttons are for.

The second, third, and fourth things you can do are practice, practice, practice. Practicing your presentation while using the technology will allow you to identify possible glitches that might occur during class.

Do you have colleagues who are comfortable with the use of media in the classroom? If so, ask them to sit through your practice session and give you tips on troubleshooting problems as they come up. If none come up during the practice session, ask these colleagues to identify some commonly occurring problems that might present themselves and the easiest ways to fix them.

On the day of class, arrive at the classroom early and test everything. Have a contingency plan to fall back on. Be prepared to switch to another tactic if the equipment fails. For example, if you are using a laptop, be prepared with a backup disk of the presentation in case the disk is the problem or an alternate technology like overheads or a flip chart that you can use in case the laptop malfunctions.

Finally, don't ever be dependent on media. Instead always be prepared to continue the lesson without it. Remember that the media you use are supposed to enhance the presentation, not be a substitute for it. So, know and be comfortable with the content you are going to deliver. If you don't rely too heavily on the media to carry you through the presentation you won't be devastated if it fails to work.

8. There are so many media available today. How do I know which one is best to use in my learning activities?

8. Whenever someone asks me a question about choosing media for teaching, I think back to a media class I took in graduate school—"The medium is the message." Those words by Marshall McLuhan, well-known Canadian communications theorist, and his work illustrate the idea that each medium creates its own environment and affects the brain in a distinct way.

Keeping that thought in mind, you want to select a medium that will not only do the job or convey the information but if possible one that will also augment the information you are trying to convey. In addition, you want to choose, if possible, a medium that will match the preferred learning style of learners. This is not always an easy task, especially if you are limited in choice by availability, budget, or portability considerations.

These are some quick notes about a variety of media to help you make better decisions when choosing a medium to use in classroom:

- Flip charts are a simple method of information delivery that are economical, portable, and can accommodate audience participation. Creating a flip chart presentation is as simple as opening up a few colored markers.

- Print is one of the oldest media available to us. It is excellent for details and reference. While some of us may believe that few people prefer this medium, it is the most traditional way of providing information and is still used today in the form of textbooks, handouts, and other printed materials that accompany other media like videos and audiotapes. Global concepts and issues are best taught using print-based charts and graphs that allow the learner to really visualize important connections.

- Video is a good choice for many younger learners who have grown up watching videos. Using video to present psychomotor skills, new strategies, and mandatory employee training works well since they are portable and don't always need an accompanying instructor. Videos (or movies), when projected on a large screen in a darkened room, can draw learners into the experience and are especially good for allowing learners to get in touch with their feelings (affective domain).

- Audiotapes are good for sound recognition like lung or heart sounds.

- Overheads are easy to create and use and are relatively inexpensive. They work well with simple images, and research has shown that instructors who use them are perceived to be approachable and down to earth. They are ideal in settings where you want to provide enough light so that students can take notes.

- 35mm slides are best to use when you need realistic color and details like in anatomy, radiology, and medicine. Since slides are presented in still frames, they are good delivery method for retention of fact patterns.

- Computers, software, and projectors are good for high-tech imagery. This is a good technology to use with the younger generation who is used to working with computers. They are flexible, can be customized, and are good for holding the learner's interest with scenarios, decision trees, illustrations, charts, and graphs. Keep in mind that computer glitches happen and cannot always be resolved during a presentation. This can be distracting to both you and the learners.

- Satellite presentations and Web presentations work well when you are trying to reach audiences who are spread out as in distance learning. For some, however, the technology represents another layer between you and the learners and can be distracting.

- Web-based activities are best for information gathering (including research), long distance mentoring, and collegiality (chat groups). Again, mastering the computer and the Web can be a challenge for some and can be more of a distraction than a learning experience.

- Audience response systems, while somewhat expensive, are good for comparison responses and for developing decision-making skills.

9. Is it ever okay not to use technology?

9. Since technology is a way to enhance the information we want to deliver, it is certainly not mandatory that you use it in the classroom. As a responsible instructor you must balance the cost of using technology in the classrooms with the objectives. Research has shown that there is no significant difference in learning outcomes when the technology used is the variable. Differences have been attributed, however, to the design and content of the program.

Consider the following questions when trying to decide:

- Do you have money in the budget for this technology use?

- How quickly do you need to disseminate the information?

- How large and dispersed is the audience?

- What type of information are you trying to convey to the learners?

- How stable is the information you need to convey?

Certainly, technology will help us disseminate information quickly to a large and dispersed audience. If the information is likely to change within a short period of time, you might consider a method of delivery like printed material with a supplemental video that you might be able to borrow or purchase as opposed to spending a good deal of money to have someone create a custom made Intranet program for the institution.

So, the bottom line is that if using technology is unavailable or not cost or time effective it is okay to do without.

10. We have a very limited budget in the institution and no fancy equipment. How can I incorporate media into my learning activities?

10. First of all, not all media are expensive. As I mentioned earlier media used in the classroom can be as simple as a good handout, a flip chart, or an overhead transparency. For the more expensive classroom media you may need to be a little bit more creative.

For many years there have been consortia between institutions that allow us to share equipment. If you don't have one set up in your area, call a few of your colleagues or ask the librarian to help you find out more information about joining or organizing one.

Most hospitals and public libraries have computers that learners can use for studies. You might want to negotiate with the librarians for time to use the facilities for a class. If this is not feasible, you might have to assign students time to visit the library individually to work on an assignment.

Most larger university hospitals have audiovisual departments and libraries from which equipment can be borrowed for use in the classroom. If the institution is affiliated with a school, college, or university you might be able to negotiate a plan that will allow you to borrow equipment for classes or perhaps allow you to conduct classes in the school's facilities.

Explore the possibility of grant or endowment monies that would allow you to purchase a few pieces of equipment for the department. Some pharmaceutical and supply companies may make money available in the form of an unrestricted educational grant.

Finally, chat with the sales representatives who visit the institution. Sometimes, they can help with loaners and possibly even equipment donations.

11. *I like using flip charts when I have to work with staff on the units instead of in the classroom. What tips can you give me to use flip charts effectively?*

11. The very first inservice education class I ever did was with a flip chart on several patient care units because of budget and staffing constraints. It was portable, lightweight, and actually turned out to be a fun experience.

Here are some tried and true flip chart tips:

- Use a flip chart stand and make sure the flip chart fits the stand. The best type of stand is the one that has a big clamp on top because it will hold any type of pad or poster board.

- Prior to beginning a teaching session, check the top of the pad to see how you will rip off the sheets if you need to (like in a strategic planning session when pages are taped around the room for future reference).

- Use a pad with grid lines if possible. The lines will help you align text as well as help you to draw straight lines if needed.

- If there is a standardized piece of the presentation you might want to write out the text or draw the illustrations ahead of time.

- If you are writing out text or drawing illustrations ahead of time begin by preparing the layout on paper first, then copy it on to the flip chart paper. Pencil in text on the flip chart before using the markers. This will allow you to adjust for spacing and figures.

- Try to use no more than six lines on each page.

- Make sure you use markers that don't bleed through the paper.

- Avoid using light colored markers since they are hard to see.

- Avoid using too many different colors since that can be confusing.

- If you make a mistake and it is small, fix it by using correction fluid. If the mistake is big, cut out two pieces of flip chart paper and tape them over the mistake.

- If you are nervous about presenting, you can pencil in notes and cues for yourself in the margins of the flip chart pages—they will not be seen by the audience. Cues penciled in at the bottom of the page will help you segue to the content on the next page. (You can also do this on the frames of overheads.)

12. Are there any rules to follow when creating a slide presentation?

- Always make sure you store and transport the flip chart properly so it will remain in good shape for future presentations.

12. While there are no hard and fast rules here are some suggestions to help you create effective slides:

- Begin by determining what information you want to convey in slides. Remember that slides will enhance the presentation, not act as a substitute for it. Also, avoid creating slides for the sake of having something for the learners to look at during the class. Spending some extra time up front deciding what information to include in the slides will help you in the long run.

- Next, select a style or "look" for the presentation. Choose elements such as background, color, and font that create an impression. You may want to include the institution's logo, which adds to the positive impression you are trying to make.

- People process information more easily if presented in short "bites" so keep slides simple. Make them easy to read. Try not to put more than five bullets on each slide. If possible, convey only one concept per slide so that it is easier for the learner to absorb the information. This will help the younger generation that has grown up with MTV and video. Their attention span is shorter, and they prefer that we get to the point quickly.

- The design of the slide should help the learner follow the natural tendency of reading left to right, top to bottom. Use arrows or other visual cues to guide the learner through the information.

- For electronic slide presentations, try using animation. It can be a powerful tool. It helps break down the information and presents it to the learner visually as you deliver it verbally. If you are going to use animation, select one type and keep it consistent throughout the presentation.

- Avoid overusing transitions, animation, and sound effects in electronic slide presentations since these can be distracting to the learner.

- Choose a print font that is simple and legible. Consider the size of the class. The bigger the class, the simpler you want the font to be. For example, if you will be presenting in a lecture hall, choose a font like Arial and avoid a font like Times Roman, which is fancier and harder to read on a screen. Be consistent with the font selection and change the font only when you want to emphasize something.

- For appropriate font size, a good rule is to use 14–16 point type for 35 mm slides and 20–22 point for screen shows.

- Keep the colors simple. Avoid using a white background. Use at least 10% of a shade like gray or blue and a contrasting color for the text.

- Always test slides by projecting them in the classroom for color accuracy, appropriate font size, and readability.

- Finally, always remember to check for spelling errors. Don't rely on spell check since an alternate spelling of a word (like "there" for "their") can be inadvertently inserted if you are not paying close attention to detail.

13. *Do you have any tips on creating exciting slides for a presentation?*

13. Here are a few tips that I have collected from my colleagues over the years:

- Keep the slides clean and uncluttered.

- Keep the information brief and to the point so it is easily absorbed by the learner.

- Use fonts effectively to create a mood. Experiment with the different types of fonts that are available in a computer program.

- Use small caps or caps on each word for emphasis.

- Use color; it adds vitality and increases the learner's willingness to pay attention. If chosen properly it can convey a message.

- Create and use tables and diagrams for emphasis.

- Experiment with using texture in the background. It will enhance the look of slides. Be careful, though, that the background doesn't distract the learner from the information being presented.

- Keep the style and color scheme consistent throughout the slides.

- "A picture's worth a thousand words . . ."—use photos,

charts, graphs, and illustrations to convey a message or feeling.

- Use animation at strategic points to add impact or to emphasize selected bits of information.

- When presenting a complex graphic, try using animated arrows for illustrating fine details.

- Try using video clips and sound to keep the audience tuned in to the slide and the information being presented.

- Experiment by using elements in different ways or rearranging their placement on the slide. For example, instead of centering the title, try left justifying it instead.

- Finally, remember that slides are supposed to enhance a presentation, not be a substitute for it.

14. What about the use of color in slides? Is it true that there are some colors that are better than others to use?

14. Colors, when used properly in a classroom, can make material vivid, interesting, and can even reinforce a message.

As a general rule, the cool colors like green, blue, and purple, which visually recede, all work well as background colors. Warm colors like red, yellow, and orange are vibrant and are good for text, accents, charts, and graphs. For slides and computer presentations, the background color is usually dark and the text and accents are light.

The opposite is true for overhead transparencies, however. Generally it is safe to use a lighter shade of a background color (about 10% shading) such as blue, green, or purple and then create text in a dark shade of the same color. This combination makes transparencies easier for the learners to read and less difficult for you to print. Take the time to experiment and consider which colors work well together.

Background Colors

- Blue is my favorite choice for background when creating slides and computer presentations. I find it calming to look at and the literature says that it communicates a sense of competence and contemplation.

- Green is associated with relaxation and money and is considered restful and refreshing. The literature says that it is a good background color for presentations that will use audience participation and feedback.

- Purple is an impressive color that denotes spirituality but promotes energy.

Text or Accent Colors

- Using the lighter shade of the previously mentioned background colors works well. It is harmonious and the text or accents will be easy to read since they won't clash with the background.

- Orange and yellow are good contrast colors and are good choices for text or accents on a dark background. Orange denotes power but is said to be cheerful enough to facilitate communication. Yellow is supposed to be stimulating and cheerful. When using these colors remember that when they are used in large areas they can be irritating and distracting to the learners and difficult to look at for long periods of time.

- White in the publishing world is considered no color. It usually denotes a clean slate or blank canvas and is a good color to use for text and titles.

- Black is also considered a clean slate and is good to use for emphasis on slides and text on overheads. It is a color that is associated with sophistication and finality. You can use this color to highlight information by creating a black box (on a color background) in which you will set important text (in a light color).

15. *I would like to use the Internet in my teaching but don't know where to begin. What should I do to get started?*

15. As with any learning activity, begin by identifying the topic, target audience, and learning objectives. Having done that, the next step should be to spend time exploring the Internet. Do a search using several different search engines and see what related information is available. Visit those Web sites, assess them, and select the ones that you believe contain the appropriate content for meeting the learning objectives. Remember to verify the source of the information and ascertain its reliability. Once you have done this, you can compile a list of Web sites that you then can present to learners for exploration.

Another approach that I like to use is to give students one or two Web sites to explore and then ask them to bring back to class one or two more credible Web sites that enhance or supplement the information you have presented in class. Then, in the classroom (if possible) students can take turns taking the class on a guided tour of the Web sites they found.

16. Some of the nurses in the institution are uncomfortable about using the computer and Internet. How can I help them overcome this feeling?

16. Most people who are uncomfortable using the Internet feel that way because they think they need to know a great deal of information to use it correctly or they are afraid that they may do something wrong that will damage the computer. I suggest that you give them the opportunity to play with the computer. Ask them to identify one of their special interests or a hobby. Then walk them through the process of conducting a search. Show them how easy it is to find Web sites related to their interest and then give them the opportunity to explore the Web sites for themselves. Allow them to make mistakes and be there to help them troubleshoot. Within a short period of time, they will see for themselves how easy it is to use the computer, explore the Internet, and find valuable information.

17. How do I know that the information that I find on the Internet is credible for use in the classroom?

17. There are several things you should look for that will help you determine the credibility of the information you find on the Internet.

- Begin by looking for the owners or sponsors of the Web site. What do you know about them? Try to find out as much as you can about Web site sponsors that are unfamiliar to you. Look for a corporate mission or vision statement and goals. That will tell you something about the sponsors.

- Next, are the authors of the content, speakers or presenters of presentations like Web casts, identified? They should be and you should have access to their biographical information.

- If there are learning activities on this site, are they offering contact hours? If so, what organizations accredit them as providers of continuing education? The same holds true for information on academic credit.

- Carefully consider the information posted on Web sites for possible conflict of interest. For example, are you looking at research information on a product that is manufactured by the sponsor of the Web site? Can this information be verified any place else? Are disclaimers regarding information posted? For example, very often in chat groups you find disclaimers regarding the information that is posted.

- Check to see how current the posted information is. When was the information on the Web site last updated?

After finding the answers to these questions, you will have a pretty good picture of whether or not you are looking at credible information. If you have doubts, do a search and try to find another Web site that verifies the information or addresses your concerns.

18. What is the appropriate amount of time the students should be interacting with technology?

18. I don't know that there is any hard and fast rule for the amount of student-technology interaction time. As adult learners, students should be able to determine for themselves just how much time they need to achieve their learning objectives.

I think we are all aware that students will process information at their own rates and that some students will need more "classroom time" than others. That is what is so wonderful about using technology in some learning settings. The students are able to review the material as many times as they want until they feel comfortable with it. They can advance at their own pace until they achieve the learning objective.

It may be that you want students to watch a video that will stimulate group discussion or that you are using slides to enhance a lecture. In that case, the students will probably have a short interaction time with the technology. On the other hand, consider the task of teaching a psychomotor skill. Think of the time it would take and how tedious your job would be if you had to demonstrate the procedure over and over again until each student "got it right." These are the students who will probably have more interaction time with the technology.

19. Is there any way to use technology to teach psychomotor skills?

19. One program that comes to mind immediately is the electronic Basic Cardiac Life Support (BCLS) and Advanced Cardiac Life Support (ACLS) program that comes complete with computer and manikins. In both cases, there is a CPR dummy that is hooked up electronically to the computer. The program, presented via CD-ROM, runs the learner though the didactic portion of the content first. Then, it provides demonstrations of the psychomotor skills and scenarios that the learner must master.

There are also electronic patient simulators that are used in nursing labs that react almost like real live human beings and react to everything the learner does or doesn't do including going into cardiac or respiratory arrest. Unfortunately, this equipment is still very expensive and often cost prohibitive.

Because of the cost, you may choose to use a less expensive type of technology, such as a video or computer to use in conjunction with hands-on teaching. The technology can be used for the repetitive part of the class. It will allow the learners to review the procedure in parts until they feel comfortable with the skill. You then work with the students to refine and master the skill.

I would imagine that unless you can find other facilities that are willing to share the cost of the expensive equipment, you will probably need to use your knowledge, creativity, and experience to put together your own technology-based psychomotor teaching unit.

20. Where can I learn more about the use of technology in the classroom?

20. I have found that the best way to learn more about the use of technology in the classroom is to interact with colleagues who use it.

First and foremost, become an involved member of a nursing continuing education or staff development organization such as the National Nursing Staff Development Organization (NNSDO). That will put you in touch with colleagues in your specialty area, many of whom are experts in technology use.

In addition to nursing continuing education and staff development organizations, you might want to consider joining a training and development organization. One organization that comes to mind is the American Society for Training and Development (ASTD). As a member, you will have access to a wealth of information related to training and development. For other organizations in this specialty, try conducting a simple search on the Internet for training associations. Remember, many of these organizations have annual meetings or conferences that afford you the opportunity to see first hand what technology is available and how it can be used in the classroom.

Another method that I find fun and have used is to browse the book and computer stores for information related to teaching and technology. Pay attention to the books that are targeted to elementary and high school teachers. They are loaded with plenty of fun and useful information and suggestions. One of my favorites is *The Family PC Guide to Home Work* by Gregg Keizer, Hyperion & Family PC, NY 1996. It has stimulated many good ideas for classroom use.

Another publication that I have recommended to colleagues and find extremely useful and thought provoking is the monthly publication, *Presentations,* published by Bill Communications, Inc., Minneapolis, MN. Each issue is loaded with technology reviews, tips, and instructions to improve presentation techniques and technology skills. They also have a wonderful and informative Web site at **www.presentations.com**.

Technology trade shows, conferences, and classes are also excellent ways to find out more about technology. Many technology trade shows are held annually in convention centers across the country. Locally, you might have access to classes offered by the companies that manufacture equipment or software. Most times, if you send in the completed warranty card for equipment you have purchased, your name is placed on a mailing list for upcoming events, classes, and special offers. Don't be shy, call, write to, or conduct an Internet search for the company that distributes the technology you are interested in learning about or talk to the sales representative. Often the sales representative can give you leads on classes available in your area.

Don't forget to check your local technical schools, colleges, and universities. Many have technology tracks or schools of continuing education that offer courses that will help you learn more.

Finally, keep an open mind, browse the Internet, have some fun, and check out some of the Web sites like **disney.com**, **hallmark.com**, or Vince & Larry's Safe City at **www.nhtsa.dot.gov/kids/** for some innovative ideas on how to use technology.

Chapter 32: *Teaching About Computer Use*

1. What is the first thing I should do when I can't get my computer to work?

1. The first thing you should try if you are experiencing problems with your computer is to close all applications, shut the computer down, turn it off, wait at least 30 seconds, turn the computer back on, and try to use the applications again. This is called a cold boot. It clears the temporary memory (RAM) so you can begin with a clean slate. If this does not help, seek assistance from an expert in the facility.

2. What is the difference between a cold boot and a warm boot?

2. A cold boot, as described above, occurs when you shut the computer down, turn it off for at least 30 seconds, and then turn it back on. This clears the temporary memory (RAM) and allows you to begin with a clean slate.

   A warm boot occurs when you use the three keys: Control, Alt, Delete simultaneously or press the reset button on the computer to shut down the operating system and bring it back up. This does not clear the RAM, and you may experience the same problems as you did before.

3. What is an effective strategy to teach computer use?

3. The most effective strategy is demonstration/return demonstration. Teaching computer use, particularly to those who have never touched a computer, requires not only cognitive knowledge but also motor skills. In order to obtain the best retention, participants need to use the equipment and practice what has been presented.

4. What models exist to teach the diverse work force about computer applications?

4. There are no models that address computer application teaching to a diverse work force specifically. The most appropriate model would be Benner's Novice to Expert. By grouping novice computer users together in a class situation, the pace of the class will be geared to the novice user and not be frustrating for the intermediate or expert users.

   Another option, used in public schools, is to pair the intermediate or more advanced computer user with a novice user in the classroom. The novice then receives some individualized attention for the basics of the computer application and the instructor can move more quickly to the information that is needed for the intermediate user. This option should only be used if class scheduling precludes grouping the classes into the same skill level.

5. *What is an appropriate computer to learner ratio?*

5. The most appropriate ratio for learning is one computer for each learner. This gives the learner the time to follow the instructor, perform the exercises, and ask questions.

6. *What kind of competency expectations should be employed regarding computer use?*

6. This is dependent upon the potential employee population. Most individuals in the younger than 35 age group have some experience with computers. Individuals over the age of 35 may have little or no experience in using computers, but they must be willing to learn.

It is important to outline the competency expectations for each job description. Once these are in place, an analysis of how to meet these expectations should be considered. Either the employee must come with these competencies or the organization needs to provide a class for the new employees to obtain these competencies.

In developing these competencies, consider that the individual must have the:

- Ability to use a mouse

- Ability to use a keyboard

- Basic knowledge of how to turn a computer on and off (reboot)

- Willingness to learn new applications

Computer applications are all moving to a Web-based format. Many employees have computers at home or have experience surfing the Web. This knowledge will make it easier to learn organization applications if they also are Web-based and use Web standards.

7. *If I have a class of novice computer users— where should I start?*

7. With a class of novices, I would start with the basics. Begin with what each piece of equipment is named, its function and how it is used. For example, explain the mouse, keyboard, central processing unit (CPU), monitor, printer, and their functions first, and then how to turn the equipment on and off. Explain Ready Access Memory (RAM), Read Only Memory (ROM), and Operating System (OS) as basics of computer functioning; then move to the specific computer software the participants need to learn.

8. *What seems to be most intimidating about the computer for new users?*

8. The most intimidating piece of computer equipment seems to be the mouse. This is difficult to understand cognitively and difficult to manipulate. Use games loaded in the computer to show participants how the mouse works, how to single and double click, how to right and left click, and allow practice time. Games make practicing the motor skills necessary to use the mouse fun.

9. **What are some common frustrations with computer use in a clinical setting?**

9. Common frustrations are usually related to the lack of time during the workday. Frustrations include multiple sign-ons and passwords, computer screens freezing up, or systems that take more than 10 seconds to navigate from screen to screen. End-users readily adapt to each system as long as it is quickly available and movement within the applications is rapid.

10. **Why do I have to enter my user ID and password so many times?**

10. With the Health Insurance Portability and Accountability Act (HIPAA) security and privacy guidelines for health care, it is necessary to make sure that patients' records cannot be accessed by just anyone walking past the computer terminal. This is the rationale behind user IDs and passwords. Not only do these make the computer record more secure, they leave an audit trail of who accessed the record with a date and time stamp.

Until very recently, technology did not allow authentication to several applications with one user ID and password. Thus, end-users must sign onto the Network, then the application, and then to various parts of the application. Many organizations are making plans for the single sign-on and password so it should be a reality in the near future.

11. **What regulations apply with a hospital clinical system?**

11. The computerized clinical system comes under the same regulations as the paper medical record. The regulating bodies include Centers for Medicare and Medicaid Services (CMS), Joint Commission (JCAHO), and the new HIPAA (government) regulation. There may also be state insurance regulations related to documentation in the medical record, privacy protection, and record retention. There also are laws related to medical record documentation and retention.

12. **What should I tell students about computer security?**

12. Computer security is necessary for the protection of the patient information contained within the computer system. Not only are there regulations to meet, but also it is the ethical and professional duty of healthcare providers to provide documentation to guide care. Protection of that documentation ensures patients that they can be honest with their healthcare provider. Honesty between patient and provider is absolutely necessary for proper health maintenance, diagnosis and treatment of illness, and the lifelong health care of people. As always, permission by the patient is necessary to share information contained in the medical record.

HIPAA regulations require a high level of security for access to patient records, an audit trail of access, and encryption of data being sent outside the institution for billing, research purposes, or referral purposes. In the future, permission from the patient will have to be obtained to transmit or share information outside the organization housing the record.

13. *There are so many ways to do the same thing in most software packages—how many of them do I teach students?*

13. Most students who are computer novices need to be taught 1–2 ways of doing the same thing in software packages to decrease confusion. Each student is an individual and has preferences about how he/she uses essential pieces of equipment. One student may prefer to use keyboard shortcuts while another student may prefer mouse clicks.

As the individual becomes an intermediate or expert at the computer system, more ways of doing the same thing can be introduced. This adds choices and may speed the use of the programs, as a new way of doing the same thing may be more efficient for some individuals.

14. *What is the best teaching method for teaching computer applications?*

14. The best teaching method is in a classroom with one computer per participant with the application in a training environment so that the real situation can be simulated as much as possible. Using case scenarios that are meaningful to the learners will enhance retention of the new information.

15. *What is helpful to individuals to take with them after they leave class?*

15. A small, laminated card with the basic steps to accomplishing the computer tasks is most helpful to individuals. This guide should also be attached to each computer workstation for reference.

16. *How can I assist students in rapidly gaining computer skills?*

16. Structuring class in the following way is the most helpful in teaching computer skills:

- Create real life case scenarios for teaching

- Explain the basics of computer equipment use

- Allow time for practice with the computer equipment (mouse, keyboard, printer)

- Explain the case scenario

- Demonstrate the steps of computer use related to the scenario

- Allow the participants to do the steps along with you as the instructor

- Have participants do 1–2 more case scenarios as practice with you answering questions and assisting them through these cases

17. What is the ideal class size for teaching computer applications?

17. In computer classes, there should be one instructor per 10-15 individuals and one expert assistant per five participants. Teaching computer applications is time intensive for instructors. There should be sufficient instructors to answer individual questions in an efficient, effective, and timely manner.

18. What function/purpose besides entertainment do computer games serve?

18. Games and other entertainment that use computer equipment make learning new skills more fun. Many of the functions of the computer/mouse interaction are simply eye-hand coordination skills that must be learned. It is less frustrating and more fun if these skills are learned and practiced using games. Using serious content can come later when the psychomotor skills have been obtained.

Many professionals are very concerned about accuracy and correctness. Using games decreases the stress of many professionals who experience these concerns.

19. What should I include in teaching materials for computer students?

19. Teaching materials should include short explanations of the purpose of each lesson, steps to each process that must be completed within the computer applications, glossary of terms, and how to obtain assistance. Screen prints of the steps to complete a computer task with arrows to the pertinent buttons, drop down boxes, or other items are a must.

20. Are some computer teaching resources on the Web? How do I find them?

20. There are many teaching resources on the World Wide Web. The American Nurses Association has an excellent site, **www.nursingworld.org,** that provides links to other nursing sites that are helpful. There is a site that puts reference information at your fingertips: **www.refdesk.com**. It includes all sorts of reference materials for the instructor. Many universities and professional organizations offer teaching information and tips.

The best way to find resources on the Web is to enter

the topic and teaching in the search box. Then choose from the resources returned from the search or select the University of your choice and search its site for information on the content you will be teaching.

21. How would you design a classroom for computer training?

21. A classroom for teaching computers should contain one or two large screens at the front of the room. The instructor should have a computer that will display on the large screen but the instructor's computer should be positioned so the instructor is facing the participants but can turn slightly to see the display screen. Each student should have a computer. The room should be narrow enough that all students can see the display screen easily.

22. What are some common computer uses in health care?

22. Computers were first used in health care for the financial and billing information. Computers are used in many of the diagnostic tools such as radiology, nuclear medicine, and laboratory instruments that interface into computers to print results. Computers are also used to produce educational materials or for self-directed learning modules. Computers can be used for staff scheduling. Human resources departments use databases to keep files on employees. The most recent use of computers in health care is for patient records. Home health, clinics, ambulatory surgery, and hospitals are moving toward an electronic medical record.

23. What is Nursing Informatics?

23. "A specialty that integrates nursing science, computer science, and information science to manage and communicate data, information, and knowledge in nursing practice" (ANA Expert Panel, 2000, p. 22).

24. I'm interested in computers. Are there jobs for nurses? What kind of jobs?

24. There is a large variety of nursing informatics job opportunities. Examples include User Liaison, Coordinator for Health Care Institutions, Installer of Clinical Information Systems for a vendor, Trainer for vendors, Product Manager, Consultant, Sales Representative, Systems Analyst/Programmer, Knowledge Engineer, and Policy Development Specialist.

25. How safe is ordering or putting information on the Internet?

25. Ordering on the Internet is usually done via a secure server connection. A Web browser will indicate a secure connection usually in the display at the bottom of the browser window. Often this display is a padlock that is closed when the connection is secure and open when it is not a secure, encrypted connection.

Many vendors sell over the Internet. You will encounter stories of both good and bad experiences. If you order over the Internet, make sure that the padlock is in the locked position when giving credit card information. Also, make sure you know the vendor with whom you are placing the order is reputable.

Information placed on a Web page on the Internet can be secured via a user ID and password just as the computer applications are secured in an organization. If you do not want everyone to see the information, use the security option when building the Web page. Otherwise, anyone surfing the Web can view the information you have posted.

Also remember that e-mail is not secure. A good rule of thumb is not to put anything in e-mail that you wouldn't want on the front page of a newspaper.

26. How do I advise patients about information they find on the Internet?

26. Advise them to look for sites of major organizations such as universities or national organizations such as the American Lung Association or the American Heart Association. The US Government maintains other good sites. The National Library of Medicine, the Centers for Disease Control and Prevention, and the National Institutes of Health have good information that is reviewed by medical personnel for accuracy and written so most people can understand the content.

Avoid sites that are maintained by an individual. If you find something interesting on a personal site, confirm the information at a site of a national organization, government site, or university site. Individuals often put opinions and personal experiences on their Web site. Any advice should be confirmed with a healthcare provider before following the advice.

27. What do I need to know to buy a home computer?

27. First decide what you want to do with a home computer. The purpose will guide the purchase. Do you want to surf the Web? Do you want to download and print things in color? Do you want to listen to things on the Web or play videos? Do you want to keep track of bank accounts, write letters, or create a mailing list? The answers to these questions will guide a store representative in assisting you with a computer purchase.

Ask questions about the service agreement and the support that comes with the computer. Is the support available 24 hours a day, 7 days a week? What if the computer has problems? Can you bring it in to be serviced onsite or will they ship it off to the manufacturer for service?

Do you want to put information on the computer that is important to keep for a long time? If so, invest in a back up system, either a tape backup or a CD-ROM writer.

28. *How often should a computer be upgraded?*

28. Computers should be upgraded as often as the user deems it necessary. If the software you are using requires the computer to be upgraded that is the time to do it. It has been my observations that if you get behind more than two versions of software, you risk data integrity by not upgrading. In order to keep data from getting lost or corrupted, use common sense. If software requires an upgrade—then upgrade the hardware. If you have data that you wish to always keep, upgrade software at least every other version and upgrade the hardware as necessary.

If you want the fastest computer, the latest graphics, the latest bells and whistles—you will be constantly upgrading and adding to your computer system.

29. *Is there specific etiquette for e-mail and chat rooms?*

29. Yes, it is called Netiquette. There are many Web sites that have the etiquette outlined. Type the word Netiquette in the browser search window and visit the sites listed by the search engine.

30. *What should I do to prevent loss of data/files in my computer?*

30. Prevent loss of data/files by having a backup system when you purchase the computer. Periodically back up files. If you use the computer frequently each week, back up once a week. If you use it less often, a monthly backup may be sufficient. If, during one session, you input a large amount of information, back up before leaving the computer session. This will save you many headaches in the future. There are data recovery companies that can recover data but they are very expensive.

31. *What can a computer offer patients and their families?*

31. If the patient's family is geographically dispersed, a computer with e-mail can keep them in touch with one another.

There are a variety of Web sites on the Internet that provide information concerning diseases, treatment options, support groups, answers from an expert, and lists of questions to ask the healthcare provider related to physical examinations and/or disease processes.

32. *Some patients are afraid that their health information will get on the Internet. What do I say to reassure them?*

32. All patient information is protected under federal and state regulations. The new HIPAA guidelines give healthcare institutions specific regulations for protection of privacy and confidentiality of patient records. Each electronic medical record must have a secure access point. If any part of the record is electronically transmitted, it must be encrypted. The medical record cannot be shared without specific permission in writing for the organization that is custodian of the records.

Assure patients that the paper and electronic health record belongs to them even though the organization is the custodian of that record.

33. *What about wireless computers? Will they interfere with biomedical devices patients need?*

33. All vendors that make biomedical devices are carefully considering the answer to this question. There has been a rare case that wireless devices such as telephones and computers have interfered with some biomedical devices. The FDA is working on guidelines to prevent this from happening. It is always best to turn off wireless devices when geographically close to patients with biomedical devices.

34. *What happens to all the patient information stored in computers?*

34. Patient record information is electronically stored at the custodial organization. It may be archived on tape or other permanent electronic storage device or it may be in a large database within the patient record application. Either way, it is accessible to healthcare providers if it is needed.

35. *What about voice recognition devices?*

35. Voice recognition devices are devices that are "trained" to recognize your voice and pattern of speech. They are dictation devices that convert dictation into a typed or transcribed document, or they can open a computer application. Some vendors claim over 90% accuracy and great savings as they eliminate the need for a transcriptionist. They are not widely used as yet, but the technology is becoming more sophisticated and probably will be used more in the future.

There is one note of caution. If you have ever tried to exactly transcribe dictation, you know that humans use slang, sentence fragments, and other idiosyncrasies that do not translate well to the written word. Dictated and transcribed documents will always need to be read and edited before becoming a permanent part of any record.

36. What is a PDA?

36. A PDA is a personal digital assistant. These palm size, hand-held devices offer many features that assist the user in decision making. These devices are powerful enough to contain book-length reference information, an address book, a calendar, access to e-mail and the Internet, and other convenient functions in a relatively small package. These devices are becoming more powerful with each development phase. Investigations are ongoing as to how these devices can be used for documentation for any job requirement. This is an exciting area of technological development. Keep watch—PDAs will become more and more advanced and valuable to the users.

RESOURCES

Gloe, D. S. (2001). *Basics of computers & nursing informatics*. Long Branch, NJ: Vista Publishing.

Graves, J. R., & Corcoran, S. (1989). The study of nursing informatics. *Image: Journal of Nursing Scholarship, 21,* 227–331.

Hebda, T., Czar, P., & Mascara, C. (1998). *Handbook of informatics for nurses & health care professionals.* Menlo Park, CA: Addison-Wesley.

National Center for Nursing Research. (1993). *National nursing research agenda: Volume I. Developing knowledge for practice: Challenges and opportunities* (NIH Publication No. 93–2416). Bethesda, MD: National Institutes of Health. (**www.nih.gov/ninr**)

Schein, E. H. (2001). *Kurt Lewin's change theory in the field and in the classroom: Notes toward a model of managed learning.* (**www.solonlin.org/res/wp/10006.htm**)

Chapter 33: *Preparing Online Courses*

1. Why should I prepare an online course?

1. An online course is one strategy to use to present content to participants. It is a popular modality that appeals to those who can learn with relative independence and can set their own schedules and deadlines.

2. How does an online course differ from most continuing education posted on the Web?

2. An online course should provide interaction between participants and/or presenters, through chats, bulletin boards, and other access to the faculty. There is continuing education on the Web that is a "straight" read or a "page turner" in the presentation of content—no interactions between participants and/or presenters.

3. What kind of education or training should participants have in order to "take" an online course?

3. Anyone considering participating in an online course should have basic computer skills—how to access the Web; download, send, and save files; how to print documents; and basic keyboarding, that is how to type, or how to begin to use a keyboard.

4. How do I develop online content?

4. First, consider content you have already developed; for instance, a self-study module, a short lecture, a poster presentation, an article written for publication, or a paper for a course. Make an outline of the content and then begin to develop a storyboard of the content. Begin with a simple, short topic. A storyboard enables you to plan for logical flow of content.

5. Are there courses or books or conferences that can teach me or help me develop a course?

5. There are courses, both online and "in person" conferences. I suggest you begin contacting schools of nursing or education and professional organizations, such as **www.nursing.iupui.edu** or **www.on-linelearning.net**.

Evaluate the course to be sure that the basic concepts of developing and managing online courses are presented. The course should prepare you to develop a module or course using a software management tool.

6. What assumptions should I make about learners who will take an online course?

6. • The learners are interested or need the content in the module or course you are going to develop.

• The learners have basic computer equipment.

• They may have limitations as to when they will access and complete the course.

• There is the rare case where someone is desperate for the credit in order to renew a license or certification.

• Some learners will experience frustration with the process due to technology problems.

7. How long should the module or course be?

7. An online course or module should be simple and to the point. Resources and references can be added and the participants can access this additional information based on their need to know and time available.

It may be necessary to develop several modules/lessons/sections, in order for the course objectives to be achieved.

Keep in mind that in a "face-to-face" conference or class, participants are usually seated for 60 to 90 minutes. Expect that the participant in an online course will only be seated and participate for a maximum of 60–90 minutes at a time.

8. How long should an online course be?

8. The course should be long enough to meet the goals or objectives. But you also have to consider how long can you hold the interest of the participant.

It has been my experience that those persons taking an online course are busy professionals who are taking a course to increase their knowledge and skills. They do not want the course to drag on and on. So my advice is to present the content in a short period of time.

Also to be considered is the amount of time presenter/faculty will be involved in the course—participating in chats, evaluating and providing feedback on lessons and activities, review of home pages, reviewing and grading tests and papers. It takes a great deal of time for presenters/faculty to be involved in an online course.

In addition to active involvement in the course, the presenter/faculty will also be involved in reviewing the evaluations of the course and in updating the course and resources linked to it.

9. What types of online courses are available?

9. Online courses may be held for academic credit and for continuing education.

There are three types of online courses for continuing education.

- The first is a course that presents content and there is no presenter/faculty interaction with the participants.

- The second type of course or module presents content and there are scheduled times for a chat or posting questions to a bulletin board for the presenter/faculty/content expert.

- The third type of course presents content and involves

chats, bulletin boards, and interchange with the presenter/faculty/content expert on an ongoing basis. This could be on a daily basis; two or three times per week; or weekly, depending on the course set-up.

10. Should I pilot test the online course?

10. Yes! Not only to establish the baseline for the determination of contact hours, but also to learn how the course can be revised or improved. The pilot test is also an opportunity for the faculty/presenter/content expert to learn how to manage teaching an online course.

11. Are there management problems connected to online courses?

11. Yes, there are several situations to be considered. First, depending on the type of course (Type 1, 2, or 3 above), how long will the participants have to complete the course? How will you handle someone who completes only part of a course? What about the participant who enrolls for the course but never participates? Who, in addition to the presenter/faculty, in the organization will be monitoring the participation those persons enrolled in the course? Who in the organization will be available to answer technical questions or handle technical problems participants may have?

12. How can I promote learning using the online format?

12. Actively involve the participants in the course. The more interactive activities the participants complete and the more contact with the presenter/faculty/content expert the more the opportunities for learning increase.

13. My agency/association really wants me to pursue online education and I'm not sure I have all the resources I need. What should I do?

13. Check with your colleagues to see what they are using. The organization can purchase the learning platform software or rent space on a university server. The main resource is faculty who are interested in the online modality and someone with instructional design skills. Time and energy are all it takes to teach using this strategy.

RESOURCES

Newby, T. (2000). *Instructional technology for teaching and learning: Designing instruction, integrating computers, and using media.* Upper Saddle River, NJ: Prentice Hall.

Novotny, J. (2000). *Distance education in nursing.* New York: Springer.

Palloff, R. M., & Pratt, K. (2001). *Lessons from the cyberspace classroom: The realities of online teaching.* San Francisco: Jossey-Bass.

White, K. W., & Weight, B. H. (2000). *The online teaching guide: A handbook of attitudes, strategies, and techniques for the virtual classroom.* Boston: Allyn and Bacon.

Chapter 34: *Delivering Distance Learning*

1. What is Distance Learning and how will it forever change my life as a provider of Continuing Education?

1. Distance learning is driven by a need to free education from the constraints of the classroom and to make learning available 24 hours a day/7 days a week! Distance learning has been used in higher education for more than 100 years and has become increasingly popular in the nursing community in meeting licensure and certification requirements. The "correspondence course" of the past has blossomed into the interactive opportunities that modern technology can provide. Increasingly, continuing education strategies strive to provide "entertainment value" desired by emerging generations including interactive elements and instant information access with an emphasis on "just-in-time" learning. Shifting trends in academic education are creating a new generation of learners who expect to continue their education at times and places that are convenient to them.

2. What are the reasons that learners seek distance learning?

2. • Convenience—available 24/7

   • Just-in-time learning—a.k.a. "What's in it for me?"

   • Basic and advanced degrees

   • Continuing education requirements to maintain licensure or certification

   • Opportunity to learn from nationally recognized faculty

   • Opportunity to participate in professional organization activities from a distance

   • Perceived lower participant costs (e.g., reduced program fees, less travel involved, less need for child/elder care, parking)

3. What methodologies are associated with distance learning programming?

3. **Print-based distance learning**

   • Independent study modules—useful for CE and staff development

   • Offered by most nursing journals and organizations—may also be available via Web-based organizations. CE quizzes can frequently be completed online with instant production of the CE certificate. This may be especially attractive to nurses who must meet licensure or certification requirements in a timely manner!

- Production of monographs can be more cumbersome than online programs because of the intensive review process and copy editing.

- Learning is passive with limited or no interaction with faculty.

Teleconference

- Opportunity to "hear" from content experts, interact with faculty via questions from the audience

- Popular with many practicing nurses who may have limited time/resources for continuing education. Teleconferences can be potential "Lunch and Learn" opportunities

- Can be enhanced with speaker slides and graphics

- Potential for archiving teleconferences for future learners accessible via organization's Web site or on audiotape

- Satellite conferencing can provide the opportunity to view the speaker and slides. Local universities or television stations with TV reception capabilities often provide this service.

Computer-assisted instruction

- Can include more "entertaining" graphics that engage the learner through video streaming and interactive technology

- Can be costly depending on the sophistication of the graphics and programming required

- Appropriate for slides and note pages from lectures presented in another venue. Frequently supported by a pharmaceutical company that may be interested in distributing this information to nurses

- Can be used to complement Web-based courses. Use of a CD-ROM in combination with the Internet may help to reduce technical problems due to low bandwidth and requirements for plug-ins.

Live chats

- Live chats provide synchronous learning that can bring together a content expert and learners from across the world. Recent live chats sponsored by the Oncology Nursing Society (ONS) and CancersourceRN were attended by nurses in Canada, Turkey, and Nepal!

- Chats may be popular with learners who may have used this technology when using the Internet for a variety of life issues (i.e., book clubs, support groups).

- Credit may be available following completion of a program evaluation with instant production of CE certificate.

- Potential to archive a transcript of the chat for learners unable to participate at the designated time.

- There is limited opportunity for discussion with very large groups in a single chat room. Live chats are most effective with groups of approximately 15–20 participants. Larger groups limit the number of questions that can reasonably be addressed within the usual time frame of 60–90 minutes.

- The technology in this area is still fairly limited. The constant refreshing of the screen and the time for information transfer by the hosting site frustrates some users. Anticipating and "scripting" frequently answered questions can help to decrease transcription time and increase the amount of content that can be presented.

Web-based courses

- University faculty with Web-based program design experience can be invaluable resources.

- Provide an opportunity for concentrated learning in a given topic with interaction between faculty and learners.

- Require significant time commitment from the organization, information technology support, and from faculty prior to launching the course.

- Provide an opportunity for enhanced interactive learning that appeals to adult learners through discussion forums via threaded chats, e-mail, problem solving, and case study exercises.

- Typically offered in collaboration with an "application service provider" such as **Blackboard.com**, **WebCT.com**, or **Certilearn.com**.

- Indiana University School of Nursing offers an excellent series of Web-based courses through its Lifelong Learning Department. The courses are focused on getting started in teaching and learning on the Web, designing Web-based courses, teaching and evaluation strategies, and development of a Web-based course **http://nursing.iupui.edu/LifelongLearning**.

4. How does distance learning compare with traditional instruction methodologies?

4. Attention to principles of adult learning is equally important in planning distance learning programs and traditional instruction offered in the classroom setting. The goal in both settings is to provide experiences that will allow the learner to use new information to change or enhance existing beliefs, patterns, or practices. Unfortunately, the result of many traditional courses has been memorization and recall with little application of content. Distance learning programs run the risk of repeating this fault if the offering is little more than a correspondence course beefed up by digital technology. Distance learning can force faculty and learners to prepare, think, and work differently. Creating a great case study can be more challenging than preparing an hour lecture. Passive attention to a teleconference or slide presentation requires less commitment than synthesizing the comments of fellow learners in a debate conducted via e-mail. Correspondence and interaction are the keys to successful distance learning!

Research has demonstrated that there is no significant difference between traditional instruction and distance learning in the ability of learners to meet course objectives.

5. What questions should be asked by a provider considering program development for distance learning?

5.
- Who is the audience? Has a needs assessment been completed to determine learner interest and/or access availability for distance learning programs?

- What outcomes are desired? How can Web-based tools help achieve these objectives?

- What distance learning strategy is best suited for this topic?

  - Controversial issues may be very appropriate for a live chat, especially time sensitive topics that may not have been addressed in formal publications.

  - Highly technical content may be better suited to monographs or slide presentations with supporting graphics.

- What are the direct and indirect costs?

- Provider expenses (e.g., personnel, marketing, CE maintenance)

- Information technology (e.g., hardware, software, technical support personnel)

- Faculty honoraria (e.g., pre-work, presentation of content, responding to follow-up questions, long term commitment as in a Web-based course)

- External production company (e.g., conference capture expenditures including travel costs for recording personnel, Web site maintenance)

• Are there opportunities for cost sharing through external funding requirements and/or participant fees?

• What technology support is available?

- Will the organization host the information or choose to partner with an application service provider?

- How will learners prepare to participate in the program (e.g., computer requirements, user-friendly programming for the "technically-challenged")?

- What technical support will be available during the course or program for users who are unable to complete the CE exam or obtain a certificate or who are "booted out" from a live chat session because of Internet access provider limitations, for example?

6. How can CE providers prepare learners to be successful in distance learning programs?

6. Learners who perceive themselves as "technologically challenged" may be difficult to attract to online distance learning programs. Using the technology must be as seamless as possible for the learner and should require minimal computer programming skills. Mastering this technology and successfully completing an online education program, however, provides its own achievements for learners.

Well-developed instructions or materials that can be e-mailed to the learner before the program, particularly related to technological requirements, can increase the likelihood that the participant successfully completes the course or program.

321

7. What are the challenges of Web-based education and learning?

7.
- Technology is still quite intimidating for many learners. The average age of the nurse today is 45, and the population is graying every year! Many nurses lack basic computer and Internet skills.

- Access to Web-based programs at work or at home may be an issue. While increasing numbers have Internet access at home, nurse learners may have to compete with younger learners in the house who are now dependent upon the computer for information access. Many nurses describe limited access at work to online educational programming because of time constraints or "firewall protections" that limit Internet use in the work setting.

- Time for continuing education. Availability of time for continuing education seems to be more of an issue than ever as other aspects of the American life-style consume discretionary time. Employer-provided resources, including time and money, for continuing education have also become increasingly limited. Popular "lunch and learns" sponsored by pharmaceutical representatives offer both intellectual and physical nourishment at a time when learners are available. Ultimately, it is the commitment of the learner that is key. The need to know belongs to the learner.

- Technology and its cost. Distance learning programs can be quite costly to develop and maintain. Many CE providers do not have the internal resources to independently offer sophisticated programs. Providers will need to seek creative funding sources. While the technology has come a long way in the past five years, the speed of transmission for complex graphics and interactive technology continues to limit Web-based training. The widespread addition of fiber optic or DSL transmission lines or group server networks will significantly enhance user access.

- Changing old habits. Faculty and learners will be challenged to move from passive to active learner processes made possible through interactive technology. Many learners still prefer to print materials from the Web to read. Providers need to be careful that distance learning programs are more than manuscripts with bells, whistles, and pretty pictures!

8. How do distance learning programs compare with traditional learning methods in terms of course preparation for faculty and student participation?

8. The development of measurable objectives and appropriate content are key components of traditional and distance learning strategies. Traditional learning environments provide faculty with the opportunity for immediate feedback regarding aspects of content that may be unclear for learners. Opportunities for reinforcement are more readily available. Obtaining feedback from learners in distance learning programs is a challenge. Providers may wish to solicit questions or feedback throughout the program and frequently remind participants to complete the evaluation. In some circumstances, however, learners who were previously quite passive in the traditional classroom setting become more participatory in the anonymous setting that distance learning provides.

Organizing content for distance learning programs may also be quite challenging. Traditional learning methods such as lectures are typically limited to the amount of content that can be presented by the speaker within a given time frame. Distance learning providers will need to consider breaking up content in units that can be "absorbed" or "digested" in reasonable segments to maximize learning and fit the available technology. For example, providing access to a Web-based article with detailed content prior to a live chat may greatly enhance the effectiveness of the discussion.

Finally, perceptions about time commitment by faculty and learners for distance learning may differ from expectations associated with traditional learning methods. Faculty will need additional time for interaction with students through review of threaded discussions, facilitating live chats, and answering learner e-mail. Learners may discount the required time to become familiar with the technical skills necessary to complete the distance learning program.

9. What techniques can be used to reduce learner isolation and increase interaction among course participants?

9.
- Opportunities for feedback—threaded discussions, e-mail

- Interaction with the audience during teleconferences, live chats

- E-mail survey to those who have registered and/or participated in distance learning programs

10. *What do you need to know about copyright laws in the preparation of distance learning programs?*

10. Copyright permission is just as important in distance learning programs as it is in traditional learning methods—perhaps even more so. Intellectual property rights and the Internet remain a tremendously gray area that is subject to creative interpretation. Financial disclosure statements become public knowledge in a way perhaps not previously experienced by some presenters. Faculty may be reluctant to "share their work" in such public venues that can be easily duplicated. Slides not limited to "read-only" files can be readily copied for others' use. Faculty need to be careful to protect human subjects whose photos may be included in Web-based programs. Application service providers frequently have detailed permission statements and faculty agreements that must be completed prior to submission of course content.

11. *How do you evaluate learner participation in distance education?*

11. A disadvantage of asynchronous distance learning programs is the lack of immediate feedback from course participants. Feedback is limited to what the learner is willing to commit to "paper" or provide via e-mail or formal evaluation forms. The non-verbal response of learners—head shaking, smiles, quizzical looks, or groans is not available. The all-important "bathroom buzz" regarding a program's success or lack thereof is also missing.

Distance learning providers may wish to follow programs with a random sample of phone interviews/personalized e-mail. A frequent reminder to complete evaluation information is necessary. Many learners may not "need" the continuing education credits and fail to complete the evaluation, thus, limiting opportunities for feedback. It is often helpful to place the evaluation in the same section as the CE quiz to facilitate feedback.

12. *What are average participant costs associated with distance learning?*

12.
- Cost depends on the distance learning modality or strategy.

- Many programs are available for free (e.g., Live chats are available through ONS Online and CancerSource RN; pharmaceutical company sponsored CE programs associated with specialty nursing organiza-tions or medical education companies).

- The average participant cost ranges from $8 to $15 per contact hour for programs offered by specialty organizations and commercial CE providers (e.g., Nursing World, Nursing Spectrum, Medscape).

- University courses typically charge a credit hour rate comparable to traditional on-campus fees.

13. *How can you use technology to create "virtual conferences" and make the most of programs presented at national meetings?*

13. Virtual conferences or meetings provide an excellent opportunity for nurses to participate in professional organizations and access content presented at national meetings! Specialty nursing organizations may consider this as a new level of service and benefit for members. Virtual meetings can reach members who are not able to participate in face-to-face programs because of travel costs or time required away from home and work.

Conference capturing can include audiotape, slides and audio, or video streaming via Web-cast that may include viewing the speaker and slides. Continuing education credit can be offered with the CE quiz and instant online production of CE certificate available at the completion of the program. This type of programming is quite costly, however. It may require significant grant support. A single live Web-cast can start at $100,000. Conference capture or virtual meetings may also be difficult for users with limited modem speed or bandwidth. Some learners simply give up because of the slow transfer of information.

14. *Will the number of participants at national conferences decrease because of participation in virtual meetings and thereby diminish potential revenue from the annual conference?*

14. This is a common concern shared by CE providers and is sometimes referred to as "fear of cannibalizing" one's efforts. Providers who have had experience in offering virtual meetings find that this feature has not reduced the number of members or attendees at annual meetings. Additional members are drawn to the organization and seek out the social interaction of peers and colleagues whom they have met via distance learning.

15. *What costs are associated with development of distance learning programs?*

15.
- Cost depends on the distance learning strategy or approach and contracts established with application service providers.

- Some estimates range from $30,000 to $100,000 per course. Live Web-casts can be significantly more.

- A potential source for information about costs: Results Direct Internet Marketing (703) 684–3932.

16. *How do you find funding support for distance learning programs?*

16. This may be the most difficult question to answer in this chapter! The pharmaceutical industry has traditionally provided tremendous support for continuing education in medicine and nursing. Restrictions by the FDA and CE providers have created some limitations on this type of funding support, however, particularly for programs that are specifically related to a particular product. Many companies request banner support on the funding recipient's Web page but are restricted from having a direct link to the company Web site in programs supported by an unrestricted educational grant. Some pharmaceutical companies perceive ads or banners as a minimal return on investment compared to the benefit of a pharmaceutical sales representative or education specialist making direct contact with a healthcare provider. Other potential sources for support include medical device companies, healthcare foundations, and Internet-based software companies.

There may be opportunities in the future to link with schools of nursing that are interested in co-providing distance learning continuing education capitalizing on the experience of faculty and information technology departments familiar with offering this type of program.

17. *What are some of the more popular distance learning Continuing Education programs for nurses that are currently available?*

17. An excellent list of online continuing education resources is available on the ANA Web site at **http://www.nursingworld.org/ancc/ceoned.htm**

Some personal favorites include:

Oncology Nursing Society
   http://www.ons.org

American Nurses Association
   http://www.nursingworld.org/ce

CancerSource RN.com
   http://www.cancersourcern.com

Indiana University School of Nursing
   http://www.nursing.iupui.edu

Lippincott Williams & Wilkins
   http://www.nursingcenter.com

Medscape
   http://www.nurses.medscape.com

Nursing Spectrum
   http://www.nursingspectrum.com

Sigma Theta Tau
http://www.nursingsociety.org

Springnet CE Connection
http://www.springnet.com/ce

18. Finally, what content should still be taught face to face?

18. While distance learning programs may be "the next best thing to being there," there remain questions about what information should still be taught face to face. A majority of educators require that hands-on skill development and competency verification occur in a face-to-face environment. Supporters of distance learning may argue that all learning is possible given opportunities for online video interaction. But it may be years before that technology is available.

The personal interaction between faculty and learners can be quite effective in the distance learning environment. It is my hope that the personal connection that occurs in face-to-face meetings will never be truly replaced by communication in a digital world.

RESOURCES

American Society for Training & Development. (2001, August). The power, paradox, and potential of e-learning [Entire issue]. *Training and Development*.

Atkinson, K. (1999). Lessons leaned in developing online education. *Convene*, 47–51.

Billings, D. M., Ward, J. W., & Penton-Cooper, L. (2001). Distance learning in nursing. *Seminars in Oncology Nursing, 17*(1), 48–54.

Gibson, C. G. (2000). When disruptive approaches meet disruptive technologies: Learning at a distance. *Journal of Continuing Education in the Health Professions, 20,* 69–75.

Indiana University School of Nursing. *Teaching and learning in Web-based courses*. [Web site course]. Accessed October 23, 2000, from **http://Webct.nursing.iupui.edu**

NursingWorld. (2001). Nursing continuing education online. *ANA credentialing center—Continuing education online* [Online]. Available: **http://www.nursingworld.org/ancc/ceoned.htm**

Chapter 35: *Collaborative Ventures*

1. *What is e-learning?*

1. The majority of registered nurses work in hospitals or healthcare systems. Thus, it makes sense that hospital staff development programs have taken a leadership role in using e-learning. For most nurse educators, e-learning has begun with content designed to comply with regulatory requirements established by federal organizations. Such regulatory compliance is often the easiest place to get administrative support and document cost savings. Assignment and tracking components assist in course assignment, tracking, and documentation. Use of the information management components of e-learning frees the staff development educator from repeating regulatory content frequently and over three shifts. Educators are then able to address issues related to new nurse orientation, precepting, mentoring, and higher-level decision-making opportunities.

2. *What questions should I ask myself before I decide if I really want to collaborate with a technology company in the establishment of an e-learning program for the organization?*

2. The decision to enter into a formal relationship with an e-learning technology company is not one that should be taken lightly. Beginning an e-learning component requires thought, investigation of options, and financial pricing. Before you launch into such a training initiative, you must carefully think through the advantages, the effects on other parts of the healthcare system, and the costs to see if such a program is right for the organization.

Here are some questions to ask:

- What am I trying to achieve? Is the goal to reduce training staff time, consolidate resources, individualize learning, or promote professional development? Be sure this goal drives all technology decisions; don't add technology just for technology's sake.

- Does it make sense to use technology to accomplish this goal? Be aware that e-learning approaches can vary from simple Internet access to elaborate information management systems.

- Am I willing to enter into a collaborative partnership? Working with a technology company requires learning and cooperation on both sides. Both organizations need to realize that the e-learning field is in its infancy. There are bound to be occasional implementation problems on both sides. These small obstacles should be viewed as challenges, not examples of incompetence on the part of the other party—unless the small obstacles grow into big ones. Good communication and risk-taking attitudes promote cooperation and the attainment of a mutually rewarding product.

- Am I willing to accept that a successful working relationship will involve "give and take" on both sides? Working with an e-learning company means a willingness to translate the abbreviations and language of one's field, as well as to clarify and document expectations so that mutual understanding is facilitated.

- Do I have realistic expectations of workload and process? Most healthcare professionals have no idea of the technical processes involved in making an educational vision an online reality. Part of this mutual working relationship is to share your vision and then receive input from your technology partner regarding whether this vision is realistic in terms of time and effort.

- These expectations must be clearly discussed and written down at the beginning of the project. Be aware that time estimates are only "best guesses," so build in some extra time and expenses as a safety net. Adding 10% for unknown expenses is a good starting point, but you might consider as much as a 25% variance on long-term or complex projects.

- Am I able to articulate my final vision? Just as you must know your destination before beginning a trip, so you must have a vision of what you want the e-learning system to accomplish. Do not expect the technology company to be able to read your mind, or worse yet, to know what you might want if you have never figured it out yourself! A good way to see your "final vision" on paper, before the project starts, is to develop a site map (or graphic representation of the site organization). Also develop a site concept (pencil sketches or computer renderings of how the site will look) as part of the organizing stage of the project.

- Do I have organizational support for engaging in this partnership? Establishing a comprehensive e-learning program in a healthcare facility will affect how, when, and where education is conducted, so be sure to have administrative support for what you want to do. One of the best ways to get such buy-in is to have your administrator speak with other administrators who have used e-learning in their organizations. After the initial setup period, most administrators are able to document learner satisfaction and cost savings.

3. *Where do I start?*

3. A good place to start is to read about the experiences of others and ask peers to share their strategies. The Internet is also a good source for identifying e-learning companies that focus on health care. Most of these companies allow interested educators to view sample courses to determine if e-learning strategies would meet the needs of their organizations.

4. *How would I locate an appropriate technology company?*

4. Once you identify several e-learning companies that you would like to know more about, you want to investigate them more thoroughly. In today's dot-com environment, you will find great variation in company size, experience, and knowledge of the healthcare area. Thus, you must use caution to ensure the company in which you are interested offers the resources and working philosophy that is compatible with your needs.

Be sure to include local companies in your search for a site developer, if at all possible. Working with a local company typically results in a stronger partnership, reduced expenses, and the ability to meet face-to-face on a regular basis. Additionally, local partners are more readily available for ongoing support and future development after the e-learning product is online.

Next, set up an appointment for a consultation or preliminary meeting. If you have not yet had an opportunity to view the company Web site, ask for the location and examples of the company's work. You should look at the company's Web site carefully before the initial meeting so you can better assess whether or not the products you have seen are compatible with your vision. You are looking for demonstrated ability—if the company's own Web site lacks professional graphics or working code, don't expect a site the company develops to be any better. Here are some things to consider:

- Attention to detail

- Style

- Clarity

- Layout

- Ease of navigation

- Intuitive layout

- Time required to load pages

- Page appearance

- Reliability of links

- Workability

This inquiry will also allow you to investigate the level of sophistication or complexity on an equivalent site. You want to determine whether the company has a really good sales approach or whether they also have a really good product. If you are not able to look at the site before the initial meeting, ask to see such sites at that time. Never let a company talk you into its capabilities—you should always thoroughly investigate the company's online references.

5. What questions should I ask in an initial meeting?

5. The first meeting is an opportunity to get acquainted. This is much like dating. Each partner may be exemplary, but compatibility and the potential for good working relationships are imperative.

Use this first meeting to ask about the processes used in providing e-learning services. Does the company translate the organization's content to the Internet, develop its own content, license content from others, or use a combination of these? Ask about the safeguards the company uses to ensure content is current, accurate, and meets defined learning objectives.

Ask the company representatives to describe prior experience in doing projects such as yours. The company's prior experience will be very helpful as you explore possible timelines and costs. You may wish to view those final projects and ask for client lists or references you may speak to about their experiences. Be sure to follow through on this step. Just as in job interviews, a few well-placed phone calls will confirm your positive impressions or warn you to investigate further to avoid future problems.

Also, elicit some information about the company's resources. How many staff do the company have? What is their expertise, especially in projects such as yours? Do not rule out a small company that might do an excellent job of meeting your needs; small companies have lower overhead, engage in fewer politics, and can change direction on a project more quickly.

Your degree of involvement in the process is a final critical area of exploration. You need to be prepared to spend time and energy on this collaborative project. A close working relationship will help the project stay on task and on time. It will also facilitate an atmosphere of synergy and collaboration.

Many companies have a content partner or a team to work with the client on all phases of the project. Explore how this process would work, how frequently communication would occur, and how (and in what format) would you provide feedback. Feedback should occur at every step of the way, not just at the time of project completion.

6. What factors may indicate that this company may be a good partner?

6. While this is a business relationship, its success will ultimately reflect the working relationship, so look for indicators of what future relationships might be like. For example, how accessible are company representatives as you set up initial appointments and have initial meetings? Is it easy to reach them by phone? Do they return phone calls or e-mail? Is the initial appointment set up in a timely way? Remember, if the company is not responsive during these early "courting periods," the representatives will probably be even less responsive in the future.

Do you and the company representative with whom you will be working share a vision of the final products and the costs required to attain that vision?

Has the company demonstrated competency in execution (i.e., can it do the job you need done or provide the service you envision, and in compliance with time and cost guidelines)?

Do you feel comfortable with the people with whom you are speaking? Do you feel that they are being honest with you about their capabilities? Do they talk with you in plain English/clear lay terms? (They should not talk down to you or try to appear smarter than you.) Are they interested in your success or just their own? In short—trust your instincts. If you have unexplainable feelings of doubt that you can't put to rest by requesting more information, do not enter into a business relationship.

7. What should I consider when negotiating a contract with a technology company?

7. Clear communication is key. Do not enter into a business relationship without a contract, no matter how well you know the company with which you wish to partner. Employees may change, so you need to be sure you have a written paper trail.

A very useful strategy is to have a contract that includes all the specific agreements you and the technology partner have made. Items to include in the contract include:

- Total cost

- Up-front costs

- Final products described in quality and quantity

- Guarantees of final product

- Arrangements for formative reviews and approvals

- Terms and timelines

- Defined relationships

- Clear contingency plans

- Decisions regarding who owns the intellectual property (content and ideas)

- Decisions regarding who owns the electronic copyright

- Provisions to ensure that materials (such as graphs, photographs, multimedia) are originals and/or not in violation of copyright laws

- Provisions for revenue sharing (if appropriate)

- Provisions for updating/re-accreditation of content

- Provisions for updating if the original author is no longer available or interested

8. What faculty issues should I consider?

8. The faculty are frequently nurses who work in the staff development department in the organization or nurses who work in specialty areas of the healthcare organization.

As you work with faculty, be aware that content used in the classroom or traditional lecture content must be modified somewhat for use in a multimedia, CD-ROM, or Internet-based format. Depending on the complexity of the project, you may wish to work with individuals who possess instructional design, graphic design, or computer programming skills. These resources may also be part of the arrangements you make with the technology partner.

• Sometimes, a faculty member develops an instructional unit or video that is used by others. In these situations, basic content is presented via the established course, but small group leaders or other staff development personnel may elaborate and help learners apply the content to a specific institution or work setting. This instructional strategy modifies traditional faculty/student or teacher/learner relationships. For example, the faculty member or author may serve as the subject matter specialist (content expert). Another instructor may serve as a guide to help learners apply content. The content may be presented in a synchronous manner (e.g., all learners are in a classroom setting and hear content at the same time). Or the content may be presented asynchronously. (An example is when learners access content over the Internet at different times.) Such flexibility in learning changes the focus from an emphasis on time spent in the classroom to attainment of competency. The nurse educator is often then freed up for expanded roles in the assessment of entry-level behaviors and competency, and in managing learning experiences that support the development or enhancement of competency.

If the employees serve as the course faculty, issues such as faculty reimbursement should be considered. Will work being done on the course under development be part of the regular workload? If not, will you pay an incentive for development? It is recommended that such incentives be paid in two stages: 1) when content is identified but the instructional design is not completed, and 2) when the entire unit has been completed, field-tested, and edited.

If the course will be marketed or licensed to others, will you be providing royalty payments to the faculty? Often royalty payments begin a year after the initial course has been developed. Royalties are usually a percentage of total revenue. Five to seven percent of revenue is a frequently used percentage.

If you have made the decision that the faculty (author) retains the copyright for the intellectual property, that generally means that the author owns the content. Or, if development of the content is viewed as part of the work responsibility, the intellectual property may stay with the author's employer. This decision serves as the basis for determining who is responsible for guidelines for usage and for periodic review. If the content is formally approved for continuing nursing education contact hours, guidelines established by the accrediting agency must also be considered.

9. What are faculty responsibilities versus production team responsibilities?

9. In situations in which the organization is going to develop its own content, questions may arise regarding actual content development applicable to Internet. The content should determine whether the information is suitable for Internet presentation or would be better delivered in a traditional face-to-face environment.

If the decision is made to use the Internet for the presentation of specific content, be aware that the process may involve production approaches that vary from the ones that the nurse educator has used previously. Frequently, the subject matter expert knows the content but needs technology experts to adapt the content for the Internet. The other members of the production team may include a producer who coordinates the process, an instructional designer who identifies appropriates size and sequence of content, multimedia developers who can add interest and depth, and a computer programmer who develops instructions for the computer.

The author would retain the final approval of content, since only the author can ensure that any sequencing changes do not adversely affect content accuracy.

10. How do we manage timelines?

10. As with most project development, the process takes longer than you think it will. Even experienced "guess-timates" cannot anticipate all possible scenarios you may encounter, so allow extra time.

The timelines should allow time for feedback throughout the process as well as at the end. Also allow time for field testing and peer review. These unbiased review processes are invaluable in ensuring that the instructional materials are clear, concise, logical, and comprehensive. Field or pilot testing is also frequently a part of accreditation/approval requirements for continuing nursing education.

11. What quality assurance measures need to be in place?

11. While a face-to-face presentation may be somewhat spontaneous, the development of instructional materials such as those available over the Internet carry a higher level of responsibility for quality control. Areas that should be subject to quality control testing by an individual who was not involved in the development process include the following:

- Copyright clearances or originals
- English and grammar
- Sequencing and instructional design
- Functionality
- Ease of navigation

Much of this data can be built into the process for field (pilot) testing or internal/external review. Inclusion of sample learners who are similar in education and background to the potential audience in the field testing will increase the effectiveness of the instruction.

12. How do we know when the project is finished?

12. A project can easily take on a life of its own. Additional information may be gained during the process or original ideas may be difficult to implement. However, hard feelings and serious conflicts can arise if you (the customer) change your mind frequently or ask for additional work beyond the scope of the original agreement. For this reason, in-depth discussions and clear contracts at the beginning of the process are critical. A well-developed vision, clearly defined objectives, mutually agreeable timelines, and measurable outcomes will let all parties know when the initial contract parameters have been met. Any additional work would most appropriately be negotiated under a contract addendum or separate agreement, with new fees involved.

13. What tracking/information management components should I consider?

13. Content development and access may meet only part of the needs of the staff development department. There is frequently a need for computerization of training assignments. Assignments are frequently done by name or by position. Assigned courses (either online or face-to-face) can be listed. Tracking functions can reveal at a glance which learner has completed which courses and which still need to be completed. Computerized tracking programs can also include report generation functions. These are particularly important in documenting compliance with regulatory requirements.

The addition of such components may require the establishment of a supportive infrastructure and technical support. The functions are frequently available through e-learning technology companies.

These components should be developed and in place prior to the launch of the e-learning activity. As with the introduction of any change in the workplace environment, a comprehensive communication plan should be developed and implemented prior to the implementation of the new program. Such "public relations" efforts help to create awareness, prepare others for the impending change, and promote participation. A few well-chosen pilot tests help provide incentives to early adapters and support others in overcoming resistance that is an inherent part of the change process.

14. What do I need to consider in reevaluating/ updating the products we have developed?

14. The content and instructional materials you develop or use in teaching may be inservice or continuing nursing education (professional development). Regardless of the category, in this rapidly evolving Information Age, content should be evaluated regularly for currency. It is recommended that these updates be scheduled on an annual basis. Significant updates require another field (pilot) testing period.

15. What issues do I need to consider related to technical assistance and maintenance?

15. Probably even more critical than the initial development of content or purchase of equipment is the provision for technical assistance and maintenance. Timely response and resolution of problems is critical when an entire e-learning operation is based on successful implementation of technology.

Technology is an evolving art, so some downtime is inevitable. However, any technology company with which you have contracted for on-going technical assistance and maintenance should be supportive and responsive. Clarify and agree to anticipated response times for potential technological problems. Be aware that such support services frequently come with an added charge, but it is well worth it.

16. What issues do I need to consider related to distribution/ dissemination?

16. Some organizations are interested in more than using instructional materials compiled by others or in developing their own materials. These organizations are frequently interested in distribution or dissemination of their materials to other organizations, as an additional revenue source.

If this strategy is of interest to your organization, some additional areas should explored. First, you would want to see if the technology company you are considering is also involved in distribution and dissemination activities. Most of them are not.

Here are some things you may wish to consider:

a) Does the company have distribution partners or an in-house sales team?

b) How will branding of your company's name be achieved? (This is most frequently done using your organization's logo). Your materials may need to go through an organizational approval process for use of the logo in this manner. Branding using a company logo is the same process as buying a "brand name" in the grocery store. Name recognition is often related to customer loyalty and increased sales. However, like a personal reputation, a brand can be destroyed quickly, so every effort must be made to ensure the image the logo is projecting is a desirable one.

c) How will branding be accomplished? Some examples include the name of the organization on the front or introduction of the instructional material or a logo at the bottom of each page.

d) How will revenues be divided between the organization and the distribution company?

e) Will the materials the organization has developed be free of charge to the organization's employees?

17. How can I convince my supervisor to approve this collaboration?

17. Your supervisor will be interested in good ideas and in your enthusiastic presentation. However, you will also need to be prepared to provide the supervisor with the appropriate business plan and rationale necessary for an informed and objective decision.

A formal needs assessment and "best business" case presentation will stimulate buy-in. Administrators responsible for healthcare risk reduction (i.e., reducing liability) will be interested in the computerized ability to document training and compliance with regulatory guidelines.

Administrators interested in education and training functions will respond to a detailing of existing training and learning capabilities and the gaps in knowledge and skills acquisition. Explain how standardization of content and use of innovative e-learning strategies reduce employee costs through a reduction in the replication of training efforts. Time saved from eliminating the need to teach the same content to employees on three shifts can be used to individualize generic content to the specific institution, as well as to address more sophisticated issues. Consistency of content and access 24 hours a day, 7 days a week will enhance employee learning and ultimately have a positive impact on recruitment, retention, and quality of patient care. Improved patient care will be the result.

Finally, address the costs of contracts with collaborating companies. Compare this with cost savings by computerizing existing content acquisition, assignment, tracking, and documentation functions. Provide an opportunity for the administrator to speak with others who have recently implemented similar e-learning arrangements to learn more about their experiences. Most importantly, include the administrator as a vital part of the project. You can learn from the administrator's expertise. In addition, the administrator's understanding and responsibility to the project will add significantly to the successful implementation of your plan.

RESOURCES

Hall, B. (1997). *Web-based training cookbook*. New York: Wiley.

Porter, L. (1997). *Virtual classroom: Distance learning with the Internet*. New York: Wiley.

Saba, V., & McCormick, K. (Eds.). (2001). *Essentials of computers for nurses: Informatics for the new millennium* (3rd ed.). New York: McGraw-Hill.

Swansburg, R., & Swansburg, L. (1995*). Nursing staff development: A component of human resource development*. Boston: Jones and Bartlett Publishers.

Section 8:

Issues in Staff Development and Continuing Education

When you move to an educator role, there is a bit of relief that you are no longer subject to the risks of working with patients. Yet challenges and incidents do occur. These are related to the training and subsequent performance of staff. Questions about staff competence, standards of practice, intellectual property, and using evidence-based practice are addressed in this section. Knowing the issues and how best to address them will make you more valuable to your employing institution.

Chapter 36: *Legal and Ethical Concerns*

1. *I like to use published cartoons in my presentations. May I use them in the classroom? May I use them online?*

1. A better way to address this is to frame the question in terms of frequency of use and scope of distribution. In any case, full and complete credit must accompany the cartoon whether published on paper or online. Without permission of the holder of the copyright, use is limited to inclusion in the presentation and prohibited from reproduction in student handouts. If it can be determined that profit is derived from the use of this work, then permission is always required.

2. *I have a great chart, but I don't remember where I got it. May I still use it in class?*

2. To start with, get in the habit of jotting down the source on documents you receive in class or at conferences. Lacking the name of the author, consider using any or all of the following: conference; the name of the sponsoring organization; the date you attended; the location; or use the phrase "source unknown." Additionally, consider building upon, expanding, or updating the chart to make it your own. In this case, you should give credit using "adapted from" or "based on." It would be quite embarrassing to you and threatening to the creator for the work to appear as your own when it is not.

3. *How do I give credit for the work or ideas of others?*

3. For the unpublished work or idea of another, give accurate credit with as much specificity as possible. An example might read, "The ideas in this four-step process are based on the work of Julie Jones, as presented at the 1995 Midwest Med-Surg Conference."

4. *I found a skills check list in a journal article; may I use it for performance evaluation in my facility?*

4. To answer this, first check the journal and/or the article for copyright information. Request permission from the publisher or the author (whoever holds copyright) to use the checklist. Some checklists state "This may be used in your facility." If permission is denied, do not use the checklist. Again, adaptation should be considered.

5. *I've been asked to collect data for a research project in the facility. I want to help! Is it okay to participate?*

5. Great question! Nurses should always be encouraged to participate in research. Two important points to consider: the first is to determine if the study has been approved by the Institutional Review Board (IRB) at the facility. This determination is most easily done by asking for a copy of the letter of approval. All studies including those which are "exempt" or "expedited" will have a letter of approval. The second important point is to clearly articulate your role and responsibilities and then make sure that credit is given to you when the research is published.

6. How do I develop policies for staff with disabilities?

6. Policies should be consistent with those of the institution and the particular job descriptions for disabled individuals. To provide confidentiality, some policies may preclude full disclosure of the nature of the disability. In this case, the staff development process should be undertaken in good faith. Implementation of the agreed upon plan for instruction may require support from community resources. Working in collaboration with the Human Resources professionals in the facility will help.

7. What kind of accommodations may I make for staff members with disabilities?

7. Reasonable accommodations may include making sure classrooms and training materials are accessible, modifying teaching schedules, adjusting testing and teaching methods, allowing extra time for testing, providing or allowing interpreters or readers, and modifying equipment or devices. The learner does have a responsibility to make you aware of his/her needs or necessary accommodations. You are not expected to guess.

8. One of the OR nurses will not attend mandatory infection control training; what should I do?

8. Mandatory education is a condition of employment. Therefore, the consequences of not meeting the requirements are best addressed by the supervisor. However, as the staff development professional, creating options for meeting the various requirements is a good idea. Patient safety is always the main concern and should, therefore, be used in decisions related to employee evaluations.

9. I went to a conference and one of the lectures included several of my slides made from material I developed! What may I do?

9. It would be appropriate to inform the speaker of the specific material used. You may request that credit be given or that the material be removed from the presentation. Ownership of the material can be supported with documents holding a copyright. The presenter could be a novice educator and will benefit from your explanation or may share your enthusiasm for a topic and end up as a collaborator on future work.

10. *A nurse manager wants to limit administration of IV medications to those who scored 95 or better on the medication administration test. Should I give her the scores? Who has the right to access staff development records?*

10. Individual facility policies vary, but they usually reflect one of two positions on record maintenance. The first position is that the employee's record has all materials related to employment, and this record is maintained by the supervisor. In this case the scores would be placed in the employee's record. Supervisor access would be allowed. The second position is maintenance of records by the staff development professional and summary documents are provided to the supervisor and documentation reflecting completion of the requirement is given to the employee. Remember, scores on tests and checklists which have not been validated by rigorous/robust research methods should not be used to influence employment decisions.

11. *Pharmaceutical representatives give me lots of teaching materials. May I use them even if we don't use their products?*

11. Materials distributed by representatives of drug companies or other medical supply companies are a form of advertising and they are usually distributed for marketing purposes. It would not be right to lead the company representatives to believe you intend to order the product if you do not intend to do so. As with any materials, if adapted for use, remember to give credit.

12. *I developed a critical care course at my previous job; may I use it again at my current job?*

12. The content of the critical care course you developed belongs to you. The associated teaching materials may belong to your previous employer. The status of ownership should be clarified at the time of development. When you develop a course for your new employer, ask your supervisor if you are free to share the materials or if they belong to the employer (a work for hire). Selling the materials is an entirely different question and should also be clarified with the employer.

13. *I want to offer some ethics classes. Where do I start?*

13. Ethics education should begin during orientation and continue on a regular basis throughout employment. Equal effort should be given to integrating ethics content into each course and providing ethics specific classes. Resources available from your community and the ethics committee at your facility could co-sponsor an ethics education program. Topics may include confidentiality, privacy, pain management, end-of-life care, maternal/child issues, ageism, sexism, conflict of interest, and ethical principles of autonomy, justice, and beneficence.

14. *I'd like to participate on the Ethics Committee. What do I need to know?*

14. To participate on the Ethics Committee, you should have enthusiasm, good interpersonal skills, and an understanding of group dynamics, as well as some knowledge of ethics. The functions of the Ethics Committee usually include consultation and education as well as policy work. Participation as an ethics consultant can be guided by the Core Competencies developed by the American Society of Bioethics and Humanities (ASBH) (1998). Education of the committee members should be a funded priority and many opportunities are available throughout the country and in most communities. Healthcare ethics classes are offered by churches, colleges, and specialty organizations. To write or review policies, current knowledge of the topic is needed. Examples of policies include organ donation and end-of-life care.

15. *Many staff members speak English as a second language. How may I help them?*

15. If English is the language in the facility then educational programs should be provided in English. Tutorials for those who need help with English might be arranged through a local college or university. Additional help may be provided just by some extra time or allowing resources to be used during the educational process; however, a common outcome standard should be used to minimize error and ensure patient safety.

16. *One of the staff members asked me to change the date on her CE certificate so she could use the credits for re-licensure. Is that OK?*

16. Rather than change the date on a certificate, it would be better to provide a letter of explanation that could be submitted with the application for re-licensure. A circumstance which might require this would be a course which begins in one year and finishes in another. Falsification of paperwork is not permitted in any circumstance.

17. *Does it make a difference who makes copies of an article? Or how many they make? Or why they make them?*

17. Single copies from periodicals, newspapers, or books may be made for use in preparation of lectures or teaching materials. Cartoons, pictures, charts, graphs, or diagrams may also be used. Copying for students may be done if the tests of brevity and spontaneity are met. This means one time use by a teacher for a class where the decision to use the work and the presentation in class are so close in time that it is impractical to request permission. Articles of fewer than 2500 words or one chart, diagram, graph, or cartoon per book or per issue may be copied. "Consumable" materials are never to be copied. Examples of these include purchased workbooks, answer sheets, and test booklets.

18. *Does it matter if I copy a whole chapter from a book to distribute in a class?*

18. Book chapters may not be copied for distribution in class. A chapter may be copied for your personal use when preparing class materials. It is preferred that you provide the bibliographic reference so that students can access the materials. You can bring the original to class for student assessment of the value of pursuing access.

19. *If I can download it from the Internet, may I use it?*

19. You cannot safely assume that material on or from the Internet is free of copyright restrictions. As with any other intellectual property, you should carefully read the information online and follow whatever guidance is given. If there is no guidance, apply the fair use guidelines and give credit with as much specificity as possible when used.

20. *Can I record a broadcast program (air or cable) and then use it in class?*

20. Broadcast programs may be recorded by non-profit educational institutions and retained for use for 45 days following the broadcast. At the end of 45 days, they must be erased or destroyed. All off air/cable recordings must include the program's copyright notice (H. R. 97–495, pages 8–9).

21. *What rules govern fair use of printed materials?*

21. The copyright act of 1976 and the doctrine of fair use (US Code Title 17, Section 107) deal with use of copy-righted works. These are accessible at: **www.copyright.gov**.

22. *Can I be held liable for the adverse actions of an employee who claims "I was never trained, oriented, or taught?"*

22. You can certainly be held liable within the scope of your responsibility. The concept of Respondeat Superior defines this responsibility. Good documentation is the best support if there is a question of what was taught or what was learned. Always include (a) content of what was taught, (b) samples of evaluation of learning, (c) rosters of attendees, and (d) results of individual perform-ance in your files. However, competency assessment is a snapshot of employee performance and observations by peers and supervisors will contribute to an overall assessment of employee ability. It's very easy to blame the educational process rather than look to the employee or work environment for an accurate explanation of poor performance.

RESOURCES

American Society of Bioethics and Humanities. (1998). *Core competencies for health care ethics consultation.* Glenview, IL: Author.

Library of Congress Copyright Office Web site: **http://www.loc.gov/copyright**

Library of Congress Copyright Office. (1995). *Circular 21, Reproduction of copyrighted works by educators and librarians.* (Available at **http://www.loc.gov/copyright/circs**)

Minnesota Nurses Association. (2000). *Nursing education and the Americans with Disabilities Act.* (Available from the Minnesota Nurses Association, Education Department, [651] 646–4807 ext. 122)

Chapter 37: *Evidence-Based Practice*

1. What is evidence-based practice?

1. Evidence-based practice is the delivery of patient care by a provider who integrates clinical expertise with the best available evidence from systematic research. Evidence-based nursing practice includes use of clinical expertise and research, but also de-emphasizes the rituals and traditions of nursing practice that are not based on evidence. Evidence-based nursing practice includes incorporation of other types of data into practice, such as quality findings, patient preferences, and non-research evidence.

2. Where did evidence-based practice originate?

2. Evidence-based practice originated as evidence-based medicine in Great Britain and Canada by physicians who realized the need to examine the evidence used to medically treat patients to ensure care was delivered in the most effective and efficient manner. Under the National Health Service in these countries, all citizens were eligible for care but the resources were unable to meet the demand. In order to ensure best practices, medical practice needed to change, since physicians were not incorporating recent evidence into their patient treatment plans and many unnecessary tests and procedures were being carried out. Groups such as the Cochrane Collaboration and the Evidence-based Working Group were formed to ensure clinical research databases were developed for healthcare practitioners to use as the basis for clinical decision making (Gray, 2001). Nurse leaders in England, familiar with evidence-based medicine, initiated evidence-based nursing practice, and formed a Center for Evidence-based Nursing at the University of York, in England. In recent years other nursing journals related to evidence-based nursing practice have been initiated, and information more widely disseminated on best clinical practices in nursing.

3. What is research utilization in nursing and how does this differ from evidence-based practice?

3. Nursing research originated when academic nursing faculty began to conduct their own research. Often the subjects of this research were nursing students or the nursing curriculum. When clinical topics were researched, the nursing investigator conducted the research and published the findings, but few practicing nurses knew about these outcomes and how to use the research in nursing practice. The nursing research utilization movement played a key role in advancing professional nursing, for it demonstrated the importance

of using research to change nursing practice to improve patient outcomes. Research utilization changed the research cycle for professional nursing from conduct - publish to actual use in practice and then completing the cycle by publishing the results of the utilization. Some significant projects that influenced research utilization in nursing were the Western Interstate Commission for Higher Education (WICHE) Project, which originally developed the research utilization model to improve nursing practice, and the Conduct and Utilization of Research in Nursing (CURN) Project. The CURN project broadened the scope of research utilization to 17 hospital sites working on 10 research based protocols, and demonstrated the significance of changing clinical practice in the areas of preoperative teaching, preventing pressure ulcers, catheterization, and many other practices (Goode, Butcher et al., 1991). While Research Utilization (RU) had certain strengths, such as bringing a clinical focus to nursing research, involving the staff nurses in the process, and emphasizing the need to use published research findings in practice, there are limitations to this process. RU is a nursing term, and other disciplines do not know the process. Patient preferences were not addressed in nursing research utilization, and other sources of evidence were not included. Evidence-based practice has broadened the view of how nurses in clinical practice use research, since it is a universal term that is widely used by many disciplines. The components of evidence-based practice include a wide range of dimensions that influence how patient care is delivered and the outcomes of patient care.

4. *What are the components of evidence-based practice?*

4. Evidence-based practice includes many components. Evidence-based medicine emphasizes the use of systematic clinical research to drive practice decisions, as well as the need to include patient preferences. Stetler (2001) addressed the importance of nursing not using traditions and opinions, emphasizing the use of other evaluation data such as quality and outcomes, as well as research. Goode and Krugman (2001) and colleagues at the University of Colorado Hospital (UCH) have developed a multidisciplinary evidence-based model that includes many data elements nurses can use and relate to their practice. The model follows:

Evidence-Based
Multidisciplinary Practice Model

© University of Colorado
Reprinted with permission.

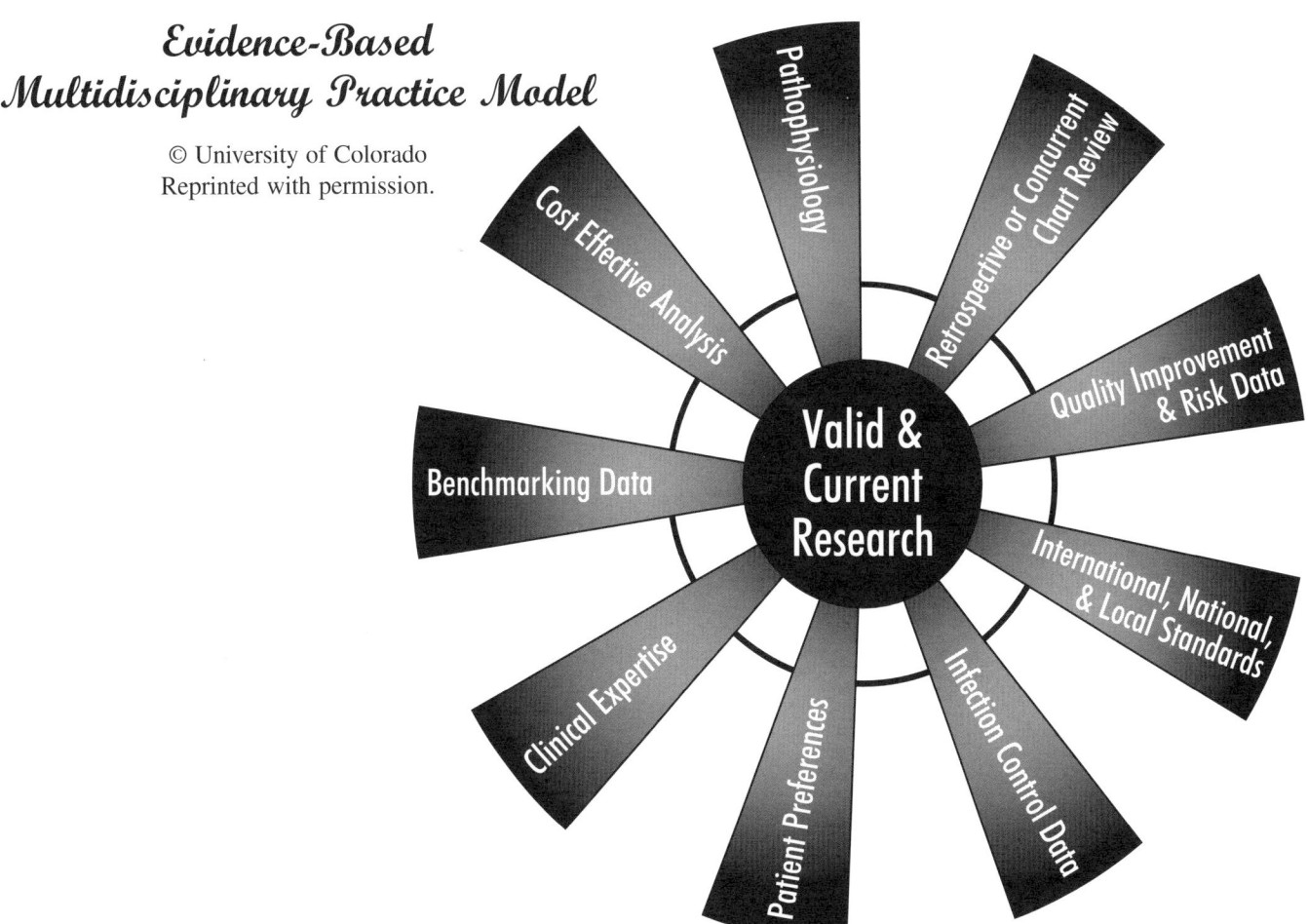

5. Is there a process involved in evidence-based practice?

5. Yes, the process involves critically analyzing the evidence, selecting appropriate evidence-based interventions, implementing them, and evaluating the outcomes. This process includes steps that nurses have learned as nursing process to deliver nursing care: assessment, planning, implementation, and evaluation. Nurses should feel comfortable with the terminology, for it draws upon the same critical thinking skills. However, evidence-based nursing practice requires nurses to rely less on traditional approaches to nursing practice. The skills needed in evidence-based practice include using critical thinking skills to examine the evidence by reading research articles, using search engines on the computer to find information, and incorporating this information into clinical nursing practice. These may be processes that are new and seem intimidating to nurses. Just remember, it is another level of depth to the familiar nursing process, so every nurse has a good beginning to incorporating the new evidence-based practice skills!

6. I am still not sure I understand evidence-based nursing practice. What are some examples of these type projects?

6. At the University of Colorado Hospital, we have used evidence-based practices in a number of multidisciplinary projects involving nurses and other care providers. For example, nursing and respiratory therapy had questions regarding the frequency of changing vents. Dr. Goode and the Respiratory Therapy Coordinator analyzed the literature and implemented new procedures, testing the outcomes of the changes. The results were published in 1999 in the *Journal of Nursing Administration*. In another example, nurse practitioners and physicians in the outpatient setting realized there were significant variations in how an uncomplicated female urinary tract infection was being treated. An evidence-based multidisciplinary team was convened to examine the literature and implement practice changes. The results were reported in *Nursing Economic$* in 2000. One evidence-based project involved acute care patients on a surgical service. A CNS/Educator became aware of published nursing research related to nurses evaluating the proper placement of nasogastric tubes. She initiated a multidisciplinary group to review this nursing research, which suggested a technique using measurement of the pH of the fluid post tube placement, rather than radiologic imaging. Members of this group, which included physicians, reviewed the evidence and decided that based on the type of tubes used at UCH, which were small bore, it was best to retain use of radiology imaging to confirm placement of the nasogastic tubes. However, during the course of these team meetings, physicians raised a question about aspiration pneumonia, asserting nurse technique during insertion of nasogastric tubes was resulting in a higher incidence of aspiration pneumonia. Chart reviews were then conducted to examine outcomes of nurse-inserted nasogastric tubes, and no relationship was found between nurse technique and aspiration pneumonia. However, a relationship was found between emergent intubation and aspiration pneumonia, which is now being further investigated. These are just some examples of clinical projects. At UCH, we also use our evidence-based model to guide assessing administrative issues and non-clinical problems as well.

7. Where do I look for the evidence?

7. Searching for the best evidence is a critical step to successfully implementing evidence-based practice. Nurses and other healthcare providers are constantly challenged to keep up with the rapidly expanding information now available for clinical decision making. Patients are now active participants in this information search, so nurses have the additional challenge of keeping up with patient questions along with their own need for information. Nurses must not only be able to search rapidly and easily for information, but also be able to evaluate the soundness of the data and know how to evaluate conflicting data. For nurses, most of the searches to examine the evidence will be found in five types of sources: textbooks, online databases, journals, special services that organize data and information, and general Internet sources such as list servs. Evaluating these sources can provide challenges! Each type of source is outlined below:

Textbooks: These become outdated quickly, so are primarily useful for information that is already tested and not changing. However, please note that at UCH, we have found even "stable" information to be potentially outdated and based on "tradition." So use textbooks with caution, carefully examining the evidence behind some of the traditional information such as procedure techniques in clinical practice.

Journals: These keep nurses up to date with the latest practice trends and information. Specialty journals are a particularly rich and significant source of data for nurses practicing in a particular clinical area. Be sure the journal you read is peer reviewed, which means other experts have reviewed the article to ensure the information meets professional standards. Nurses have a tendency to read only nursing journals. Consider reading some of the widely regarded medical journals, such as the *Journal of the American Medical Association* (*JAMA*) and the *New England Journal of Medicine*, to keep up with trends that significantly influence nursing practice. Look for articles that have analyzed many articles using statistics for significance (meta-analysis), or integrative reviews that provide an in-depth examination of many articles on the same topic.

Bibliographic Databases: Most nurses are familiar with CINAHL (Cumulative Index to Nursing and Allied Health Literature) or Medline (National Library of Medicine). If you are not aware of these or do not know how to use them, you definitely should take a course at a local library or community college on how to search the literature using these type databases. While journals and textbooks have their place in the search for evidence, databases are by far the fastest and most up-to-date method for keeping up with changing information and the evidence. Usually using CINAHL and Medline work for everyday needs, but more in-depth searches may be needed using EMBASE and other types of databases. Specialty organizations and disciplines have their own databases, which can be most helpful if you have a particular question related to pharmacy or mental health, as examples.

Consolidated or Aggregated Data Sources: These sources can be very helpful for obtaining the most up-to-date information on abstracts of research organized by others, with a critical appraisal. Some examples of these sources are Evidence-based Nursing, Evidence-based Medicine, Evidence-based Mental Health, or the ACP (American College of Physicians) Journal Club. These sources include high quality of studies that save you time; you don't have to sort out what is important and what is not, since experts have already done this for you. You get systematic reviews by experts, and the latest information. The largest collection on helping evaluate clinical research systematically is the Cochrane Collection, an international network of healthcare professionals committed to producing and maintaining reviews of effects of healthcare interventions. These reviews are available from the Cochrane Library, and are included at most major libraries associated with health science centers.

Internet: While the Internet offers high-speed access, the sources may be questionable and require the nurse (and patient!) to evaluate the sources carefully. Quality is difficult to assess. It is important, therefore, to use sites which are known to be valuable or screened, if the nurse is accessing them on behalf of patients. Often specialty organizations, such as the Oncology Nursing Society or the Cancer Institute at the National Institutes of Health, will have reviewed sources that are considered of quality for a particular disease process. The Internet is a wonderful addition for nurses to communicate informally with one another. Each specialty has **Listservs**, which are ways to "talk" to other nurses who have the same specialty interests, such as informatics, critical care, education, neurology, and others. You will need to equip yourself with access to a good computer, take classes to learn the tools, and give yourself time to explore some of the many sources of information available as resources for evidence-based practice.

8. How do I evaluate the evidence?

8. Nurses want to know, "Can I use this new information in my practice?" Evaluating the evidence is a very important step toward developing skills in evidence-based practice. There are three questions that need to be answered:

1. Can the information in this article/project/research be transferred into clinical practice?

2. Will implementing this practice change result in improved patient outcomes?

3. Will this change close a gap between research and practice?

All types of research and information should be evaluated for potential contribution. If you go back and review the UCH Multidisciplinary Evidence-based Practice Model, you will note that research is at the core of this model. Always start by looking for research based evidence. This research may be either quantitative or qualitative. Most commonly, the medical literature related to evidence-based practice will emphasize the need to have randomized controlled clinical trials (RCTs). While this method of research constitutes the "gold standard" of the highest level of evidence, some types of data lend themselves to descriptive research. An example of this is the data nurses have collected related to stresses and problems of families who have a loved one with Alzheimer's disease. Nurse researchers have contributed important information that has served to guide the development of public policy related to this disease, data that could not have been obtained through randomized clinical trials. Sometimes there is no research available to review related to a specific clinical issue. As the model shows, many types of evidence can be used to determine best nursing practice: infection control data, quality and outcomes, and patient preferences to name just some of the elements that comprise the evidence. Not all of the evidence is research based. For example, patient preferences may be related to one individual patient's response to a condition, and may not be typical of other patient responses to that

9. How do I know the evidence is valid and reliable, if I am not trained in research?

disease. You may begin to collect your own evidence on a clinical issue, such as quality data or preferences data. You will want to evaluate to be sure the data are scientifically sound, have been or could be replicated, and causes no harm to patients. You should not make changes in practice, however, based on one study with one small sample.

9. First of all, you need to learn what validity and reliability mean and understand the concepts (Burns & Grove, 2001):

Validity: The degree to which the instrument used to provide the results measures what it is supposed to measure. For example, are you trying to determine whether or not an article about nurse job satisfaction is valid? If the author measured nurse job satisfaction by using an instrument that measured critical thinking, you would not be learning about how satisfied nurses were with their jobs! Measuring skin breakdown requires a valid tool such as the Braden Scale (Bergstrom & Braden, 1998) so you know all of the potential dimensions of skin breakdown are included as content categories on this scale.

Reliability: The degree to which an instrument is consistent and precise. So, if you were looking at job satisfaction, and the author used an instrument measuring job satisfaction, would the instrument show consistent measurement over time so you could compare job satisfaction rates yearly? If you were looking at skin breakdown, would the assessment tool provide consistent rating results over many types of patients, so you could count on the score results being accurate over shifts and clinical services? The Braden Scale has been tested repeatedly across patient populations, with the content consistently measuring skin reliably.

One of the ways you can find evidence and determine its strength is by reading integrative reviews and meta-analysis reports by researchers who have done the work to determine validity and reliability. These types of articles are a valuable contribution to the literature and help those who are not as skilled in research techniques. Unfortunately, these articles may not exist on the clinical problem you desire to study. Be sure and look first for these, however, before assuming there are no resources. Another way you can begin to learn is by reading about reliability and validity in nursing research textbooks. You can also take a beginning course on research and statistics. Learning the language of research is just like learning French or Spanish. You have to read about it, study it, and practice it. The more you practice and learn about it, the more comfortable you will feel. You can learn about reliability and validity by working with a knowledgeable colleague, either within the discipline of nursing or another discipline, who understands the scientific literature. It is good to find someone you feel safe with, who will encourage and promote your learning and give you feedback and information. All of these ways of learning about validity and reliability help build your confidence to better understand medical and nursing literature.

10. What if my healthcare institution doesn't know anything about evidence-based practice? How can I make a difference?

10. Many institutions are not "tuned in" to evidence-based practice. You can be a leader for a hospital or healthcare institution by starting in very modest ways to bring evidence into practice. The easiest way is by starting with clinical policies and procedures. All policies and procedures in a hospital or healthcare setting need to be updated regularly to meet JCAHO or State Health Department accreditation standards. Begin by taking policies and searching for the evidence to reference these policies. Share this approach and activity with others serving on the policy and procedure committee. If other colleagues on such a committee take key policies and begin searching for the evidence, the content of these policies will improve, and the skills of those reviewing them will also be improved. This activity begins to change the culture of the institution, setting the tone for how important evidence is in policies to "back up" why a particular procedure is done in the way described. You can also begin by using the terms in a meeting, when clinical issues are being discussed, by saying, "What is the evidence for us to do one procedure rather than the other?" Using the vocabulary starts others thinking about the evidence to validate actions and activities related to patient care.

11. Are there any tools available to help me learn how to critique and analyze the evidence?

11. At the University of Colorado Hospital, we use a modified tool that was initially developed by Goode, Butcher et al. (2001) and modified further at the University of Colorado Hospital (Research Report Critiquing Form available by contacting Mary Krugman at mary.krugman@uhc.edu). This tool is very helpful for practicing how to analyze the literature. Nursing research textbooks also provide criteria for analyzing the evidence. Each of the criteria or categories for analysis has cues that ask questions about the different aspects of the nursing or medical article, and take staff through each step of the review process. Use the analysis criteria to work in groups, to teach one another and begin to feel more comfortable with the process. The more you practice, the better developed will be your skills! It is no different than learning how to manage pumps or vascular access devices, just another dimension to nursing practice that requires practice, practice, practice.

12. Why is evidence-based practice important to staff development?

12. For years, nurses considered research to be an "extra" or " add on" to practice and something only learned by those who were intellectual, not practicing nurses. Now we realize that unless all nurses understand and know how to seek evidence, they are not empowered in their practice. Research and evidence-based practice are *essential* for nursing practice, and can only be developed properly if staff development incorporates these principles into institutional practice through orientation and continuing education programs. Since staff development plays such a critical role in how nurses are socialized into the institutional setting, we should be leaders in evidence-based practice, and viewed as resources for this important dimension in professional practice. Staff development needs to model the principles and practice of evidence-based nursing practice in all courses and programs, as well as developing special programs just in this area of practice to educate nurses.

13. How can I start using evidence-based practice in staff development?

13. Start with incorporating evidence into the foundation of staff development programs. This means you will have to be convinced, like I am, that evidence-based practice is one of many basic competencies nurses need to know and demonstrate continually. Research and research based evidence needs to be valued by a healthcare institution. Would you want a physician practicing in the hospital or clinic who did not have a scientific basis for his or her practice? Of course not! Then why would you expect anything less of practicing professional nurses? Nurses should also have a scientific basis for their practice. If nurses are to be colleagues with other disciplines, and full participating members in the healthcare team, they need the same skills and background. Nursing plans of care should be based on evidence, just like physicians use their knowledge and evidence to develop and implement the medical plan of care. This means competencies for evidence-based practice need to be on skill lists for orientation, just like checking off pumps, policies, and other such skills. For example, at University of Colorado Hospital, nurses in orientation are provided a tour of the Health Sciences Center Library and receive a library card, which sends the message up front about our expectations for continued learning. Orientation for nurses also includes a session on our computer gateway page, showing them how to access the search engines and resources on a computer to look up patient conditions right on the clinical unit. They are oriented to policies and procedures online, and the procedure for referencing all policies with citations, and why that is important. That is just the beginning of how we set the stage for socializing them into the culture of evidence-based practice. We then continue, during orientation, by reviewing the job description and performance standards for professional registered nurses, which both identify the expectation for nurses to know evidence-based practice and research in the performance of their staff nurse position. Newly hired nurses are given examples of the expectations for research and outcomes, along with the technical and clinical skills outlined for their job. So, orientation can be framed as professional orientation, where research is valued along with the technical skills to perform the position. These are only a few examples of how staff development educators can begin to demonstrate the importance of evidence-based nursing in practice.

14. *What are some examples of continuing education offerings related to evidence-based practice?*

14. Staff development departments have a big job in this area, since frequently nurses come to the clinical setting from education programs that do not provide this type of foundation. However, I believe healthcare organizations have to start at the top, with nursing leadership. Unless nursing leadership understands and uses these concepts, and models them in their own meetings and actions, all the expectations in the world will mean nothing for staff nurses practicing clinically with patients. It will feel like a double standard to them, since those evaluating them will not be using the tools. So, at UCH, we started with basic courses in evidence-based practice and required it of three levels of leadership: nursing directors/managers, clinical educators (who are staff development personnel), and permanent Charge

Nurses. All of these personnel have been required to take a four-hour foundational course called Introduction to Evidence-based Practice. For those members of the nursing leadership team who do not have strong skills in analyzing the literature, we next have them take Clinical Research for the Novice Nurse, an eight hour class that includes more depth to understanding how to analyze the literature, as well as four hours with a librarian learning how to conduct searches of the literature.

For many staff nurses who are advancing levels in the clinical ladder, these classes become very important to their success in participating in outcomes related projects, either on performance improvement, research, or evidence-based teams. Clinical staff nurses can take these two classes, and obtain credit on their yearly performance appraisals for these activities. All leadership and clinical nurses are encouraged to attend the annual Research Symposium, which also counts as part of their continuing education and provides them with a window into the world of research and evidence-based practice through podium and poster presentations. We try to pair up staff nurses with others more expert such as a principal investigator on projects, so they can learn how to do a poster presentation at a conference and gain confidence in these skills and activities.

15. What is the role of journal clubs in evidence-based practice and staff development?

15. Journal clubs are one of the most essential ways for clinical nurses to learn about using evidence in practice. A journal club is the single most powerful tool to incorporate the values and skills of evidence-based practice into the everyday work of nursing. A journal club is a meeting of staff nurses, or multiple disciplines together, to critique literature and share knowledge about a particular practice issue. The purpose of a journal club is to promote awareness of current research and provide a mechanism for updating information about patient care issues. It is a group discussion format to explore different viewpoints and stimulate critical thinking about care. Staff development educators can teach staff nurses how to participate in journal clubs, and help journal clubs get started. The most effective journal clubs are held on a specific service, with staff choosing the article and meeting at a time convenient to them, so they have control over the process and feel ownership of the event. Usually there is a facilitator, who is one of the staff taking a turn leading the group. This provides staff nurses with experience doing this activity, and is one of the ways UCH staff nurses meet their research performance standards. Teaching staff nurses how to lead and participate in journal clubs is one of the most satisfying ways of increasing professionalism and development among registered nurses. When nurses gain confidence with journal club skills by practicing with one another, they can then participate with other disciplines and experience collegiality and be viewed as a full member of the professional team. Journal clubs are one of the most effective ways to teach critical thinking skills. We start with new graduate nurse residents, teaching them journal club skills during their residency orientation. Staff development educators can shape the level of staff nurse professionalism through journal club participation.

16. *I am a solo educator in a small hospital. How can I start evidence-based practice in my institution, without any resources?*

16. The most important resource for starting evidence -based practice is with yourself as a staff development expert! Your conviction and valuing of the importance of learning and practicing using the techniques of evidence-based practice are the single most important action to make this happen. Dr. Colleen Goode, a national expert on research utilization and evidence-based practice, began her career in a small community hospital of less than 100 beds in Ida Grove, Iowa. She requested articles and books on research utilization from the local library, and taught herself and her staff, together, how to do research utilization. At the time she had a BSN, and most of her staff were Diploma and Associate degree nurses. From these beginnings, she returned to school to continue her education, and she and the staff even developed a video and educational materials to help others, based on their own self-learning. This story shows how any one of us who takes the initiative to learn can do these activities. Of course, resources are terrific if you have them! Partnering with a local community college nursing faculty or a colleague from another discipline who has these skills can build your confidence and ability. Now that we are so easily linked to the Internet, you can gain support and partners across the country without relying on the local scene. The Web sites on evidence-based nursing practice provide support "long distance" to answer questions and help with program implementation. Starting with policies and procedures, journal clubs, basic classes, and putting expectations into job descriptions and performance standards are all ways to begin that do not require significant resources. The most important requirement is your own learning and conviction as a place to begin the process.

17. What kind of resources can staff use to learn about evidence-based practice?

17. The most current and up to date resources on evidence-based nursing practice are accessible on the Web and Internet. All you need is a computer with access to online service to the search engines and Web sites. Additionally, there are some books that are considered expert references in the field of evidence-based practice to help you. One is by Gray (1997). While this book is physician-oriented, it will provide a good start for learning about evidence-based medicine. Nursing resources include a primary Web site and information from the Evidence-Based Nursing Center at the University of York in England at **www.york.ac.uk/depts/hstd/ centres/evidence/ev-intro.htm** In the USA, there is a journal called the *Evidence Based Nursing Journal*, which serves as a good resource for monthly articles. Best Evidence is a distilled version of a bibliographic database (available on CD ROM), and includes material from both medicine and nursing related to evidence-based practice. This reference is an excellent time-saver. Grateful Med (**www.nlm.nih.gov/databases/ fremedl.htm**) is a free service from the US Library of Medicine which provides an effective and easy method to search for evidence.

18. What is an evidence-based program in staff development and continuing education?

18. In contrast to offering a single class or course, or just engaging in evidence-based activities on a random basis, a program of evidence-based practice involves purposeful planning and program development. Activities in evidence-based practice are designed to meet specific educational and programmatic needs according to the American Nurses Association's definition of staff development. A program of evidence-based practice would include the following components:

a. Courses designed after conducting a needs assessment of nurses to determine level of learning needs and knowledge deficits. These courses would include a basic or introductory course to evidence-based practice, and additional classes in the series to provide more in-depth learning regarding research and literature review.

b. A variety of educational activities and media to further the learning options. These include the following examples:

- Written materials, such the *UCH Practice Outcomes Manual*

- CD Rom program on Research Utilization to help staff learn some basic principles of nursing research use (Goode et al., 1991)

- Specific competency activities to ensure staff are meeting yearly performance expectations related to knowledge and use of research. These activities can include posters with post-tests or a requirement to attend a journal club, as examples.

19. What are some ways to incorporate evidence-based practice into current staff development and continuing education offerings?

19. The easiest way to do this is to start by referencing any materials you use with citations. Are you giving credit to those whose work you are using when you lecture and teach? Do nurses know where diagrams, charts, and other materials come from that you use? That is the most important step you can take in the introduction of evidence-based practice . . . show that you know and are using actual evidence in your own instruction. A second important step to take, which was mentioned early in this chapter, is to ensure ALL clinical policies and procedures are updated with actual references and citations to source. In this way, nurses begin to learn that a certain way of doing a procedure is based on standards such as those from ANA, or the Oncology Nurses Society, or other such national or specialty organizations. Nurses need to learn they must use evidence in daily practice, and this is an important way to begin. A third way to incorporate evidence-based practice is to talk about it, refer to it in your teaching, and use examples that highlight nurse research in the course you are teaching. For example, teaching a course on neonatal care? Don't forget to mention the nurse researcher who was instrumental in bringing kangaroo care into neonatal intensive care units, putting premature neonates skin to skin to improve their growth rate and stabilize their temperature control and their heart rate. Teaching oncology? Be sure and mention the outstanding research oncology nurses have conducted in relation to pain management, symptom management, and others. In other words, nursing research can be referred to frequently and often to let nurses know and be proud of their profession, and begin to realize there is a world out there filled with outstanding professionals who are helping build a scientific basis for the care they deliver.

REFERENCES

Bergstrom, N., Braden, B. J., Kemp, M., Champagne, M., & Ruby, E. (1998). Predicting pressure ulcer risk: A multi-site study of the predictive validity of the Braden scale. *Nursing Research, 47*(5), 261–269.

Gray, J. A. M. (2001). *Evidence-based healthcare.* New York: Churchill Livingstone.

Goode, C. J., Butcher, L. A., Cipperley, J. A., Ekstrom, J., Gosch, B. A., Hayes, J. E., Lovett, M. K., & Wellendorf, S. A. (1991). *Using research in clinical practice* [CD ROM]. Ida Grove, IA: Horn Video Productions.

Goode, C., & Krugman, M. (2001). Evidence-based practice: A tool for clinical and managerial decision making. In J. McCloskey- Dochterman & H. K. Grace (Eds.), *Current issues in nursing* (6th ed., pp. 60–68). St. Louis: Mosby.

Nicoll, L. H. (2001). *Nurses' guide to the Internet.* Philadelphia: Lippincott.

Stetler, C. B. (2001). Updating the Stetler model of research utilization to facilitate evidence-based practice. *Nursing Outlook, 49*(6), 272–279.

RESOURCES

Burns, N., & Grove S. (2001). *The practice of nursing research.* Philadelphia: Saunders.

Mulhall, A. (1998). Nursing, research and the evidence. *Evidence Based Nursing, 1*, 4–6.

Chapter 38: *Standards of Practice*

1. Why is the term Nursing Professional Development (NPD) used rather than staff development and continuing education?

1. Nursing professional development encompasses both continuing education and staff development. The goal in developing the new term was to try to bring out the similarities in the roles rather than the differences. Educators in both staff development and continuing education provide educational opportunities for nurses to continue their professional development.

2. How have the NPD Standards evolved?

2. The first educational standards published by the American Nurses Association (ANA) in 1974 were titled *Standards for Continuing Education in Nursing*. This was followed by *Guidelines for Staff Development,* first published in 1976 and revised in 1978. In 1984, ANA published revised standards for continuing education in nursing and in 1990 published the *Standards for Nursing Staff Development*. In 1992, ANA published a document called *Roles and Responsibilities for Nursing Continuing Education and Staff Development Across all Settings*. This was a necessary component for the certification exam in Nursing Continuing Education and Staff Development. The term nursing professional development was first used with the standards that were revised in 1994. Since these standards replaced both the continuing education and staff development standards, those terms were still included in the title. The latest revision of the standards, published in 2000, replaces both the 1992 and 1994 publications, since it includes both the scope of practice and standards. In this latest revision, the terms continuing education and staff development are not included in the title.

3. Who develops these standards?

3. The American Nurses Association is responsible for the development and publication of standards. When there was a Council on Continuing Education, typically the executive board of the council was involved in the revision of standards. Sometimes a specific task force or work group was appointed by the American Nurses Association to revise these documents. With the latest standards, a workgroup of nine nurses with various backgrounds and expertise was pulled together to revise the standards.

4. How can someone get a copy of the standards?

4. The standards are available through the American Nurses Publishing Company, publication number NPD–20; the cost is $11.95 for ANA members and $14.95 for non-members. The standards can be ordered by contacting

American Nurses Publishing at 600 Maryland Avenue, SW, Suite 100 West, Washington DC 20024–2571, by calling 1(800) 215–3727 or online at: **www.nursingbooks.org**

5. *How often are the standards reviewed/revised?*

5. ANA determines the frequency of the revision of the standards. Typically, every 5–10 years the standards are reviewed and revisions made.

6. *How can individual educators give feedback on proposed revisions?*

6. Every time the standards are reviewed, there is a process for a field review of the standards. Each constituent member association (CMA) of the ANA receives a draft of the proposed revisions, as well as each member of the Nursing Organizations Liaison Forum (now together with the National Federation of Specialty Nursing Organizations [NFSNO] known as the Nursing Organizations Alliance [the Alliance]), a group of specialty nursing organizations. In the case of the nursing professional development standards, the National Nursing Staff Development Organization (NNSDO) also received the draft, since it was a collaborating group in the development of the certification exam. The NNSDO Executive Board, as well as committee chairs, all received draft copies of the latest standards. In addition, an article appeared in *TrendLines*, the NNSDO newsletter, offering opportunity for input from all NNSDO members.

7. *Who is responsible for being aware of/adhering to these standards?*

7. All educators in any setting need to be aware of and adhere to these standards. The standards can be used in legal proceedings to determine if an educator acted appropriately. Standards delineate the roles and responsibilities expected of professional nursing development educators in any setting.

8. *What happens if my institution or staff members do not meet these standards?*

8. The standards provide a guide for practice, and represent the ideal situation. Especially in terms of the qualifications of educators and administrators, there may be reasons why an institution does not meet the standards. The standards indicate the educator should have a master's degree, with either the bachelor's or master's degree being in nursing. If there are not master's programs in the immediate area, some institutions may not be able to meet that portion of the standards. However, the standards can be used to justify the need for someone with those qualifications. If specific staff members are not following the guidelines outlined in the standards, you should look at that and try to determine why.

9. Why are the NPD standards important?

9. The standards provide a basis and framework for practice. They outline specific responsibilities of our role, and provide guidance on role expectations and scope of practice. By meeting these standards, we help contribute to quality educational programs, which ultimately help promote quality patient care. The standards are also used to identify what is expected in any legal action.

10. Are these standards for the educator or learner?

10. The workgroup that revised the last standards struggled with this question. The learner has specific responsibilities for his/her professional development; however, the standards focus on the role of the educator. The educational process is outlined in the first part of the standards, and the second part of the standards deals with standards of practice for the educator. In the appendix of the standards there is a section that outlines responsibilities of the individual nurse.

11. How do the standards relate to the quality of care?

11. Everything that we do as educators ultimately should influence the quality of care. Whether we are orienting new nursing personnel, going over new equipment/procedures, or teaching nurses new skills, the ultimate goal is to assist them to provide quality care. All professional development activities should assist individual nurses to document continuing competence, which promotes quality care.

12. How do the standards define continuing competence?

12. With the increasing focus on competence, the work group that revised the latest standards had that as a central theme or framework of the standards. Many definitions of competence were reviewed, but the one selected for this publication was the one developed by ANA in 2000. Continuing competence is defined as "ongoing professional nursing competence according to level of expertise, responsibility, and domains of practice as evidenced by behavior based on beliefs, attitudes, and knowledge matched to and in the context of a set of expected outcomes as defines by nursing scope of practice, policy, Code of Ethics, standards, guidelines, and benchmarks that assure safe performance of professional activities" (p. 3). Although this definition is fairly long and involved, the key components are:

- Based on expertise, responsibility, and domains of practice

- Focused on safe performance

• Defined by policies, standards, guidelines, and benchmarks

13. How can I use the standards in my practice?

13. The standards can be used to document that you are following the steps of the educational process in the assessment, planning, implementation, and evaluation of educational activities. They can also be used to show how you are meeting the standards of professional performance. Criteria from the standards can be incorporated into position descriptions, can be used to justify the need for additional resources, and also can be used to justify hiring qualified personnel for the educational role.

14. How do the standards relate to the certification exam?

14. The standards provide the basis for the certification exam. One of the requirements of the American Nurses Credentialing Center is that there are standards and a scope of practice outlined for all certification exams. When item writers develop and/or revise questions for the exam, the standards and criteria in the standards are used as a basis for those questions.

15. How does academic education fit in with the standards?

15. Academic education consists of courses taken for undergraduate or graduate credit in an institution of higher learning that may or may not lead to a degree or completion of a certificate program. In this publication, academic education refers to those courses taken in colleges or universities after the basic nursing education program. Academic education is one way of achieving nursing professional development.

16. What's the definition of staff development in the standards?

16. The definition of staff development in the standards is "Staff development is the systematic process of assessment, planning, development, and evaluation that enhances the performance or professional development of health care providers and their continuing competence" (ANA, 2000, p. 5). Staff development activities include continuing education, orientation, and inservice education.

17. How is staff development different from continuing education?

17. Continuing education activities can be a part of staff development, or they can be offered by independent agencies, entrepreneurs, or universities. Typically, staff development activities are provided by a specific institution or agency for the personnel in that setting, although they may be opened to others outside the institution for a fee. Continuing education includes any systematic professional learning experiences designed to augment the knowledge, skills, and attitudes of nurses and, therefore, enrich the nurses' contributions to quality health care and their pursuit of professional career goals. Continuing education programs typically provide contact hours for completion.

18. What is the relationship between staff development, continuing education, and academic education?

18. These are all avenues nurses can take to achieve their professional development goals. There is some overlap in these areas as individuals determine the best way to meet their professional development needs. Staff development can include continuing education activities, academic education, or activities designed to assist someone to prepare for a specific role. Continuing education can be a part of staff development, part of a formal academic program, or simply taking activities to enhance one's professional development. Academic education can also be part of staff development or continuing education activities. The new framework has three overlapping circles to show this interrelationship.

19. What are the roles of the NPD educator?

19. The roles of the NPD educator as outlined in the latest standards are:

- Educator

- Facilitator

- Change agent

- Consultant

- Researcher

- Leader

Specific information about each of these roles is included in the standards.

20. Who is responsible for nurses' professional development?

20. The individual nurse has a personal responsibility to identify and select professional development opportunities to meet learning needs. However, the employer also has some responsibility to ensure that personnel in that setting can competently deliver care. The employer provides an environment and assists employees to maintain and increase competency. Regulatory bodies, such as individual boards of nursing, and agencies such as the Joint Commission on Accreditation of Healthcare Organizations, may establish guidelines or specific criteria that nurses or agencies must meet to maintain licensure or demonstrate competency of staff.

21. *How do the standards address advanced practice?*

21. A joint task force of the ANA Council on Nursing Professional Education and Development and NNSDO was established in 1995 to look at advanced practice in continuing education and staff development. This Task Force conducted a modified Delphi study to determine if there was advanced practice in these areas, and, if so, what was included in that. They concluded there were advanced practice competencies. The standards workgroup looked at the work of the joint task force, as well as Benner's novice to expert framework, and concluded that all the standards were on a continuum. An individual's level of expertise would be a factor in determining how these standards were met.

22. *What responsibility does the employer have to provide NPD opportunities?*

22. The employer has to meet certain requirements of regulatory agencies to ensure that its employees are competent to function in their role. Employers must validate appropriate credentials and provide an environment for the provision of safe quality care. Many employers provide educational opportunities for staff, either through in-house programs, sending people to outside workshops, or through tuition reimbursement programs for ongoing professional development. The employer is not obligated to provide continuing education programs to assist staff members meet requirements for relicensure or renewal of certification, but many do provide these opportunities.

23. *Why is a PhD suggested for the administrator of the NPD program?*

23. We are dealing with a very complex nursing and healthcare environment today, and the administrator must have the educational and management expertise to deal with that environment. Optimally the administrator should have a PhD, but minimally a master's degree is required. The suggestion for educational preparation for the educator role is a graduate degree in nursing or related specialty. If the graduate degree is in a related discipline (e.g., education), then the baccalaureate must be in nursing. Both educators and administrators need to have expertise in testing and outcome measurement and evaluation, learning theories and principles, methodologies of delivery, and knowledge of teaching.

24. *What is the difference between standards of practice and standards of professional performance?*

24. Standards of practice deal with the specifics of planning and presenting educational activities, including assessing and diagnosing educational needs, identifying outcomes, planning, implementation, and evaluation. Standards of professional performance deal with those aspects relating to performance of the educational role, such as continuing professional development, ethics, collegiality, monitoring the quality of practice, and leadership.

25. Why don't the standards address specifics about contact hours of credit?

25. Specific criteria relating to the provision and awarding of contact hours for educational programs are developed and published by the American Nurses Credentialing Center's Commission on Accreditation. Since that group reviews and revises those criteria, it was determined that the standards should not include that specific information.

26. What is a portfolio and how is it used?

26. A portfolio is "material documenting the professional development, career planning, demonstration of learning, and maintenance of continuing professional nursing competence of the individual nurse" (ANA, 2000, p. 25). The format of this material can vary, and often includes self-reflection or analysis of additional learning needs. Portfolios can be used in a variety of ways, including:

- Documentation of continuing competence

- Description of job-related skills and accomplishments

- Confirmation of professional development

- Annual performance evaluation

- Verification of meeting criteria for clinical ladder promotion

27. How do the standards address new technology (e.g., distance learning)?

27. The standards recognize that a variety of methods are needed to meet the educational needs of a diverse population. Distance learning occurs when instruction is provided and the learner and educator are not in the same place. The instruction may either take place synchronously (at the same time, such as interactive video) or asynchronously (at different times, such as online or correspondence courses).

28. How are the standards used by entrepreneurs or other non-traditional educators?

28. The educational process is the same, regardless of who is applying that process. All educators, regardless of setting, go through a similar process to provide educational activities. Typically, entrepreneurs are more concerned about the overall costs of programs, but the educational process is the same.

RESOURCE

American Nurses Association. (2000). *Scope and standards of practice for nursing professional development.* Washington, DC: American Nurses Publishing.

Section 9:
Staff Development as a Career

When asked if you might consider a job opportunity in Nursing Professional Development (NPD), you might offer to try it for a while, maybe a couple of years. After all, you can always go back to clinical practice. Yet once you start in the position you find that you like it and as with any specialty in nursing you'll want to be as good as you can be at your job. So what opportunities are out there for your continued development? How can you become certified? Are there graduate programs to help you gain more credentials? Can you make a living from speaking, writing, or consulting?

This section is especially close to our hearts as NPD has been our focus for the majority of our careers. We love what we do and hope this section gives you some tools to continue in NPD after we're long gone.

Chapter 39: *Preparing for Certification*

1. Why did you become certified in Nursing Professional Development—NPD (formerly Continuing Education and Staff Development—CESD)?

1. When the certification exam was first introduced in 1992 (as CESD), I had no doubt I would take it and be successful. It was my fourth certification. The hospital where I grew up as a nurse really valued certification both financially and professionally. I've always believed it is important to celebrate nursing, demonstrate competence, and offer the patient the best staff care possible. Becoming certified in this specialty allowed me to accomplish all three goals. As long as I practice staff development, I'll maintain that credential, a "good housekeeping seal of approval."

2. Why should I become certified?

2. Regardless of agency recognition of excellence, certification affords you the opportunity to affirm your knowledge and skills in continuing education and staff development. It becomes a benchmark for general practice. Success indicates an ability to operate in both the staff development and continuing education environment, regardless of your practice setting. When asked your nursing specialty, you can proudly say you are an *education expert*. Personal satisfaction and goal attainment are reasons as good as demonstrating achievement to healthcare professionals and the public.

3. Has certification made a difference for you?

3. I believe that it has. I've signed my name RN,C since attainment of the designation, from a sense of pride in nursing, and as a sign of achieving a standard. (With recent changes, the credential is now RN,BC.) I believe that the healthcare system acknowledges this achievement, much like patients seek care from board certified physicians. I know the baseline information of other NPD certified nurses, creating a common bond and an education community.

4. What are the resources I can use to prepare for certification?

4.
- NNSDO *Core Curriculum*
- NNSDO resource consultants
- Kelly Thomas and Abruzzese textbooks
- Certified nurses
- NNSDO certification review course (live)
- ANCC manuals
- Institute for Research, Education, and Consultation (IREC) certification review course (taped)

- *Journal for Nurses in Staff Development & The Journal of Continuing Education in Nursing* articles

5. Is there one source that's best?

5. Based on your learning style you can choose one that suits you. Reading texts and manuals is effective if you are able to apply the information to multiple choice test items. Listening to a tape may work best for the auditory learner or to reinforce other methods, while a live review or use of an expert provides an opportunity for interaction, validation, and clarification. Don't underestimate your experience; those 1100 nurses who successfully took the first certification exams in the specialty in 1992 had only their experience to support their knowledge.

6. How do I decide when to pursue certification?

6. You are eligible to take the exam after five years or 4000 hours of practice, and 20 hours of continuing education in education-related topics within the past two years. The fee is discounted for members of ANA or NNSDO. Depending on your role or scope of practice, there may be gaps in your experience that should be supplemented prior to testing. Large departments may have segregated responsibilities, so some cross training is helpful. Allowing sufficient time for preparation is necessary. Although your manager may suggest certification, you should pursue it when you feel ready professionally to wear the title, are ready based on your knowledge and experience, and are just enough uncertain of everything to use your critical thinking skills. It is a generalist, not an advanced practice examination.

7. Who can I ask for help?

7. Use a local NNSDO affiliate or educator's group to access already certified nurses. If you are isolated in your practice, you can access the forum at **www.nnsdo.org** or phone NNSDO at 1(800) 489–1995 for a certified member near you.

8. How do I develop a study plan?

8. A study plan can be developed once you have selected a test date. Depending on which resource you choose to use, allow enough time to read the texts, schedule a review course, or gain experience in an unfamiliar area. Two to three months is generally enough study time. Check your knowledge using the practice questions that come when you've registered for the test. Practice answering multiple choice test questions. Take a few days off and relax before taking the certification exam.

9. *I haven't taken a test since nursing school. What do I do to be successful?*

9. Again, using the practice questions may help; however, there aren't enough for you to get a rhythm. Check out a NCLEX-RN practice question book so that you can practice answering questions and can tolerate sitting through 175 of them. Another strategy to prepare that is also developmental for you is to practice writing test questions that you would expect to see.

10. *I'm already certified in another specialty. Why should I get this certification?*

10. Nursing is a wonderful profession, with many opportunities to specialize. As your career path changes, so does your expertise. Each certification you attain represents expertise. Many certifications build on previous ones. However, a certification only represents one specialty practice. To be fair to colleagues and consumers, certification should accurately represent your specialty.

11. *What about recertification? What's involved?*

11. Recertification is a voluntary process every five years. An application, fee, and appropriate documentation are submitted for review. Continuing practice within the specialty, participation in continuing education within the specialty, and contributions to the body of knowledge are necessary for recertification. Retesting is an option; however, continued competency is appropriate to obtain certification. Requirements for recertification can be met through continuing education credits, academic credits, presenter credits, publishing credits, or preceptorship credits.

12. *What can you tell me about review courses?*

12. There are currently two review courses available. The NNSDO course is 16 contact hours with a live certified faculty. An average of 60 participants take this course at the annual NNSDO convention. It was most recently revised in 2001. The IREC course is an independent study booklet with 13 hours of tape. It includes information that goes beyond the test plan: evidence-based practice, pain management, and ethics. This course was copyrighted in 1998.

13. *What can you tell me about textbooks?*

13. Both Roberta Abruzzese and Karen Kelly Thomas produced two editions of their textbooks in the 1990s. There are no plans by these authors or any major nursing publisher to revise these texts. These are excellent resources and useful in either edition for all information except use of ANCC guidelines for approver and provider. These guidelines are available directly from ANCC and were most recently revised in 2001. NNSDO has produced two editions of its *Core Curriculum*, the most recent one in 2001. These and other NNSDO publications are useful for test preparation.

14. What can you tell me about the test plan?

14.

	Questions	Percent
Foundations of Practice	42	28.0%
Educational Process	43	28.6%
Management of Activities	44	29.3%
Roles	21	14.0%

175 questions; 25 new items introduced each year. 150 items scored. Passing score determined after test administration.

15. What happens when I'm successful?

15. You'll feel a sense of accomplishment, success, and competence. You can sign your name as RN,BC (Board Certified). You are now in a position to encourage and support others through certification.

16. What happens when I'm not successful?

16. While I've worked with many people to help them prepare, I personally do not know anyone who has not been successful. Good preparation and confidence will serve you well. In the case of failure, you can reapply to test again on the next testing date and prepare based on the gaps identified in the scoring report you are sent. Seek out assistance and try again.

17. I'm not involved in the CE provider or approver process. How can I learn about this?

17. The manual can be accessed on the World Wide Web at **www.nursingworld.org/ancc** or purchased. The best approach is to spend time with someone who uses the process regularly. Examples include:

School of Nursing Continuing Education Director

ANA Constitutent Member Association Continuing Education provider

Specialty Nursing Organization program planner

18. Do you think that employers will ever value certification?

18. The annual Omni Credentialing Conference sponsored by the American Nurses Credentialing Center is working on precisely that issue. Watch for updates through **www.nursingworld.org** and participate in activities that help validate the value of certification. Let your employer know your knowledge level and marketability as a result of your certification.

RESOURCES

www.nnsdo.org

www.nursingworld.org

Chapter 40: *Advanced Education*

1. If I want to move into staff education, what type of degree(s) would I need?

1. According to the *Scope and Standards of Practice for Nursing Professional Development* developed by the American Nurses Association, the minimum level of education for the nurse in staff education is a graduate degree in nursing or a related specialty. If the graduate degree is in a related discipline, then the baccalaureate must be in nursing.

2. Can I get an advanced degree in nursing from a National League for Nursing (NLN) approved School of Nursing from the Internet?

2. Absolutely! In this age of super connectivity and high-speed communication, there are now a variety of NLN-approved programs for nursing education, ranging from the bachelor's in nursing to a variety of graduate degrees. Some of the distance learning programs, such as the one at University of Delaware, offer the MSN program with a concentration in health services administration completely online except for a two-day seminar that takes place on campus. As of this writing there are over 44 schools of nursing offering degrees ranging from BSN to Doctoral via the Internet.

3. What kinds of scholarships are available for nurses who want to go back for an advanced degree?

3. Scholarships abound for nurses who want to go back to school. If you are a member of a nursing specialty organization, such as the Emergency Nurses Association, there are educational scholarship funds set up through the organization's foundation. For some graduate programs, the schools provide a stipend for the students, and/or offer scholarships to enrolled students. Some cultural, religious, or ethnic groups, such as the National Association of Hispanic Nurses, offer scholarships (**www.thehispanicnurses.com**). Use the Internet to search for scholarships available. Try such sites as **www.collegefunds.net** or private trusts or organizations, like the March of Dimes, Florence Rogers Trust, John Hartford Foundation, and many more. Many of these require that you pursue education in specific fields of nursing to qualify for the financial assistance. If you belong to a professional nursing sorority such as Sigma Theta Tau International or Chi Eta Phi Sorority, Inc., check out their scholarship opportunities as well.

Don't forget to check with the nursing school you plan to attend to see what types of financial aid and scholarships are offered to incoming or enrolled students. Your hospital or healthcare system may also be a source of scholarship or may have tuition assistance programs established. There are over 90,000 Internet sites alone related to nursing scholarships. Another site to check out is **http://kcsun3.tripod.com/id77.htm** where you can search nationally, internationally, or selected states for scholarships and loans. Other places to check may include such agencies as the Utah Department of Health (if you live in Utah and have a Utah RN license), which will give up to $15,000 per academic year for the nurse pursuing a graduate degree.

4. Would it be better for me to become a Nurse Practitioner?

4. The nurse practitioner role was originally developed for practice in an expanded role to provide health care to individuals, families, and/or groups in a variety of settings. If the path you want to follow involves hands-on patient care, you would want to focus on the clinical aspects of nursing and patient care issues, not necessarily staff development.

5. Should I go back to school for an advanced degree in nursing or education?

5. YES! To quote Bob Richards (**www.cybernation.org**), "You are what you think. You are what you go for. You are what you do!" Whether it is an advanced degree in nursing practice or in education, not only will you personally benefit from the experience and the knowledge gained so will your patients and colleagues. Either way you will make an impact on patient outcomes. By becoming an educator you will directly influence the providers of health care and their practice, ultimately affecting (in a positive way, of course) patient outcomes. With the advanced degree in nursing practice, not only will patient care be enhanced, but you will serve as a role model to your colleagues in the clinical setting.

6. How can a graduate degree help me in my role as an educator?

6. Going back to school to obtain an advanced degree gives you the opportunity to grow both personally and professionally. In the majority of graduate programs related to nursing or education, there are components on philosophy, integrating research and practice, and educational theories and opportunities to practice communication techniques that will enhance your ability to function in the role of educator.

7. What place does continuing education have in my development, rather than another degree?

7. Continuing education, as defined by the American Nurses Association (**www.nursingworld.org**), is "those professional experiences designed to enrich the nurse's contribution to health care." Continuing education is a way to build upon the skills you have, and can enable you to comply with the ANA's *Code for Nurses*, which requires competencies in nursing practice, and assists, in some states, in achieving certification and maintaining licensure. While you are making the decision about if and/or when you will go back to school, remember that as a life long learner you must continue to seek out those opportunities to enrich your knowledge about nursing, your specialized field of interest, and your role in the healthcare industry.

8. *After I get my degree as an educator, what are the other options I have for a career?*

8. Once you receive your degree as an educator, whether it is a Master's in Nursing or a Doctorate in Nursing or another field, you can pursue a career in higher education serving as an instructor/professor at the community college or university level (depending on which degree you have). You can work in the hospital setting in an administrative role or an advanced clinical role. You can become an entrepreneur or intrapreneur and set up business as an educator and/or consultant.

9. *What are some non-traditional methods I can use to obtain an advanced degree?*

9. The traditional methods of face-to-face learning no longer meet the educational needs of the many people who want to pursue a degree in nursing. Schools of nursing have recognized this fact and are adapting their curricula to meet the needs of this type of student. Programs are now offered via distance education using the Internet (either partially or completely), video conferencing, video taped lectures, and a variety of other self-study methods. Clinical sites for the hands-on training are set up locally by the school using hospitals or other agencies that are approved sites for training, with approved preceptors. The fees vary for distance education, but most are comparable with tuition fees for regular on-campus students.

10. *What types of preparation do I need to have before I go back to school?*

10. The preparation you will need to do prior to going back to school will depend on the type of program you are enrolled in. For many advanced degree programs you will need to take the Miller Analogies Test (MAT), Graduate Record Examination (GRE), College Level Examination Program (CLEP), American College Testing Assessment (ACT), or other types of examinations. You can attend preparation courses or buy a self-study book to prepare for the exam. You may have to meet specific criteria such as a 3.0 GPA from your

previous education, submit college and/or high school transcripts, letter(s) of recommendation, and even have an interview prior to being admitted to the program.

Some schools may not accept college courses taken more than five years prior, and you will need to retake those courses. Others may allow you to challenge those courses or even give you "life experience" credit for the time you have already been a practicing registered nurse. You will also need to look at your life-style. What changes in the home/family life will need to be made to accommodate your reentry into school? Will you need childcare? If you will be completing your degree via distance education do you have the hardware necessary to "attend" the classes?

11. How do I decide which school to go to if I have more than one program offered in my home area?

11. The first thing you need to do is to assess your learning needs and what will work best for the life-style you have. What type of program do you want? Are you looking for a Clinical Specialist or Nurse Practitioner career after completion, or are you interested in management or nursing informatics or any of the other types of degrees out there? Will you need to work either full or part-time while you complete your degree? If you work a Monday to Friday job, there may be weekend programs available in your area whereby you attend classes anywhere from Friday evening through all day on Sunday. What is the flexibility of courses if you are working every other weekend, or a variety of shifts? Check out the school's references. Is the school accredited? Ask nurse colleagues for recommendations of one program over another. Visit the schools and speak with someone in the nursing program to find out if this school will meet your learning and life-style needs.

12. How long will it take me to complete my degree?

12. It can take you anywhere from twelve months to seven years or more to complete your degree depending on the type of program you are pursuing and whether you attend school on a full or part-time basis. At Duquesne University, the online BSN program can be completed part-time in five semesters. The University of North Carolina School of Nursing recently began an accelerated degree program for qualified candidates with a bachelor's degree in a non-nursing field to attend campus classes over a period of 14 months to graduate with a BSN.

13. Can I get an MSN if I only have an Associate's Degree in Nursing?

13. Many states now provide opportunities for nurses with an Associate's Degree in Nursing (ADN) to obtain a Master's in Nursing. In some programs, you will take courses that fulfill the requirements for the BSN at the same time you are completing the Master's program.

14. If so, where do I get it?

14. More and more schools are recognizing there is a need for the non-BSN prepared nurse to access the Master's level program. A school such as Texas Christian University, Fort Worth, Texas, is one of these schools. At this institution, students with an Associate's Degree in Nursing are admitted to a year-round, three-year accelerated program, whereas the BSN-prepared nurse can complete the program in two years.

15. What is the difference between a PhD in Nursing, DSc, EdD, or ND as far as the educator role?

15. The PhD, Doctor of Philosophy, in Nursing, or Doctor of Philosophy is designed for individuals who in most cases have a MSN degree and will focus their sights on research, concentrating on organization and development of knowledge essential to nursing practice. The focus may include health outcomes, ethics, and or health policy.

The DNSc, Doctorate of Nursing Science, such as the one at Columbia University, prepares the nurse to work with refining, reshaping, and evaluating the healthcare industry. This type of degree is heavily based in research as well.

The Doctorate in Education, EdD, does not require a degree in nursing. However, you must have a Master's degree to qualify for the majority of programs. This degree provides the individual with training in educational techniques, theory and practice, philosophy of education, and research.

The ND, Nursing Doctorate, such as offered at Case Western Reserve University provides a four-year program during which the first two years prepare the bachelor's prepared individual (not a BSN) to sit for the NCLEX exam and the second two years to prepare those students for advanced practice and clinical research in nursing.

16. How does belonging to a professional nursing organization(s) help me when I decide to pursue an advanced degree?

16. The majority of professional nursing organizations offer information on what types of advanced degrees might be applicable to that specialty. If your interest lies in emergency nursing, then an advanced degree as a Clinical Specialist or Nurse Practitioner in Emergency Nursing might be the ticket for you.

383

17. *Is it worth my time and effort to go back to school? I've got kids, bills, and a full-time job.*

17. Only you can be the judge to answer this question. You will have bills, kids (maybe), and a job whether or not you go back to school. If a degree is a stepping stone to advance your career or climb the clinical ladder, or a requirement for your position, you may not have a choice. Continuing your education, learning something new, is *always* worth the time and effort.

18. *Do you think an advanced degree really makes the difference for a staff development position?*

18. With all the mergers and partnerships that hospitals and health systems are developing, now more than ever, it will take someone with advanced leadership skills and training to participate in designing and measuring educational activities. An advanced degree does not guarantee that one has those skills; however, the additional educational experience and training you would receive through this type of degree will only serve to enhance your role in staff education and development.

REFERENCES

Richards, B. (n.d.). Motivation. Retrieved February 12, 2002, from **http://www.cyber-nation.com/victory/quotations/authors/quotes_richards_bob.html**

American Nurses Association. (n.d.). Glossary. Retrieved February 12, 2002, from **http://nursingworld.org/ancc/accred/provider/glossary.htm**

RESOURCES

American Nurses Credentialing Center: **http://www.nursingworld.org/ancc/**

Peterson's College search for distance education programs in nursing: **http://www.petersons.com/**

Nursing Scholarships: **http://www.411scholarships.com/NURSING/**

Chapter 41: *Making Presentations*

1. What special skills should I develop to make presentations exciting?

1. I think you must find your sense of humor because it will serve you well in all presentations from bad to perfect. Explore your talents and capitalize on those that make you unique and will benefit those who hear you. I suggest you find your "best self" and be there as much as you can. Practice the presentation until your anxiety is manageable. If you can share your excitement of the topic to the audience, your presentation will be exciting.

2. How can I market myself as a keynote speaker or presenter?

2. If I knew this, I would be a millionaire! From my experience, it is a challenge. You must continue to market yourself daily. Make contacts with as many other people as you can. Create opportunities to network. E-mail and ground mail information on your presentations to groups that may use your services. Hire a marketing person to find leads for you. There are speakers bureaus around the country that you can market to, but most specialize in full time, high profile speakers with many years of experience.

3. When are props appropriate?

3. I find props are particularly appropriate when making a point called an "object lesson." This is when the prop is used in an analogy that makes the point clearer than words. For example, one of the topics I teach is motivation to learn. I ask for three volunteers to come to the front of the room and select one of these three items: a koosh ball, an squoosh earth ball, or a rock. I then ask the group to raise their hands and vote for the item they think would bounce highest in a bouncing contest. Most people vote for the earth ball or the koosh ball, not the rock. I then conduct a bouncing contest for all to see. The rock wins every time because it is made of super ball material, but it looks like a rock. I then ask the group to compare the balls to learners and the bouncers to the educators. What are the factors that affect learner motivation or how high the balls bounced? This begins a concrete discussion of a hard to grasp concept. I find kinesthetic learners love using props, so I use as many as possible including tape flags, markers, and toys.

4. What audiences require special treatment?

4. All audiences require special treatment if you want to be invited back. Each time you plan a presentation, personalize it to the needs of that particular group. That might mean you must do your homework ahead of time

and talk to some key people before the date of your presentation, even if you have done it hundreds of times before. I also suggest that, once you begin, if you sense the audience is not with you that you check in with some of them during break and change the presentation if necessary.

5. *I talk to many analytical audiences. How do you get them on board when they perceive your presentation as "touchy feely" which they hate?*

5. Start out with something the analytical audiences will like. I like to use a brainteaser or problem solving challenge to begin. Use algebra, chemistry or physics problems. I like the game Mindtrap™. It provides many problem-solving situations. After they are involved in this sort of activity, I present about ten minutes of lecture before I ask for their involvement again. To me the key to success is starting with something they like or are interested in and then asking them to come out of their comfort zone. I also give the analytical reason for everything I do that looks "touchy feely" so they see its purpose.

6. *How do you develop a keynote speech?*

6. First, you must discover what you know that you feel passionately about that could be of benefit to others. Do research and get good content. I believe a keynote needs to be more than just information delivery. It must deliver emotional impact as well. That's where the passion link comes in. You must not be afraid to show how you feel on a topic to a crowd of many. Keynotes are a delicate balance between information and emotion. The best keynotes I have experienced have included belief and audience emotion as well, all headed toward a common goal and feeling at the end.

7. *How do I best present at meetings?*

7. Discover the purpose and time frame involved and plan for that. I find it best to start out with a brief opening activity to put everyone at ease before I go into my material. I also ask for involvement at meetings as I do in my keynote and other educational sessions.

8. *What if I get to the location of my speech, and my notes, props, and wardrobe don't?*

8. Immediately shop at the nearest variety store for the props and wardrobe. Recreate the notes as best you can. In the future carry the notes with you. You can fake the wardrobe and props, but the notes are harder. I would suggest you really learn your information so that all you need is an outline to prompt you. No one likes to have someone read to him or her when presenting anyway. See it as an opportunity to try something new and learn from what discoveries you make.

9. How can I improve my presentation skills?

9. Audiotape yourself at least twice a year. Listen to the tape with someone you trust and ask for 3 things you might do better next time. Videotape yourself at least once a year. Look to improve one thing each time you present. Focus on the positives and try to do more of them and less of the negatives. Get a mentor or coach who will work with you to make you better. Pick someone you admire and work with that person. Go to conferences that teach you something new.

10. I was told I would be giving an hour presentation. When I got there, the intro and announcements took 20 minutes that were supposed to be mine. How do I prevent myself from running long when I present at a conference and this happens?

10. Plan a 40-minute presentation, with information you can use that is extra if the intro only takes ten minutes. That way, you will never run over. Running over at a conference messes up the schedule of many, which is inconsiderate to everyone, including your host.

11. How should I dress for a keynote speech?

11. Dress one level up from the audience. That means if they are all in scrubs, you might wear a nice skirt and blouse with a lab coat at a facility. If they are in business casual, wear business formal, such as a suit. If they are at a pool party in swimsuits, you would not want to wear a business suit because it will seem you are "out of touch" with your audience. You might then appear in an informal casual sun dress. Try not to wear anything that is sexy or risqué.

12. What are some essential marketing tools I must prepare to be seen as credible?

12. I would suggest putting together the best marketing tools using a brief biosketch, a list of services, a list of past clients, some testimonials, and make it something they will want to keep. It does cost money to design and print high-end materials, but the initial impression to potential clients is in the materials if they have not seen you.

13. How do I get to do what you do?

13. Start small. Send proposals to every local, state, and national conference you can on a topic you know and are comfortable teaching. Keep your full time job. Present on vacation time. When you get busier, work each job part time. Then when you have enough business, you can do it full time. I meet many people who say they are going to hang out their nurse entrepreneur shingle on Jan 1st and quit their full time jobs and they will suddenly have a successful business. It has been my experience that business builds slowly over the years, and there should be a plan until that day comes.

14. Should I offer my services for free to groups who can't afford to pay anything for my services?

14. It depends. You might want to look for other means of compensation that are valuable such as free advertising in the group's newsletter, a referral to another group the client is affiliated with, or that they buy your book or materials for the presentation. I do believe there is a benefit to the client to provide even a small honorarium, because there is a perceived value associated with it. They will be more likely to have good attendance and be less likely to cancel if there is money involved.

15. What is the best audiovisual media to use with a group during a presentation?

15. I think the best audiovisual media to use is the one you are most comfortable with and fits the size of the group so all can see it. That means if you are using power point, slides, overhead projector, or a flip chart, you want to practice and use it many times before you try your skills in front of a group. It's always best to have a backup plan. That might mean you have all your power point screens or slides on transparency as well just in case of a computer problem.

16. What is the worst experience you have had?

16. The worst experience came from breaking my own rules. I did not mix up a hostile group once and they "ate my lunch!" They were schooled in intimidation techniques; the host said I couldn't mix people in teams at the facility, and I let them fluster me and they knew it. I learned so much that day; it reminds me that failure is always possible if I don't follow my own beliefs but instead go by the beliefs of others. I learned to be true to myself and not doubt my instincts.

17. What is the best experience you have had since you started?

17. There are so many wonderful ones; it is hard to say. I had an amazing experience at a national conference in Anaheim about five years ago. I was told to expect 700 attendees total at both of my presentations and had brought that number of materials. Instead I had 700 at the first and 350 at the second of the sessions, and somehow, they all had materials. To me it was a nice little miracle, and it was an amazing session in my growth as a presenter in many ways because I trusted it would all be okay and it was.

18. *How long do you need to set up before your speech?*

18. Ideally, I like to have an hour to an hour and a half before any attendee arrives.

19. *How do you deal with the challenge of travel to all different locations?*

19. Traveling is indeed an exhausting activity. It can disturb your ability to sleep, eat, and be physically comfortable. It is important to take the best care of yourself as possible when traveling. Take some comfort items from home with you so you can simulate familiar surroundings. Eat right; schedule some down time. It is important to have a backup plan in mind; never take the last flight anywhere and carry all essential items with you; do not check them.

20. *How can I assure everything will be perfect for my presentation?*

20. You can't. You can, however, come early, prepare, and do all you can to make it the best it can be. I also believe that if things aren't perfect, I must pretend to myself and the audience that it is, unless it is obvious to them. I try to make lemonade from whatever lemons I find. I've become a better lemonade maker every time something not perfect happens, so it actually is a learning experience for me.

21. *What have you learned in over eleven years of making presentations nationally?*

21. I have learned that national standards are very high, and that I must strive to continually improve what I present to stay on top of the game. I have also learned there are two types of people at this level. One group is very self-focused. They are in it for the fame and glory and are very competitive and unwilling to share with others: they have an inflated sense of self. The other group is the warm, caring, mentoring people who revel in others' success and want to help others succeed. I avoid the first and seek the second.

22. *How do you deal with bad evaluations of your sessions?*

22. I learn from every group and every evaluation I receive. I have a small rule that I follow that works for me. After a presentation, I do my own evaluation of how I felt it went that day. I do not read the written evaluations until the next day. I find this helps me not to over focus on the negative things that come on some evaluations. In the past if I got 150 excellent evaluations and one that was not I would focus on the one that was not excellent until I drove myself into the ground. It would consume and overwhelm me. Now I find if I wait until the next day I am more objective and improvement focused. And now I know the old saying is true, "You can't please all of the people all of the time, but you can please some of the people some of the time."

RESOURCES

Deck, B. (2001). *Prop up your presentation.* Metairie, LA: Tool Thyme for Trainers.

Deck, M., & Deck, B. (2001). *Live to train another day.* Metairie, LA: Tool Thyme for Trainers.

Chapter 42: *Publishing*

1. *Why should I write for publication?*

1. Writing for publication is a great way to advance your career. You can obtain opportunities to present at conferences, consult, and write additional articles, or even a book on the topic. Sometimes career advancement in your employment setting depends on activities such as writing: the "publish or perish" phenomenon in academia is an example. Career ladders or career portfolio programs often require an individual to publish. Writing for publication also can be a great source of personal satisfaction.

2. *What keeps people like me from writing for publication?*

2. Most people say it's time, although they find time for other activities that are important to them. I believe many nurses are afraid they don't have the expertise to write for publication although they perform these activities about which they can write best every day in their practice. I think, too, many nurses believe they need advanced education (e.g., a master's degree or a doctorate) to write. That's simply not the case! Manuscripts reviewed for publication do not contain any author identification, so no one knows the identity (or the credentials) of the author.

3. *What are some strategies I can use to overcome my barriers to writing?*

3. I suggest you make time to write. Set an appointment with yourself that you treat with every bit as much respect and attention as an appointment with a physician or dentist. Find a private place where you won't be interrupted, and have everything related to your writing easily accessible, so if time is limited, you won't spend it just getting organized. Too, think about the personal benefits of writing to motivate yourself.

Get help from a content expert, an already published author, or an English major in college if those are areas where you need help. You may also want to consider enrolling for a continuing education or academic course on writing or search out an online course on writing or publishing.

4. *How does writing for publication differ from other writing I'm doing?*

4. Writing for publication is like writing for colleagues —people just like you in your practice setting. It differs from charting, or writing reports for administration, or school papers because you're basically writing for yourself and your colleagues, not for someone else like a supervisor or a teacher. Writing for publication follows the same general guidelines for spelling,

grammar, punctuation, and style as other writing: it's professional but not necessarily what someone else (e.g., teacher, administrator) wants you to write, but rather, what you want to write.

5. Where do I get ideas for writing?

5. The best place to get ideas for writing is from what you do most often and best: work! What do you like to do at work? What don't you like to do? If you could help one of your colleagues do something better, faster, easier, cheaper, what would that one thing be? What have you tried that works? What have you tried that didn't work? Writing about something that didn't work may keep a colleague from making the same mistake you did or from reinventing the wheel. You can also get publishable ideas from reading and listening at conferences, from Internet searches, discussions with colleagues, or interactions with others in your employment settings or participants in the classes you teach.

6. What are some publishable ideas?

6. In staff development and continuing education, we're always looking for new and better ways to orient nurses and others to the employment setting. The increase in numbers of healthcare workers with English as their second language points out the need for literature on cultural diversity. The current—and projected nursing shortage—should spawn a great deal of writing on solutions! Look for ideas that represent "trends" in a specialty area of practice, not the fads that come and go. Write about what you know best!

7. How will I know I have a publishable idea?

7. Actually, the best way to know whether your idea is publishable is to write it up and submit it; but, before you do all that work, you may want to ask some colleagues for their feedback about the idea. Tell several people, those with whom you work and those from other facilities, if possible, about your idea and ask for their feedback. Be open about what they tell you; perhaps they'll suggest a different slant or give you some rationale about why your idea wouldn't work in their facility. Adding content related to the feedback you receive may strengthen the idea. Even negative feedback can be useful. Offering solutions to the potential problems identified by a colleague strengthens your argument for your approach.

8. How do I search the literature?

8. A literature search can be easily done via computer, using key words related to the topic. An invaluable source of assistance is a medical librarian who is skilled in conducting searches of the healthcare literature. Even a community librarian, however, will be familiar with resources. Include the most relevant literature related to the topic in the manuscript. Sources in the healthcare literature should be less than 5 years old. There are "classic" sources that should be cited, such as Benner's book, if the topic describes a "novice to expert" approach. Look at the journal to which you intend to submit your manuscript to get an idea of how many references are average for each article and then conform to that number.

9. Should I have an outline of my manuscript?

9. Some authors do better with outlines than others. An outline does help organize your thoughts, but beware of tinkering with the outline rather than writing the manuscript. If you want to help organize your writing, jot down the major ideas you wish to cover, then fill in the details. Some authors find it helpful to use index cards or Post-It notes to help them develop an outline.

10. What if I see my topic already published elsewhere?

10. Even if you see the topic published elsewhere, don't despair. Often you'll have a different perspective on the topic, and that will be publishable too. Then, too, if the article is about a trend, it will bear repeating in the literature. Review the already-published article carefully to determine how best to slant your idea differently. If you can't find any differences, abandon the topic and choose another.

11. How can I be sure I cover the topic completely?

11. Begin by deciding what readers absolutely need to know to replicate your idea exactly in their work settings. Try to eliminate the "nice to know" aspects that may lengthen the article without adding much substance. Then, turn to colleagues again to review the manuscript and provide feedback about what to add, delete, or change.

12. What journal shall I publish in?

12. Depending on your area of practice and the audience for your topic, there will often be several journals from which to choose. In staff development and continuing education, the two primary journals are the *Journal for Nurses in Staff Development* (published by Lippincott Williams & Wilkins) and *The Journal of Continuing Education in Nursing* (published by SLACK, Inc.). A librarian is a good source of ideas for journals in other nursing practice areas.

13. What's a query letter and should I write one?

13. A query letter is used to ask the Editor of a journal whether the journal is an appropriate venue for your topic. Writing a query letter gives you practice in specifying your idea, and gives the Editor the opportunity to provide feedback on its suitability for publication. Address the letter to the Editor of the journal and describe your idea in a few sentences. Be as specific and clear as possible, so the Editor doesn't have to try to figure out what you'll be writing about. If you've prepared an outline or an abstract, you can include it, but it is not generally necessary. You should receive a relatively prompt response from the Editor (usually within two weeks). If you don't hear from the Editor within this time frame, keep working on the manuscript and submit it when it is completed. You can write a query letter to more than one journal at a time, but submit a completed manuscript to only one journal at a time.

14. *How do I know about the article format to use?*

14. Usually the topic of the manuscript will dictate the format to use. A research study lends itself only to a formal presentation of the question researched, and the methodology used to research it, followed by the conclusions and the implications for practice. A description of a successful project or program needs a "how to" approach describing what we did, why we did it, how we did it, and what others should do to do it too. A case study approach or a review of the literature on a specific topic follows naturally from the idea contained in the manuscript.

15. *How do I prepare the manuscript for submission?*

15. Follow the journal's "Instructions for Authors." These generally are contained in the journal or can be requested from the Editor or downloaded from the journal's (or publisher's) Web site. Follow the instructions exactly to expedite review and publication of the manuscript. If you have any questions about the instructions, do not hesitate to call the editorial office for clarification.

16. *Do I need to edit the manuscript?*

16. You should make an attempt to edit the manuscript for spelling, grammar, and punctuation. Often someone in your work setting (e.g., a librarian, a public relations staffer) can be of assistance with this. Review the manuscript carefully to eliminate excess words (e.g., very, quite) and jargon. Asking colleagues to read the completed manuscript often is helpful. A reader unfamiliar with the manuscript often can identify poor transitions and areas that should be more clear.

17. *What about getting permission to use someone else's materials?*

17. If you use someone else's work that has been copyrighted, you will need written permission to include it in the manuscript. That includes figures and tables from other published works, or such information as Bloom's taxonomy of objectives, for example. To obtain permission, write the copyright holder (generally the publisher, not the author) and request permission to use the copyrighted material in the manuscript you are writing. You may be required to include the letter of permission when you submit the manuscript. Again, if you have questions about obtaining copyright permission, or whether it is necessary to do so, contact the Editor of the journal to which you plan to submit the manuscript.

18. How long does the manuscript review process take?

18. When a manuscript is received in the Editor's office, it is logged in and then sent to several reviewers who may or may not be members of the journal's Editorial Board. Most reviewers need approximately 3-4 weeks to review a manuscript since they read it several times before making a final recommendation. Generally, the journal's Editor will acknowledge receipt of the manuscript and let you know when to expect a reply. If you haven't heard back by the stated time, allow another two weeks or so to pass, then contact the Editor and politely inquire about the status of the manuscript. Occasionally, delays do occur in the review process, but most take no longer than 8 to 10 weeks.

19. What happens when a manuscript is reviewed?

19. Typically, a reviewer reads the manuscript at different times and looks for specific elements: Is the manuscript describing an original idea? Is the idea well supported by the literature cited in the manuscript? Is the topic relevant to the specialty area? Will it make a difference to readers?

20. What can I expect to hear from the editor?

20. Once the manuscript has been reviewed, the Editor will contact you with one of 3 decisions: accept, revise, or reject. Each of the decisions will be accompanied by information on what to do next. In the case of manuscript acceptance, which is highly unusual for novice authors—and even for many experienced ones—you'll probably be told to release copyright to the publisher (if you weren't required to transmit copyright when you submitted the manuscript for review). In the case of revision, you will be sent the reviewers' comments or the Editor's summary of what the reviewers said about the manuscript. In the case of rejection, you may or may not receive the specific reasons. In the event the reason is vague (e.g., "Sorry, the manuscript doesn't meet our editorial needs at this time."), you may wish to contact the Editor and ask in general terms why the manuscript was not accepted (e.g., "Can you advise me how to improve or rewrite the manuscript so it will be suitable for publication?"), as this is valuable information. In either case, revision or rejection, make certain you do something else with the manuscript—do not just file it away!

21. What shall I do if revisions to my manuscript are recommended?

21. If revisions are recommended, review them alongside a copy of the manuscript to see where changes are needed. It may be that changes are minor, such as expansion of some of the content or clarification of the idea. Make every effort to address those criticisms of your work that you consider valid. If you have problems, either ask a trusted colleague to review the manuscript and the suggested revisions, or call the Editor and ask him/her to "walk you through" the necessary revisions. A previously published author of your acquaintance may be able to help as well. If you choose not to address some recommended revisions, indicate those changes you did not make and provide a rationale when you send the manuscript back to the Editor. It often is the case that no additional revisions are necessary after those you make the first time. Sometimes, however, a manuscript will be sent for review again and that may result in some additional, minor changes that need to be made. Responding promptly and thoroughly to requests for revisions will help ensure final publication.

22. Do I have to transfer the copyright to my article to the publisher?

22. In each instance where you submit a manuscript for publication, the publisher will want to hold the copyright. This means that the publisher owns the manuscript as you wrote it, not the ideas in the manuscript. So you are free to use the ideas in other presentations, projects, and writings, just not the manuscript as you wrote it for the specific journal.

Some journals require that you transfer copyright when you submit the manuscript; others wait to request copyright transfer until the manuscript has been accepted for publication. The Information for Authors will tell you when to transfer copyright.

23. How long will it take to get my article published?

23. Publication times vary depending on the journal's backlog of articles, but a safe guess is about 1 year from the time of acceptance to publication. Most journal editors will provide information on when the manuscript will be published and will update you if changes in that schedule occur.

24. What if I want to write a book instead of an article?

24. Writing a book is a large task; often authors find it easier to write a series of articles first to get the hang of publishing. A book idea requires a proposal to a potential publisher, outlining the book's content, planned length, audience, potential market, and often several sample chapters. Review books in the specialty to identify the publishers; then, contact these publishers for specific information on book proposals.

25. What is a really easy way to get started writing for publication?

25. If you're looking for an easy way to get started, consider volunteering to review books or other media for a journal. That way, you get to critique someone else's work rather than starting with your own. Once you've done a book review, check the printed version to see what changes were made in your writing and use that information to improve your next review. Then, tackle an article for a newsletter published by a professional association at the local, state, or even national level. The more you write for publication, even letters to the editor, the more skilled you'll become, and tackling that first journal article won't seem so daunting after all!

RESOURCES

Barnum, B. (1995). *Writing and getting published: A primer for nurses.* New York: Springer Publishing Company.

Oermann, M. H. (2001). *Writing for publication in nursing.* Philadelphia: Lippincott Williams & Wilkins.

Sheridan, D., & Dowdney, D. L. (1997). *How to write and publish articles in nursing* (2nd ed.). New York: Springer Publishing Company.

Chapter 43: *Entrepreneurship*

1. *How did you have the courage to become an entrepreneur?*

1. It was never my intent to be the co-owner of a business. It just seemed to happen!

I had been working for 17 years in the same hospital—first as a faculty member in the School of Nursing, then in Staff Development as well as taking clinical shifts during part time schedules and during grad school. Part of my responsibilities in staff development was the management of CPR training for about 1700 clinical employees and the coordination of that training with about 75 CPR instructors. Sharing the next cubicle space was Diane Byrum. Part of her staff development responsibilities was the management of ACLS training and instructors. In the fall of 1994, the phone rang a couple of times with callers asking about whether or not there was someone at the hospital who could come to their office or group to teach CPR. I remember asking Diane what I should charge and thought it was pretty neat to be able to add to the budget for that son in college! Then Diane received a couple of calls for ACLS needs. We found ourselves talking about money again. And she went out and added to her college fund too! As we talked we realized that there were some other ideas and skills that we could probably "sell"! We gave this joint effort a name—Innovative Solutions.

Much later, I realized how naive we actually were… no business plan, nothing in writing… although we did look in the phone book to check that no one else was using the name! Diane also took advantage of a group of retired business people who are available to evaluate ideas and assist small businesses to begin. Their response was positive. They weren't very sure what we actually would be doing but that there certainly seemed to be a market.

2. *How much money did it take? Did you have to get a loan?*

2. We were able to begin our business without borrowing *any* money and actually have *never* used any out-of-pocket money. We were able "borrow" the equipment for the first couple of classes. To purchase the first set of manikins, and to pay for those first office incidentals, we each taught a couple of classes and didn't take any money for it, but put it into the business

There may be grants and/or very low interest loans available for women beginning a business as minority business owners. Check with a local bank, Women in Business Association, or college/university for potential funding for your business.

3. How do you pick a partner?

3. I have had many co-workers and friends who know both Diane and me say that it's hard for them to picture Diane and me as business partners. Yes, our personalities are different—very different. We knew that in the beginning—and know that now. But we feel that these differences create a "dynamic duo"! While Diane may jump headlong into a project (without too much thought to detail) I am more cautious—sometimes too much so. So the positive part of this partnership is that we complement each other—Diane pulling me when she needs to and me begging for more details some days. We understand and accept that we can drive each other nuts pretty quickly—but have found that the combination works well—at least on most days!

My advice—don't look for a partner just like yourself. Look for someone with complementary skills.

4. Where are your offices and classrooms?

4. Now, six years later, we both have fairly normal offices in our homes. A bedroom is now a real office and Diane has also created a real office in her home.

One of our biggest business challenges is the fact that we live about 45 minutes apart. In the beginning, when we felt the need to celebrate business opportunities or to agonize about whether to try this or that, this proved to be a difficult situation. As we have become more comfortable with "who does what," we have overcome this challenge—most of the time. We *do* spend quite a bit of time on the phone, with e-mail, and when traveling together spend time concentrating on "business." We also "call a meeting" on occasion at some half-way point, such as gas stations, fast food restaurants, and lately in the food court of a mall.

Classes are typically held at a location provided by the group requesting the class. We have also located several classrooms made available to us at no cost, such as a conference room at a nurse staffing agency. These have promoted positive relationships because they can "show off" their companies to healthcare providers while we use their space.

5. When you were getting started, how did you market?

5. In the beginning, we didn't realize that we had a business so we really didn't do any marketing. Marketing is still a piece of this business puzzle that we acknowledge that we need to work on. Marketing, even now, is still mostly word-of-mouth, although we have identified "markets"

that we know we should/could be targeting. We have been lucky to have several sustaining agreements at area facilities as well as a strong connection with the American Heart Association that sends us contacts as well.

We have attempted at least a couple of mailings related to a variety of courses that we could make available—with only minimal success. For products such as books, games, self-study programs, and class preparation materials, we have found exhibiting at nursing education conferences, such as NNSDO, to be our market for both sales and networking. Sales at conferences rarely, if ever, cover the cost of travel, vendor booth fees, or shipping of booth supplies, but in the past exhibiting has been a wonderful resource for networking and has offered us the opportunity to travel and present at a variety of conferences all over the country.

6. *I would love to work for myself! Isn't it great to be able to work whenever you want?*

6. It is nice! If I want to stop working at 1:00 in the afternoon to do something with my daughter—or work until noon in my nightgown—I can. BUT what I've also had to learn—and continue to have to attempt to control—is turning work "off." I find myself nearly every night at my desk at 10:30 p.m. "just handling one more piece of mail" or putting that deposit together or more often than not, getting ready to teach the next day. Just recently I heard the best description of owning your own business from someone else who has also "been there." She said, "Owning your own business means getting to *choose* the 60 hours a week that you work!"

I must admit that I also enjoy not dealing with the "politics" of working in a department setting. I am one of those personalities who find confrontation uncomfortable. I can now just go into my office and really close all of that out.

One of the biggest adjustments for me has been to work out of my home in relationship to "separation of home and office." I have found it difficult to be working in that home office and know that there is a pile of dirty clothes that I could just put in the washer—or to just take 15 minutes to empty the dishwasher. I am getting better at this, but when there are pressing family things to do, it is hard to make that separation!

Another challenge is to let others around you realize that even though you are at "home" you are at "work."

One other challenge for me has been the fact that I am now working mostly on my own. My experience has generally been in a group in an education department. I miss that networking and "using others' brains." Diane is a wonderful sounding board and assistance when I need ideas about how to teach a class or see those business processes that can be done differently.

I can certainly say that I do enjoy having my office in my house and working there on my own! I do have control. I just sometimes need to remember that.

7. Innovative Solutions seems to be everywhere we go these days! You must be making a lot of money?

7. I am still not making what I was making—financially—six years ago in that cubicle in that hospital staff development position.

I consider myself financially conservative and until last year continued to work at least 20 hours a week part time as the clinical educator in a large multi-physician practice. I was fortunate that this job allowed a great deal of flexibility. It was difficult for me cut ties with a predictable income, even while my husband, family, and Diane were encouraging me to work for Innovative Solutions full time. I began to work full time for Innovative Solutions 18 months ago, about four years after the business began. The salary is now reasonable and I can certainly see the potential for an increase each year.

8. How do you decide who does what?

8. The division of responsibilities seemed to just evolve. In the beginning, it was easy. We were the CPR and the ACLS queens. As the company changed and became more multi-focused, we each have developed our own focus. When we got the first ACLS contract and set up 20+ annual classes the coordination of those classes became one of my responsibilities—even though I am not an ACLS instructor. We were able to find individuals to be the lead instructors, and others to help out with the other parts of the class. Diane rarely is actually there at a class but continues to be the resource for questions related to format and technical information. The numbers of subcontracted instructors varies from year to year and we have agreements with them for payment and to use the teaching format that we prefer.

As we began to exhibit our products at conferences, that began to be Diane's role. She updates the games, reproduces and assembles the books, works with the conference planners, and manages all aspects of the exhibit.

We both enjoy the conference presentation and special classes part of the business. Diane generally is the one to send the abstracts, create the handouts, write the objectives, and put the visual part of the presentation together. Meanwhile, I am in the office and take care of the everyday mail, e-mail, phone calls, and accounting, as well as coordinate the Training Center and the daily repetitive types of classes; for example, first aid, OSHA, and medication administration.

The financial income is then divided with percentages calculated by who taught the class, created the product, or who had the most responsibility. For example, if Diane teaches a class for a special group, then she receives the higher percentage of the profit. I also receive a percentage and Innovative Solutions receives a percentage. Therefore, our monthly salary varies from month to month in relationship to how much business we have done.

9. What kind of equipment does it take?

9. Innovative Solutions now owns both class equipment and basic office equipment. Each December we have a business meeting to look at the money in the bank and equipment needs.

We started out bare bones, using our own computers. Because my home had two phone lines, the line previously assigned to the modem became the "Inno" phone. As our offices developed, we have each added the normal office supplies—as well as each having a computer paid for by the company. Our predictable monthly bills now include the telephone, computer purchase payments, and Web site expenses. Each of us use prepaid telephone cards for long distance and each has a credit card for travel and other business expenses. The everyday office equipment gets added on an as needed basis.

Equipment for CPR and ACLS is expensive! We are finally at a point where we have all of the equipment to do each of these classes without having to borrow anything. Not many other people I know drive around with a defibrillator in their trunk! We are only missing a couple of items of PALS equipment; that will be the next purchase. We do understand that this equipment needs to be continually updated/repaired and, as the business grows, we budget for those expenses.

10. How do you grow a business?

10. As we have grown and changed, we have tried different approaches as we have learned about time and costs. For example, we had a game that we created for review of ACLS medications. It included a set of about 200 questions, a game board, and dice. We originally built it as a standing poster with colorful boxes—each with a piece of Velcro "glued" on with hot glue. As we sold games and "burned" off our fingerprints, AND spent late nights in motel rooms cutting up game cards—each a different size—it became obvious that when we sold a game we probably were making about $3 an hour! We changed to cards that could be made with perforated business cards and a game board that is an overhead. Now we have a "better" game AND one that can at least cover the costs of supplies!

We tend to travel together about three or four times a year—usually meaning pretty extended periods of time closed up in a car together. We have found that time very effective for brainstorming about new products, new topics to present, and new approaches to the business. That confined space seems to make us able to really think well.

We have also been lucky to have a strong group of instructors who teach with us. They have supported us in planning classes, as well as marketing our business to groups that need classes. Since they truly represent "us" in the classroom, we do believe that we have to pay them well and support them well. One of us typically coordinates the class—sometimes I call it being the "hostess"—keeps the equipment in good working order, supplies all of the paperwork, and pays the instructors as close to the class time as possible.

11. How many proposals should you have out at one time?

11. This seems to be a constant challenge for us. After having created a fairly predictable class schedule, we now know which months will be particularly busy and which ones will be more manageable. But we still get surprised! Just recently we ended up having four ACLS classes and one PALS class in the same week. No, we didn't plan it that way—but with some creative scheduling I believe that we were able to keep all of our clients and instructors happy. Again, because Diane and I don't work out of the same office, we sometimes double book a class day inadvertently. That may make for some long teaching days, and many phone calls to instructors and a renewed check of the calendar before we give available dates to a client.

What has become a problem for me as we have grown is having very little "office time"—and when I have that time feel overwhelmed by the phone calls, mail, e-mail, and class coordination (cleaning manikins, registering participants, sales tax, accounting needs). But the hardest thing to find is what I call creative time—the time to create self-study books, or new presentations. I am finding that I need to subcontract some of those basic classes that I would normally teach to other instructors and to actually schedule office time in order to have more control over the time that I spend in the office.

12. What about the uncertainty?

12. I have already admitted that I am a bit conservative with money—so the uncertainty of a regular income can become a stressor for me. As the company has grown, income has become more predictable. I know now that during the first few months of the year my salary will be lower and that the fall months are higher income months. This has evened out somewhat—but it feels a bit like those first few years of my marriage when we lived on commission and really didn't know about salary from month to month—that chicken today, feathers tomorrow life-style. It's not my favorite life-style but I am feeling more comfortable with having a baseline income and what's above that is extra!

As the business has grown, the months have evened out—and I don't become panicked if we only have three classes scheduled in a week instead of four or five. There are those other projects to be created, and that office time of which I have become so protective.

13. If I wanted to do this where is a good place to get some experience?

13. My "standing in front of a classroom" education experience began with becoming a CPR instructor. As I worked as nursing school faculty and then in staff development I had the opportunity to learn from some of the best nurses and educators in my area. I believe that most presenters create their own style by watching others—the good and the not so good. I also had the opportunity to take some presentation seminars and attend presentation techniques sessions at conferences. I would suggest being in a classroom as frequently as possible, trying out different approaches to the same topic, networking with others about how to teach a topic, and stretching yourself in topics and different groups—

14. What if one or both of us decided that we've had enough?

15. What does the future look like?

this sounds like staff development, doesn't it? What a great place to learn!

14. To be perfectly honest that is one of those "business plan" issues that we need to determine. From strictly a financial viewpoint the "business book" would say that the purchase of one person's share from the other would be related to percentage of business performed, annual salary earned, and what would be a fair share of the assets (equipment). The questions that would also have to be dealt with would need to include competition issues and customers. We have actually never had a focused discussion on these points—but realize as we continue to grow that there is a need to have these plans in writing.

15. If our present growth continues, it is obvious that some present business practices will need to be adjusted—more instructors assisting with classes, more office support and so on. The accounting system that we are using was not designed to handle the size of our business and it is presently being upgraded to a new and more formal system. But the future does certainly look bright! As the hospitals in the area continue to reformulate their education departments we are able to present ourselves as an option. As we have identified different markets, such as managing the educational needs of employees of area group homes, we seem to fill in more and more days of our calendars.

As we send e-mail to each other with more class opportunities we often close those with ". . . and the beat goes on"—and that certainly seems to be reflective of the growth and success of Innovative Solutions!!

RESOURCES

Puetz, B. E., & Shinn, L. J. (1996). *The nurse consultant's handbook.* New York: Springer.

Zagury, C. (1992). *Nurse entrepreneur: Building the bridge of opportunity.* Long Branch, NJ: Vista.

Index